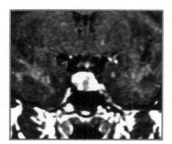
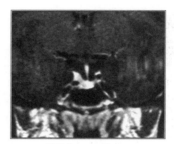
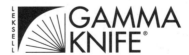

Second Edition

The second edition of the Pituitary Patient's Resource Guide was compiled and published in Los Angeles, California by the Pituitary Tumor Network Association (PTNA). Executive editors: Shereen Ezzat, M.D., F.R.C.P. ©, F.A.C.P. and Robert Knutzen, MBA, PTNA Chairman.

All editorial and graphic contributions to this Guide are used by permission from the authors.

All rights reserved. Written permission must be secured from the publisher to reproduce any part of the book for sale or commercial distribution.

Anyone wishing to contribute professional articles to future editions may do so by submitting them to the PTNA at:16350 Ventura Boulevard, Suite 231, Encino, California 91436. (805) 499-2262. Inquiries are welcome.

Important Notice

This publication is intended to function as a patient/physician peer guide, not a medical journal, and should in no way be considered an endorsement of any particular organization, physician, treatment method, or medication. The information contained within this book represents the contributions and opinions of various individuals, and while the information has been reviewed by the PTNA editorial committee for appropriate content, *neither the PTNA, its members and advisors, nor the editors and publishers and their staffs are responsible for the accuracy of any of the information contained herein.*

As always, you must be responsible for your own life, health and medical care. We urge you to investigate, ask questions and make your own informed decisions.

In addition, neither the PTNA scientific advisors nor the medical members of the PTNA have been responsible for the compilation, placement or wording of the information contained within this guide.

The Editors and Publishers of
The Pituitary Patient Resource Guide

The Pituitary Patient Resource Guide™

Second Edition

This book provided to you courtesy of:

Published by
Pituitary Tumor Network Association

Second Edition

Table of Contents

Second Edition

Pituitary Patient Resource Guide

Second Edition

Pituitary Patient Resource Guide

Second Edition

Pituitary Patient Resource Guide

Second Edition

Introduction

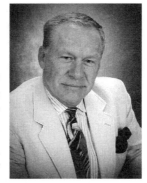

It is with great pleasure that we bring you this second edition of the *Pituitary Patient Resource Guide.* Larger, better, and more complete than ever before, it is our answer to your calls, letters and demands for more information, deeper knowledge, and better explanations!

Patients and physicians alike loved the first issue; this one should go "under the pillow!" The information in these chapters is the total sum of the authors professionalism, love of the healing arts (and sciences), a caring for their "fellow-man" and patients , and a dedication to making this world a little better for their having been here. Authors -- we salute you with deep gratitude; physicians and patients alike. Patients, in this edition, have contributed knowledge and experience from their hearts as well as their scholarly minds.

Some of you were concerned earlier that we were compiling another "phone book" of physicians, surgeons, and medical centers. We are extremely pleased to point out that the leading members of the endocrine and neurosurgical community, along with esteemed colleagues in psychiatry, ophthalmology, reproductive endocrinology, radiology, dentistry, etc., have joined us in selective numbers so that we, the patients, may find our way to better care through informed choices. Pharmaceutical and equipment companies share information, hospitals and universities are letting you know about their services and skilled professionals.

As before, however, **you and you alone** must interview the physicians into whose hands you entrust your treatment and satisfy yourself that this is your course and your decision. The PTNA can only make the physicians known to you; **you** must make all the other choices.

Much has happened since the first edition of the *Resource Guide* in 1995. New medicines have been approved, new methods and modalities have been tried and implemented (or discarded). The medical and patient-care communities and insurance companies/HMOs are under attack regarding cost and government regulations as never before, and not just in the U.S. But as is always the case, we the patients, are paying for it, in more ways than one. Patients are denied services and medicines in many countries because it is just not "cost effective."

However, we know this with certainty: more pituitary patients are being "discovered" earlier and treated better than ever before. By using this book, our newsletter, the website, and other PTNA materials, they are being listened to and taken seriously by their physicians and their HMO's - and hopefully - their governments.

We have a long way to go, but with your help, the next two years will hopefully allow us to achieve greater goals than in the last two.

For those of you who are new to the PTNA; we are not here to offer sympathy - we exist for the sole purpose of helping you get better and heal!

Our mission statement is clear and to the point. "Research!" With the strides being made today, we'll hopefully know half the needed answers in the next ten years. And that, in medicine, is lightning speed.

For the first time, in this edition, we are introducing articles by physicians and patients alike driving home the points we have made for years; the emotional and sexual aspects of pituitary

Pituitary Patient Resource Guide

disease need and deserve more attention! These subjects have been virtually neglected since they were first described by Dr. Harvey Cushing, the teaching pioneer in pituitary disease. We have elected to place these issues squarely in the middle of the table for all to see.

They will not go away, and they will not "cure" themselves. Examine these issues, come to terms with them, deal with them! They constitute the missing 30% of pituitary patient care. Now let's get to work!

By the time the next issue of this book comes out, we will expect that all universities, hospitals, and medical centers which offer quality pituitary care will remember this wish and desire: **Any pituitary center which considers itself a "center of excellence" will not be considered so unless it also offers psychological/psychiatric care, and sexual and family counseling through professionally-run support groups!**

To our authors, thank you! To our Editor-in-Chief Dr. Shereen Ezzat, from my heart, thank you. To my wife, Rosemary, and my children, goes my heartfelt thanks for believing in the cause and supporting my "crazy notions" of what is the right thing to do. Mitchell for his creativity and hard work, Anne-Christine for her secretarial assistance, Suzanne for professional proofing and editing, and Timothy for caring and sharing. My thanks also to Lee Hinderstein for his tenacious wrestling with technical issues and computers, Brenda Janda for her cheerful 'traffic direction', as well as Pat Gantenbein and Joanne Abelson for always "counting the pennies."

Hopefully, all who read these pages will feel uplifted, emboldened and enlightened! Tomorrow will indeed be a better day and each succeeding day better yet!

To your very good health!

Robert Knutzen
Chairman, CEO
Pituitary Tumor Network Association

Introduction

9

Second Edition

Overview

Overview

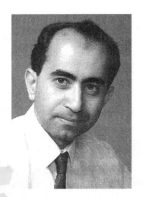

Thus far, pituitary disorders have been considered to be rare and mostly "benign conditions." Such a belief left physicians, investigators, and patients frustrated in a world of relative isolation. It was only two years ago that the first edition of the Pituitary Patient Resource Guide came to life. Prior to this, as physicians, we could only refer patients to medical textbooks intended mostly for use by student physicians. A great deal has happened in the last six years since the inception of the Pituitary Tumor Network Association. Exciting progress is developing on the medical front with research elucidating the cellular and molecular mechanisms involved in pituitary tumors, design of more selective and effective medical, surgical, and radiotherapeutic approaches to pituitary disorders. The significance and impact of such developments, however, can only be fully realized if they are accurately translated and communicated to the public. We hope that we have moved closer to this target in this second edition of the Resource Guide.

We are grateful to the many contributors to this edition. Patients have been generous in sharing their experiences and messages. Physicians have provided us with glimpses of their invaluable experiences in caring for patients with pituitary disorders. Investigators reviewed for us some of the recent advances in pituitary research and what to expect in the near future.

While much of the impetus to put this patient-oriented Pituitary Handbook came from the patients themselves, it was Robert Knutzen's dedication and enthusiasm that allowed it all to happen. The fact that thousands of copies of this book found their way into the hands of patients and health care providers speaks volumes about its success. We have heard mostly positive comments from patients and physicians alike. We encourage you all to continue to give us your feedback. Let us know how we can continue to grow to meet your needs.

Best wishes to all,

Shereen Ezzat, M.D.
Toronto, Canada

Foreword

Endocrine disorders are often subtle in their early signs and symptoms. They often progress so slowly that it is difficult even for the patient or the patient's family and friends to remember exactly when the changes first began. Some of these disorders are sufficiently unusual that the average family practitioner, internist, or gynecologist may not see a single patient with the disorder in any given year. Disorders caused by pituitary tumors, unfortunately, fit all three of these descriptions. I cannot remember how many times my patients were first told that they probably had acromegaly or Cushing's syndrome, for example, by a friend or acquaintance rather than by their physician.

In my experience as a physician, as a patient, and as the relative of patients, I have found that the better educated you are with respect to what's ailing you and what your options may be, the more likely you are to receive appropriate care. This collection of essays by well-known endocrinologists serves that purpose well. They provide concise descriptions of the clinical manifestations of the various tumors of the pituitary gland and related disorders of other endocrine glands, how the disorders disturb normal hormonal homeostasis, what diagnostic tests and procedures are usually required, what treatment options are available, and what you may expect from the treatment. Finally, it includes a section in which the diagnostic and treatment referral centers around the country are identified.

Use this volume and the many other resources that are available to you, such as The Endocrine Society's toll-free telephone number (1-800-HORMONE) or website (http://www.endo-society.org), to inform yourself about your disease. You will find that there is often consensus about the overall approach to pituitary disorders, but there is sometimes significant disagreement about details of diagnosis and treatment. In part this reflects our current state of knowledge - or ignorance, if you prefer - and emphasizes the need for additional basic and clinical research to find the answers. In part it reflects the fact that there may be two or more paths leading to the same goal.

Knowing as much as you can about your disease enables you to provide your physician with information you might not otherwise have considered important. It allows you to ask your physician intelligent questions about proposed diagnostic procedures or therapy. It makes you an active partner in your health care. Any physician or surgeon whom you want taking care of you should welcome your involvement and be happy to answer your questions, to explain possible alternatives and to assist you in obtaining a second opinion, should you desire one. Your physician should offer the most informed advice and provide the best possible care for you on the basis of what path you choose but you are ultimately responsible for your own health.

David N. Orth, M.D.
Vanderbilt University Medical Center
President, The Endocrine Society

Acknowledgement

The directors and volunteers who direct the operations and work of the PTNA are deeply indebted to the many, many individuals and firms who made the book possible.

First and foremost, to the many authors who, because of a love of their noble professions and a belief in the cause of the PTNA, wrote exclusively for us or made the material available for our use and for your edification. We hope you understand that no such gathering of data has ever before been undertaken for pituitary patients.

Our deepest gratitude to:

- Sylvia Asa, M.D., Ph.D.
- Douglas C. Aziz M.D., Ph.D
- Ariel L. Barkan, M.D.
- Bengt-Ake Bengtsson, M.D., Ph.D.
- Francoise Brucker-Davis, M.D.
- P. Michael Conn, Ph.D.
- Lisa Bensmihen
- David M. Cook, M.D.
- W.T. Couldwell, M.D,
- W.W. de Herder, M.D.,
- Antonio A. F. De Salles, M.D., Ph.D.
- Endocrine Nurse's Society
- Richard C. Eastman, M.D.
- Shereen Ezzat, M.D.,
- Yvette Ficekova, M.D.
- Delbert A, Fisher, M.D.
- Dan Freed
- Keith E. Friend, M.D.
- Robert F. Gagel, M.D.
- Ron Grunstein M.D.
- Morton A. Hirschberg M.D.
- Ken Ho M.D.
- Sandy Hotchkiss, MSW, BCD
- Laurence Katznelson, M.D.
- Anne Klibanski, M.D.
- E. A. Koller, M.D.
- George T. Koulianos, MD,
- Edward R. Laws, Jr., MD,
- Michael J. Link, M.D.
- Cheryl A. Muszynski, M.D.

Pituitary Patient Resource Guide

- David N. Orth, M.D.
- Tara Pritchard
- K. M. M. Shakir, M.D.
- L.G. Sobrinho M.D, Ph.D
- Nicoletta Sonino M.D.
- Ladislau Steiner, MD,
- Constantine A. Stratakis, M.D.
- Carey B. Strom, M.D.
- Eric C. Sung, D.D.S.
- Phyllis Taylor
- John M. Tew, Jr., M.D.
- Michael O. Thorner M.D.
- J. M. Treese.
- M. L. Vance, MD,
- Christina Wang, M.D.
- M.H. Weiss, M.D
- Michael A Weitzner M.D.
- Charles B. Wilson, M.D.
- Kathleen Wong

As in all endeavors of modern times, the PTNA requires financial support to get the job done. The following organizations have made an extra effort to accommodate our needs and we salute them: Alza Corporation, Sensus Drug Development Corporation, Eli Lilly and Co., Mallinckrodt Nuclear Medicine, Novartis, Quest Diagnostic Laboratories and Electa Gamma Knife. And of course, every single pharmaceutical and equipment company listed in the book.

Finally, we would like to thank every physician, surgeon, hospital, university, and medical center from across the world who helped us identify themselves so that you, the patient, family member, or thoughtful health professional would know where to find expert help. Their listings mean they truly do care.

Thank you, **EVERYONE!**

The Publisher

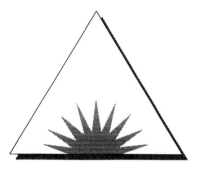

Second Edition

Recognition

Editor-In-Chief:	Shereen Ezzat, M.D.
Book Design & Layout:	Mitchell Knutzen
	Lee Hinderstein
Copy Editor:	Suzanne Pajot
Marketing Coordination:	Mitchell Knutzen
Computer Coordination:	Lee Hinderstein
Editorial Coordination:	Robert Knutzen
Administrative Coordination:	Brenda Janda
Sales:	Robert Knutzen
Records & Bookkeeping:	JoAnne Ableson
	Pat Gantenbein
Administrative Assistance:	Anne-Christine Knutzen
Publisher:	Pituitary Tumor Network Association
	Robert Knutzen/CEO

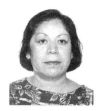

Board of Directors

Herrera, Olga
Nursing Home Administrator
4328 N. Cedar Avenue
El Monte, California 91732

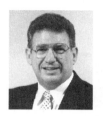

Hornbaker, Lawrence, Ed.D.
Executive Vice Chancellor, Pepperdine University
24255 Pacific Coast Highway
Malibu, California 90263-4891

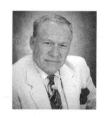

Knutzen, Robert, M.B.A.
Chairman of the Board, CEO
38 S. Wendy Drive
Newbury Park, California 91320

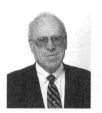

Miles, James S.
Attorney at Law – Retired
P. O. Box 944
Taylor, Texas 76574

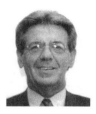

Seitzinger, Jack, Ph.D.
Compaq Computers
P. O. Box 69200
Houston, Texas 77269-2000

Editor-In-Chief

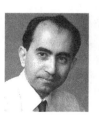

Ezzat, Shereen, M.D.
Wellesley Hospital, University of Toronto
Division of Endocrinology & Metabolism
160 Wellesley Street East, Room 134 Jones Building
Toronto, Ontario Canada   M4Y 1J3

Scientific Advisory Panel

Scientific Advisory Panel

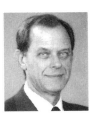

Besser, G. Michael, M.D.
Professor of Medicine
Departments of Medicine and Endocrinology
St. Bartholomew's Hospital
West Smithfield, London EC1A 7BE

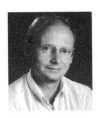

Christiansen, Jens Sandahl, M.D.
Professor of Medicine
Department of Endocrinology and Diabetes,
Aarhus University Hospital, Kommunehospitalet
DK-8000 Aarhus C, Denmark

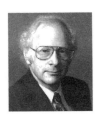

Conn, P. Michael, Ph.D., Associate Director,
Oregon Regional Primate Research Center
Special Assistant to the President, Oregon Health Sciences University
Oregon Regional Primate Research Center
505 N.W. 185th Avenue, Beaverton, Oregon 97006-3499

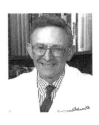

Frohman, Lawrence, M.D.
Edmund F. Foley Professor and Head
Department of Medicine
The University of Illinois at Chicago, College of Medicine
840 South Wood Street, Chicago, Illinois 60612-7323

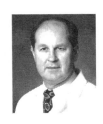

Gagel, Robert F., M.D.
Professor of Medicine
Chief, Section of Endocrine Neoplasia and Hormonal Disorders
The University of Texas, MD Anderson Cancer Center
1515 Holcombe Boulevard, Houston, Texas 77030

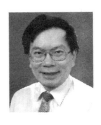

Ho, Ken, M.D., F.R.A.C.P.
Garvan Institute of Medical Research
384 Victoria Street
Darlinghurst Sydney,
NSW 2010 Australia

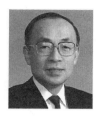

Imura, Hiroo, M.D.
President
Kyoto University, Japan
53 Kawahara Cho Syogoin
Sakyo-Ku, Kyoto 606, Japan

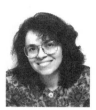

Klibanski, Anne, M.D.
Professor of Medicine, Harvard Medical School
Chief, Neuroendocrine Unit, Massachusetts General Hospital
55 Fruit Street – BUL457B
Boston, Massachusetts 02114-2696

Lamberts, Steven W., M.D., Ph.D.
Professor of Medicine
Erasmus University, The Netherlands
Molenlaan 172, Rotterdam, 3055 GJ
The Netherlands

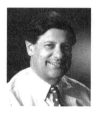

Melmed, Shlomo, M.D., Chairman
Director, Division of Endocrinology & Metabolism
Cedars-Sinai Medical Center
8700 Beverly Boulevard
Los Angeles, CA 90048-1869

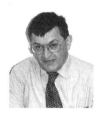

Thorner, Michael O., M.B., D.Sc.
Chair, Department of Internal Medicine
Interim Chief, Division of Endocrinology and Metabolism
University of Virginia Health Sciences Center
Charlottesville, Virginia 22908

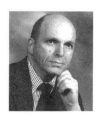

Weiss, Martin H., M.D., F.A.C.S.
Chairman, Department of Neurological Surgery
University of Southern California School of Medicine
1200 North State Street, GNH 5046
Los Angeles, California 90033

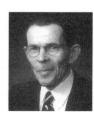

Wilson, Charles B., M.D.
Department of Neurosurgery
University of California San Francisco
533 Parnassus Avenue, Room U-125
San Francisco, California 94143-0350

Scientific Advisory Panel

Second Edition

Our Mission

Our Mission

To Support, pursue, encourage, promote, and where possible, fund research on pituitary tumors in a sustained and full-time effort to find a cure for these illnesses. PTNA will disseminate information helpful to the medical community, the public, pituitary patients and their families on matters regarding early detection, symptoms, treatments and resources available to patients with pituitary tumors.

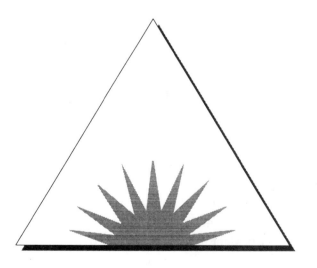

The Pituitary Gland & Its Function

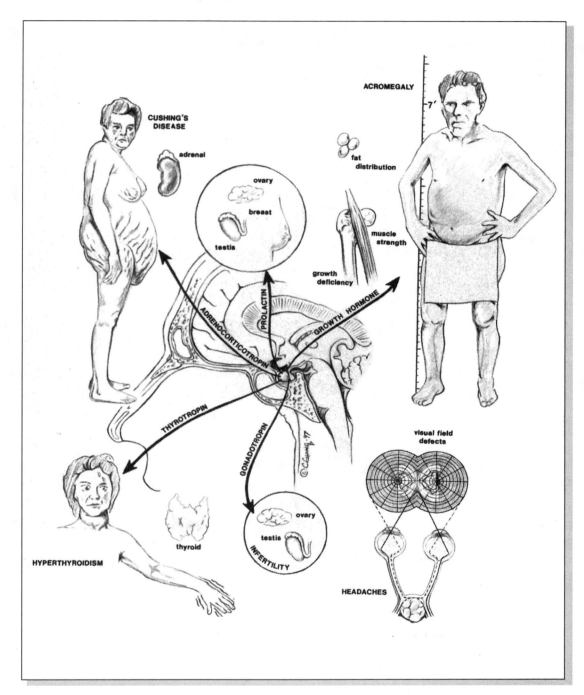

This illustration shows patients in the most advanced stages of acromegaly, Cushing's disease, and hypothyroidism. We know that with better knowledge and understanding of these conditions, patients can be diagnosed and treated long before ever reaching this point in their disease.

With our sincere thanks to Sylvia Asa, M.D., Ph.D, who commissioned and provided us this overview.

Second Edition

Pituitary Issues Overview and Position Statement

The pituitary gland has long been recognized as the master gland of the human body. It influences or regulates most of the vital metastatic functions of the body.

Not until the mid-1960s, however, was it possible for medical scientists to begin to measure (assay) pituitary hormone levels in the blood, and for the study of hormonal function to start in earnest.

Hence the delayed knowledge of pituitary issues and the explanation for the lack of information about pituitary issues within the patient community, the public at large, and too often, the general medical community.

The pituitary plays a primary role in thyroid function, adrenocortical (adrenal) function, gonadal (reproductive/sexual) function, growth, and water and food intake. When tumors are present, it can affect appetite, sleep, mental activity, mood, and muscle function.

The pituitary sits at the base of the brain in a bony structure called the sella turcica or "Turkish Saddle." It is small, about the size of a peanut, with the anterior and posterior portions responsible for different functions.

When things go well and a person is healthy, the pituitary is rarely thought of or appreciated. When it malfunctions, it generally manifests itself in the form of a benign tumor (adenoma), and only very rarely as a malignant cancer (carcinoma).

In 1938, in an autopsy series at the Mayo Clinic, it was determined that 22.4% of the population develops pituitary tumors in their lifetime. Age, sex, gender, race or national origin have apparently no influence on who will develop the tumors, most of which, fortunately, are clinically silent and cause no symptoms.

Today, with our longer lives, nearly 30% of the world's population may develop pituitary tumors. It is estimated that between 1% and 2% of the world's population develops clinically significant tumors if we take into account infertility, impotence, emotional problems, vision problems, etc.

The number of estimated cases of pituitary tumors climbs every year, not because of an actual increase in their number, but because of greater awareness, better detection and diagnostic methods and a clearer understanding of cause and effect.

By far the greatest number of pituitary patients, however, are still undiagnosed and, therefore, untreated or under treated.

Pituitary disease (and tumors) and their clinical consequences date back to Goliath in the Bible and Akhenaten, the Egyptian Pharaoh, and before. It is also known that genetic links and therefore a tendency for susceptibility to the tumors is often passed from parent to child.

Though certainly not an issue of an epidemic proportion, pituitary disease, disorders and tumors are sufficiently prevalent to warrant intense studies as a major public health issue.

The far-ranging, very destructive and often fatal outcome of pituitary disorders demands nothing less.

Pituitary Tumor Backgrounder

Patient Population
It is estimated that between 1% and 2% (60 million to 120 million people) of the world's population harbor clinically significant pituitary tumors. Approximately 22% of all adults have been found to harbor pituitary adenomas (tumors). While most of these tumors are thought to produce no symptoms, it is, in fact, unknown to what extent most of these tumors affect the hosts. Much still remains to be learned about pituitary functions and disease(s).

Overview
The pituitary is a peanut-shaped gland located just below the brain behind and between the eyes. The pituitary gland, long referred to as the "master gland," secretes a number of hormones that govern growth, urine output, and many other functions. Both the thyroid and adrenal glands are regulated by the pituitary gland. Pituitary tumors are usually not cancerous, but they do cause severe medical problems by pressing on the optic nerves, or by pressing on the normal pituitary, disrupting the pituitary's secretion of hormones.

The symptoms of pituitary tumors vary depending on the size and location of the tumor and whether or not the tumor secretes hormones. The majority of pituitary adenomas are nonmalignant and grow slowly within the pituitary gland, inside the sella turcica, but the more aggressive and invasive of these tumors grow rapidly. They can cause blindness, increased intracranial pressure and life-threatening endocrine abnormalities.

Some pituitary tumors stem the gland's secretion of growth hormone (GH) and cause growth arrest in children. These tumors may also limit the pituitary's secretion of the gonadotropic hormones (FSH and LH), which govern the development and function of the ovary and testis. Men may manifest testicular atrophy, decreased body hair, decreased libido, impotence and infertility. In females, the tumors often cause breast shrinkage, cessation of menstruation, decreased libido, and infertility.

Tumors that foster a lack of adrenocorticotropic hormone (ACTH) may cause low blood sugar, as well as low blood pressure, weakness and fatigue. Extreme cases can be life-threatening by causing the body to go into shock. Tumors that limit the secretion of thyroid stimulating hormone (TSH) may stunt growth and induce tiredness, constipation, dry skin, sensitivity to cold and hoarseness. Lack of normal secretion of pituitary hormones is called hypopituitarism. If all hormones are lacking, it is called pan-hypo-pituitarism.

Other tumors induce specific symptoms by releasing an excess of pituitary hormones. Tumors that secrete the hormone prolactin can prompt the abnormal production of breast milk and the lack of menstruation in women and impotence in men. GH-secreting tumors often boost growth excessively, so that, if untreated, children may reach giant-like proportions (gigantism), a few attaining heights greater than eight feet tall and shoe sizes in the 30s. In adults, excessive GH secretion results in acromegaly. Acromegaly causes the feet, hands, nose and jaw to grow, in addition to enlarging internal organs. Gonadotropin-secreting tumors usually produce inactive hormone fragments and are associated with hypogonadism, a condition of testosterone absence or deficiency in men and estrogen deficiency in women.

ACTH-secreting tumors result in over activity of the adrenal cortex (Cushing's Syndrome), with excessive weight gain, weakness, high blood pressure, and diabetes as some of its effects. Some patients may inherit a common pituitary tumor called a craniopharyngioma. This tumor often disrupts vision by pressing on the optic nerve. Craniopharyngiomas also prompt a lack of most pituitary hormones, thereby causing a combination of many of the symptoms previously described. It often is found in children and is very difficult to treat. Rathke's cleft cyst is a close cousin of the craniopharyngioma.

Treatment: Should only be undertaken by highly skilled and experienced endocrinologists and neurosurgeons. Successful outcome often rests on their specialized training.

Physicians treat pituitary tumors with surgery, radiation therapy, drugs or a combination of these treatments. Surgery is the first treatment of choice for most tumors that enlarge rapidly and threaten vision, followed by medication and finally, if other methods fail, radiation.

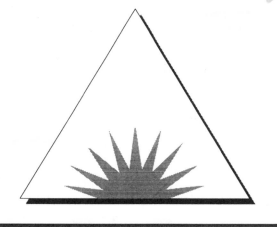

"*A turn in the road is not the end of the road unless you fail to make the turn.*"

Symptoms of Pituitary Disease

Do not attempt to diagnose yourself. Please see your physician if you have symptoms of pituitary disease. This list of symptoms is not meant to replace a visit to your doctor.

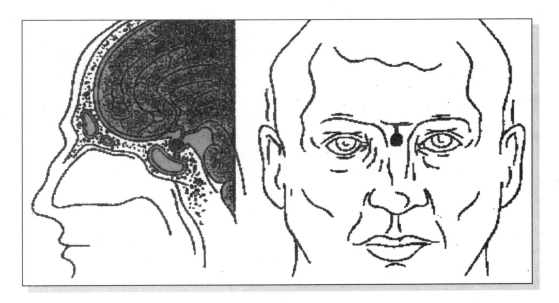

Symptoms of Prolactinomas
(prolactin = milk hormone)

A prolactinoma is a tumor on the pituitary gland that secretes the milk hormone. The tumor is benign (non-cancerous) over 99% of the time. It is the most common of all pituitary tumors (28%). The cause of the tumor is unknown.

Symptoms are:

- Changes in menstrual cycle or loss of cycle (amenorrhea)

- Milk discharge (galactorrhea)

- Reduction in sex drive

- Pain on intercourse/vaginal dryness

- Headaches

- Visual field disturbances

- Male hypogonadism/impotence (shrinking testicles) and milk discharge

- Mood changes and depression

Symptoms of Acromegaly
(akron = extremity, megas = great)

Acromegaly is chronic, insidious, debilitating disease, resulting in serious cosmetic changes and metabolic complications. Apart from the coarsening of facial features, the metabolic abnormalities associated with GH (Growth Hormone) hypersecretion are mainly responsible for morbidity and increased cardiovascular mortality, complication that warrant effective GH lowering therapy.

Symptoms are:

- Soft tissue thickening (flesh) palms of hands
- Oily skin
- Coarse facial features
- Excessive sweating
- Low vitality (fatigue)
- Headaches
- Carpal tunnel syndrome
- Osteoarthritis
- Potency decrease
- Hypertension
- Loss of sexual interest (libido)
- Enlarging hands (ring size)
- Enlarging feet (shoe size)
- Enlarging head (hat size)
- Enlarging jaw (underbite)
- Spreading teeth (food gets caught)
- Interrupted menstrual cycle
- Impotence
- Depression
- Sleep apnea
- Vision defects (peripheral)

Symptoms of Cushing's Disease/Syndrome
(Named for Dr. Cushing, pioneer physician)

Cushing's Syndrome is caused by prolonged exposure of the body's tissues to high levels of the hormone cortisol. Cortisol is normally produced by the adrenal glands, which are just above the kidneys.

Scientists think that normal cortisol levels:

- Help maintain blood pressure and cardiovascular function

- Help slow the immune system's inflammatory response

- Help balance the effects of insulin in breaking down sugar

- Help regulate the metabolism of proteins, carbohydrates, and fats

- Help the body respond to stress

Symptoms of Cushing's Syndrome are:

- Rapid/unexplained weight gain with rounding of the face (moon face)

- Increased fat in the neck and above the collar bone

- Skin changes -- cheeks often red

- Easy bruising

- Bluish red stretch marks on thighs, abdomen, buttocks, arms, armpits, and

- Menstrual disorders in women

- Decreased fertility or absent libido (sex drive) in men

- High blood pressure

- Muscle and bone weakness

- High blood pressure

- Severe depression

- Mood and behavior disorders

Symptoms of Craniopharyngioma
(cranio = skull, pharynx = throat, oma = tumor)

Craniopharyngiomas are intercranial tumors that can occur at any age, but are most commonly found during childhood or adolescence; they account for about 10% of all central nervous system (CNS) tumors in these younger age groups. Craniopharyngiomas are usually not discovered until they impinge upon important structures around them. For this reason, although they are almost always benign, they are frequently quite large when detected, ranging from an average of about one inch across to more than four inches across.

Symptoms are:

◆ Growth failure

◆ Delayed puberty

◆ Loss of normal menstrual functions

◆ Loss of sexual drive

◆ Fatigue

◆ Constipation

◆ Dry Skin

◆ Nausea

◆ Low blood pressure

◆ Depression

◆ Piuitary Stalk Compression can also increase prolactin levels enough to cause a milky discharge from the breasts

◆ Visual disturbances can occur. Also obesity, increased drowsiness (somnolence), body temperature regulation problems, and water balance (thirst-urination)

◆ Other symptoms may include personality changes, headaches, confusion, and vomiting

Section I

General Issues

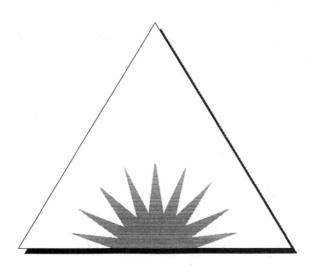

Second Edition

The Endocrine Society is "In This Fight With You"

P. Michael Conn Ph.D, Past President, The Endocrine Society.
Board of Directors, The Hormone Foundation.

The Endocrine Society is composed of nearly 9,000 scientists and physicians worldwide, involved in the research and treatment of diseases of chemical messengers - hormones. If you are reading this, the chances are that you or a loved one have such a disease. We know that it can profoundly influence your life. We also know that there are things you can do now to ease this burden.

In this note I want to tell you about research that is being conducted by members of our organization and about free services that we have available for you and for your doctor.

In 1997, the Endocrine Society established the Hormone Foundation, which is involved in making available information on hormonal diseases to the general public. There are several ways that the Endocrine Society and the Hormone Foundation can help you. You may request printed information (Fact Sheets), written in non - medical language. These can help you understand your disease and will tell you about the research underway to help in its treatment. You may also consult our web site. At the time I am writing this, our web site is designed for our members, endocrinology professionals, although plans are underway for the Hormone Foundation to establish a web site for lay readers. Our web URL is listed below and is linked to the PTNA site. The Endocrine Society can also direct you to physicians in your area who treat your disease. If your doctor is not an endocrinologist, our services may help him (her) identify other professionals who can be of assistance to you.

Endocrinologists are interested in all aspects of hormone disease; how genes express themselves, how molecules interact with one another, communication between cells and organs, and most important, the diagnosis and treatment of disease. By understanding molecular and cellular processes, we learn about your disease and its causes and can focus on its treatment.

Every day we are learning more about the causes of your disease although, as Robert Knutzen has pointed out, "more is not known than what is known about the function of the pituitary." Although we have few absolute cures available, many new treatments exist which can deal with the symptoms of your disorder and can move you closer to a normal life. We are in this fight with you. It is less than 25 years since the first drugs were available, designed for treatment of pituitary tumors. Thanks to research in animals and other laboratory models and funding by federal and private dollars, you should expect to see advances in your lifetime that will materially aid in your disease.

To reach us -

Toll free: 1-800-HORMONE or Tel -301-941-0200 Fax -301-941-0259
By mail: 4350 East West Highway, Suite 500
Bethesda, Maryland 20814-4410
Through our web site: http:\\www.endo-soc.org

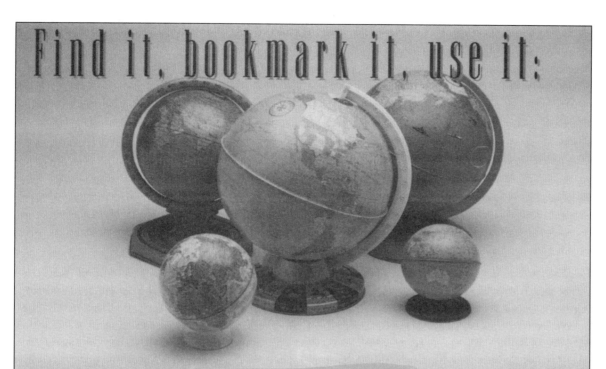

The Cause of Pituitary Tumors:
The Known and the Unknown

Sylvia L. Asa, M.D., Ph.D., Associate Professor of Pathology
Department of Pathology & Laboratory Medicine, Mount Sinai Hospital
Department of Laboratory Medicine and Pathobiology, University of Toronto

The pituitary is an intriguing yet confusing organ that is essential for life. This tiny bean-shaped tissue, hidden within the cranial cavity and well protected from external insult, is responsible for the production of hormones that determine growth and development, sexual maturation, reproductive function and lactation. It regulates thyroid and adrenal function that in turn are responsible for maintaining all bodily functions from protein, carbohydrate, fat and water metabolism, to blood pressure, sleep cycles and immunity. Its importance is obvious, yet it is the site of common pathology. Despite our advances in medical science, we remain ignorant of the cause of most pituitary diseases.

Descartes was the first to recognize that the brain was an organ integrating the functions of the mind and body in 1649. The association was reinforced by Zander who noted in 1890 the connection between the adrenals and the brain, referring to observations on the absence of the adrenal cortex in anencephaly as recorded by Morgagni in 1733, Soemmering in 1792, and Meckel in 1802. It was only in 1849 that direct evidence of a role for the hypothalamus in endocrinology was provided by Claude Bernard when he demonstrated that injury to the floor of the fourth ventricle, the "piqûre diabetique." caused excessive urination; subsequently, numerous studies in the late 19th century and early 20th century confirmed that the hypothalamic-posterior pituitary system was the site of production of an important substance that regulated water retention.

Galen (129-201 AD) had described the pituitary as the site of drainage of phlegm from the brain to the nose and throat. Soon after the description of acromegaly by Pierre Marie in 1886, the association of acromegaly with pituitary tumor was noted by Minkowski in 1887, and the recognition of endocrine functions of the pituitary followed rapidly thereafter, with major contributions by Cushing and Simmonds.

The early part of the 20th century saw the identification, isolation and characterization of the hormones of the anterior pituitary. Their regulation by the hypothalamus was the subject of the landmark monograph by Harris in 1948, "Neural control of the pituitary gland."

Since these major discoveries, the identification of hypothalamic-pituitary hormones has led to three Nobel Prizes, in 1954 for du Vigneaud and for Guillemin and Schally in 1977. Despite these tremendous advances in physiology, however, the study of pituitary pathology has lagged well behind the volumes of information that have clarified the basis of disease in many other organs.

As a Torontonian, I am proud of the history of research in this field in my own city. The 1960's saw Dr. Calvin Ezrin attempting to identify the pituitary cells involved in various pathological processes; I hope that Dr. Ezrin still proudly wears the golden pituitary tie-clip that he richly deserved.

The 1970's and 1980's were the era of tumor classification by the reknowned husband and wife team, Dr. Kalman Kovacs and Dr. Eva Horvath, who truly live in the "casa pituitaria" and whose lives have been devoted to this work. They devised a classification scheme that remains the basis for our understanding of pituitary tumors (Table 1).

Today, the story goes yet another step. We now recognize the cells of the pituitary; we are able to study their hormonal activity at the individual cell level with such tools as immunohisto-chemistry and reverse hemolytic plaque assays. We can accurately determine their structural alterations with the electron microscope. We can dissect the reasons for their ability to produce one hormone or another by analyzing the intricacies of transcription factors at the molecular level. We have been able, by careful analysis, to determine that pituitary tumors are very common as incidental findings at autopsy, and the latest technology has given us magnetic resonance imaging (MRI) to identify even tiny tumors in the living. We can administer natural and synthetic hormones to replace damaged glands and maintain endocrine homeostasis; we can medically and surgically reduce problems of hormone excess, such as acromegaly, hyperprolactinemia with its resulting sexual dysfunction, and Cushing's disease with its resulting cortisol excess. Surgical technology allows experts to microdissect tiny pituitary tumors as well as to resect large ones that compress the optic nerves, causing visual deficits, and invade the brain; all this can be done through a small incision in the nose or mouth that will never even leave a visible scar! It almost seems like we can accomplish miracles!

But we have failed to answer the most important questions: Why do people develop pituitary tumors? Why are they so common and why do only some wreak havoc on their host? How can we identify those at risk before the disease becomes clinically manifest? How can we predict which tumors will grow aggressively and which will recur after surgery? The answers to these questions are the objectives of current research in this field.

A number of studies have started to shed light on these problems. We know, for example, that these tumors, even small ones, are monoclonal proliferations. This means that there is a genetic basis, a molecular abnormality involving a gene, that predisposes a single cell to grow when it should not and when its neighbors are behaving in their normal regulated fashion.

We know that the major oncogenes and tumor suppressor genes are not involved in most pituitary tumors. The large body of literature on cancer has identified a number of key genes that when mutated, can play an important role in the development of a tumor. Investigators have examined these target "culprits" in the pituitary, and have found that they rarely or never are involved. This is probably good news - when they are implicated, they can cause malignant transformation, the development of true "cancer." But the bad news is that we are still looking for the culprit.

Recently, one of the most sought after culprit genes was cloned and studied. It had been recognized since the 1950's that members of certain families were predisposed to the development of pituitary adenomas along with parathyroid disease and pancreatic endocrine tumors. These families displayed an autosomal dominant pattern of inheritance of a gene that was implicated as the cause of Multiple Endocrine Neoplasia Type 1 (or Wermer Syndrome, after the initial description by Wermer). Although it was long ago mapped to the long arm of chromosome 11, the exact gene remained elusive until April of 1997 when it was finally identified. Finally, here was the gene that caused pituitary tumors! We hoped that it would be abnormal in the far more common sporadic tumors.

Sadly, this is not the case. Just as with the BRCA genes that, when mutated, cause familial breast cancers, it appears that the MEN1 gene too is altered (deleted or mutated) in only a small proportion of patients with sporadic pituitary tumors. So we are still looking for other culprits.

We have suspected for a long time that the pituitary had a unique susceptibility to be driven proven that continuous and excessive hormonal stimulation can cause a pituitary tumor. But the vast majority of patients with pituitary tumors are not in the rare group of the chronically "hormonally challenged." For most, the story is a totally unsuspected tumor arising in a totally unsuspecting patient. There is no evidence of hormonal stimulation as the cause of most tumors.

Other potential factors that can play a role in tumor development, and that have been implicated in the development of tumor growth in other tissues, are members of several families of "growth factors." These hormone-like substances stimulate cell replication and differentiated cell functions, like hormone production. They are the subjects of investigation and early reports suggest that there may be abnormalities of these growth factors or their receptors in pituitary tumors, and that the degree of abnormality may determine the aggressiveness of tumor growth.

Studies such as these will hopefully lead to answers to the really important questions. We hope to identify the genes that will allow us to predict who will develop a pituitary tumor and will allow us to identify those at risk before the disease becomes clinically manifest. It is likely that there are several genes, and only some are responsible for making the tumors grow so quickly that they wreak havoc on their host. Those will be the culprits that we need to identify so that we can predict which tumors will grow quickly or recur, to determine which patients need more aggressive therapy.

We are all in this together. Patients, their families, endocrinologists, neurosurgeons, pathologists and basic scientists who work in this field have learned from the lessons of Descartes, Cushing and Simmonds; it is now our responsibility to work towards a common objective - the early diagnosis, treatment and cure, perhaps even the prevention, of pituitary disease.

Clinicopathologic Classification of Pituitary Adenomas

Clinically Functioning Adenomas	Clinically Nonfunctioning Adenomas
GH-PRL-TSH Family	
Adenomas Causing GH Excess • Densely granulated somatotroph adenomas • Sparsely granulated somatotroph adenomas	Silent somatotroph adenomas
Adenomas Causing Hyperprolactinemia • Lactotroph adenomas • Acidophil stem cell adenomas	Silent lactotroph adenomas
Adenomas Causing TSH Excess • Thyrotroph adenomas	Silent thyrotroph adenomas
ACTH Family	
Adenomas Causing ACTH Excess • Corticotroph adenomas	Silent corticotroph adenomas
Gonadotropin Family	
Adenomas Causing Gonadotropin Excess • Gonadotroph adenomas	Silent gonadotroph adenomas Null cell adenomas oncocytomas
Unclassified Adenomas	
Unusual plurihormonal adenomas	Hormone-negative adenomas

The Laboratory Assessment of Pituitary Gland Function

Delbert A. Fisher, M.D., President, Academic Associates
Quest Diagnostics, San Juan Capistrano, California

The human body is composed of a variety of specialized tissues which must function in an integrated fashion. This integrated control is accomplished by two major systems of communication: the brain and nervous system and the endocrine system. The nervous system conveys electrochemical signals to and from the brain and the body tissues. The endocrine system, composed of a series of endocrine glands, releases chemical signals called hormones which act by way of hormone receptors in responsive tissues.

The pituitary gland, a unique endocrine gland in a thimble sized pocket of bone at the base of the brain, serves to link these important communications systems. It functions as an endocrine transducer system in that it transduces (or converts) nervous system signals into hormonal signals and provides the brain with a direct pathway to influence endocrine gland function. The hypothalamus at the base of the brain contains nerve cells which produce small protein molecules which are transported in small blood vessels to the pituitary gland where they act to regulate production of one or more of the anterior pituitary hormones. The anterior pituitary hormones, in turn, regulate body metabolism directly or by controlling the activity of other endocrine glands. The anterior gland hormones and their functions include:

Growth Hormone (GH)
Regulates growth in children and has effects on protein, sugar, and fat metabolism in adults and children.

Prolactin (PRL)
Involved in regulation of breast milk production.

Gonadotropins
Regulates the sex glands, including the testes in males and ovaries in females. Two gonadotropins are involved: luteinizing hormone (LH) and follicle stimulating hormone (TSH).

Thyroid Stimulating hormone (TSH)
Regulates function of the thyroid gland.

Adrenocorticotropic hormone (ACTH)
Regulates function of the adrenal gland.

The hypothalamic hormones include growth hormone releasing hormone (GHRH) and somatostatin which regulate (stimulate and inhibit, respectively) GH release; prolactin inhibiting hormone (PLH) which regulates PRL release gonadotropin regulating hormone (GnRh) which influences LH and FSH secretion; thyrotropin releasing hormone (TRH) which modulates TSH secretion; and corticotropin releasing hormone (CRH) which modulates ACTH production.

A posterior pituitary gland composed of nerve fibers from the hypothalamus produces other small protein molecules, the Posterior Pituitary Hormones, These include:

Vasopressin (VP)
Also called antidiuretic hormone (ADH), modulates water excretion by the kidney to maintain body fluid volume and composition.

Oxytocin (OT)

In females OT stimulates uterine muscle contractions and is involved in labor and delivery; it also stimulates breast milk secretion during breast feeding. OT has no important role in males.

The pituitary gland has been referred to as the "master" (endocrine) gland because its hormones are regulatory for a number of the important endocrine glands. These glands, sometimes referred to as "target glands" include:

The Sex Glands, or Gonads
The testes in males produce the male hormone testosterone when stimulated by LH. Both LH and FSH in males regulate sperm production. In females, FSH stimulates growth of ovarian follicles, estrogen production and maturation of the female eggs or ova. LH in females regulates progesterone production which is important for growth of the egg in the uterus after it is released from the follicle and fertilized by a sperm.

The Thyroid Gland
This gland at the front and base of the neck is stimulated by TSH to produce the thyroid hormone thyroxine (T4) a small iodine-containing hormone. T4, in turn, is converted to the active hormone triiodothronine (T3) by removal of one of the 4 thyroxine iodine atoms. T3 acts on various body tissues to regulate the level of energy production (metabolic rate). It is also critical for normal childhood growth.

The Adrenal Cortical Glands
These paired glands lie just above the kidneys. When stimulated by pituitary ACTH, they produce the hormones cortisol, aldosterone and several weak androgens. Cortisol is required for normal body metabolism and adrenaline and noradrenaline are critical for the body's response to stress. Aldosterone helps regulate body fluid volume and blood pressure by regulating salt (sodium) excretion by the kidney. The adrenal androgens are testosterone-like molecules of limited significance unless secreted in excess in females.

The Role of the Laboratory in the Diagnosis and Management of Pituitary Divider
During the past three decades, we have witnessed development of highly sensitive and specific immunoassay methods for the direct measurement of all of the hypothalamic, pituitary, and target organ hormones in blood. See Table 1.

Table 1.		
Hypothalamic Hormones	Pituitary Hormones	Target Hormones
GHRH	GHRH	Insulin-Like Growth Factor 1 (IGF-I) produced in liver-IGF Binding Proteins produced by liver: IGF-FP2, IGF-BP3
PLH	PRL	No target hormone, but PRL suppresses LH, FSH and gonadal function
GnRH	LH	Testosterone Progesterone

Hypothalamic Hormones	Pituitary Hormones	Target Hormones
GnRH	FSH	Estrogen
TRH	TSH	Thyroxine Triiodothyronine
CRH	ACTH	Cortisol Aldosterone Adrenal Androgens
VP		No target hormones can measure urine concentration
OT		No target hormones

Physicians now have the ability to directly measure the levels of these hormones to assess the level of activity of the pituitary and target endocrine glands. An important characteristic of pituitary-target organ interaction is "feedback regulation." The target organ hormone levels in blood circulate or feed back to the pituitary gland and participate with the hypothalamic hormones to regulate the production of the pituitary hormone. For instance, TSH stimulates the thyroid gland to produce thyroxine. The circulating blood levels of TSH are stimulated by hypothalamic TRH and inhibited by increasing levels of circulating thyroid hormones so that the blood thyroid hormone levels are maintained within a narrow normal range. Damage to the thyroid gland reduces thyroid hormone levels with the result that pituitary TSH production is increased and blood levels of TSH are increased. Such feedback control also is operative for the GH, IGF-I, the LH-progesterone or testosterone, the FSH-estrogen, and the ACTH-cortisol systems. Thus simultaneous measurements of the pituitary and target endocrine gland hormones allows an assessment of feedback regulation and proper pituitary target organ interaction.

Pituitary tumors usually involve specific anterior pituitary cell types and this may produce excess amounts of one of the pituitary hormones. Acromegaly is due to excess GH secretion; Cushing's Disease is due to excess ACTH secretion; other less common tumors secrete TSH or LH/FSH. In these cases, the tumors are "autonomous" or self-controlled so that feedback regulation is abolished or diminished and the excessive, continuous stimulation of the target gland results in the classic signs of the target organ hormone excess (Acromegaly = IGF-I excess; Cushing's Disease = cortisol excess; Hyperthyroidism = thyroid hormone excess).

Many pituitary tumors involve cells which have lost hormone producing capacity. These tumors enlarge and destroy function of other pituitary cells with the result that target organ deficiencies may occur. Even the specific hormone secreting tumors may damage other pituitary cells if they grow large enough. Moreover, damage to functioning pituitary cells may occur during the process of treatment of pituitary tumors by surgery or radiation. Pituitary tumors involving posterior pituitary hormones have not been described, but tumors in the area of the hypothalamus can alter production of VP and alter the ability to regulate water (and urine) excretion. Large anterior pituitary tumors sometimes can do this.

It is believed that at least some pituitary tumors are due to the chronic overproduction of the specific hypothalamic regulatory factors (or hormones) which stimulate their respective pituitary cell types. In normal circumstances their circulating levels of hypothalamic hormones are low because they are not secreted into circulating blood (only into pituitary system blood).

However, tissues in various parts of the body are capable of producing small amounts of the hypothalamic hormones, and on occasion excessive amounts can be produced by tumors in the abdomen or chest. Such "ectopic" production of GHRH or CRH has been a rare cause of Acromegaly or Cushing's Disease. This can be detected by measurement of these hormones in peripheral blood. Finally, it is important to recognize that a pituitary tumor or pituitary dysfunction is not usually cured. Long term surveillance and management are essential. Thus, the physician and the patient must depend heavily on the laboratory for initial diagnostic assessment of the pituitary and target hormone activity and for ongoing surveillance of disease activity and treatment management. Many of the hormone measurements are available only in specialized laboratories and some tests require special handling of the specimens and special timing of their collection. Additionally, the physician may conduct scheduled stimulation or suppression tests to assess the responsiveness of the pituitary or target glands or the function of the feedback control systems.

The physician will maintain records of these test results, but it is also important that patients maintain an ongoing record of therapy and test results. Such records may be very important during travel; accidents may occur and the physician records may not be readily available. Having records available in the event of a move or job change may avoid problems. It is also helpful to know the laboratory source of your test results so that recent data can be retrieved in the event of travel or accident.

The Oral Presentations of Pituitary Tumors

Eric C. Sung, D.D.S., Section of Hospital Dentistry.
UCLA, School of Dentistry, Los Angeles, CA.

The pituitary is considered the master gland of the body. Individuals with pituitary tumor have many medical needs, and require lifelong medical *follow-up*. It is often crucial to recognize the signs and symptoms early to initiate the necessary medical treatment. Along with the physical findings that one may have, there are also many findings that may present in the oral cavity. This article will review the oral presentations of pituitary tumors, and the oral complications of some pituitary tumor therapies.

The initial presentations of pituitary disorders are highly variable. They depend on hormone over or underproduction or may cause mechanical problems by impinging on neighboring structures. Clinically, the tumors may cause galactorrhea, hypogonadism, short stature, gigantism and acromegaly, Cushing's, hyperthyroidism, and visual field disturbances. However, the oral presentations can also be significant detected by dentists. In patients with acromegaly, the initial presentation may include the patient's inability to chew properly with their front teeth. The patient may also present with temporomandibular joint dysfunction or myofacial pain. Much of this is due to the continued and abnormal condylar growth which leads to extreme prognathism. In severe cases, it may result in very unstable occlusion with only the molars touching. If growth hormone overproduction occurs before development of the adult dentition is complete, generalized macrodontia (large teeth) can be seen. Other oral facial findings include thick and full lips and macroglossia. The pressure of the enlarged tongue on the dentition are reflected as indentations on the sides of the tongue. With the prolonged tongue pressure, tipping and displacement of teeth may occur. In the edentulous patient, they may present themselves to the dentist with complaints of continued ill fitting dentures. The continued growth of the mandible may change the dimension of the mandibular arch and lead to changes on occlusion. Other common head and neck findings include thickening of the skin, enlargement of the supraorbital ridges, enlargement of the nose, exaggerated nasolabial folds, and increased head size.

In the congenital condition where there is a deficiency in pituitary and thyroid function, the decrease in size of the mandible is often observed. The face is wide and fails to develop in the longitudinal direction. The dentofacial changes seen in cretinism are related to the degree of thyroid deficiency. With regards to the dentition, both the size of the crown and root may be diminished. In addition, the exfoliation of the deciduous dentition is delayed, along with the eruption of the adult dentition, and the wisdom teeth are often congenitally missing. With regards to the soft tissue, edema is common and may lead to enlarged tongue. Again this may lead to malocclusion. In adults with pituitary and thyroid deficiency, the dentofacial changes are typically limited to the soft tissue of the face and mouth. The tongue may become edematous and it may interfere with occlusion and compromise speech articulation.

In patients with Cushing's syndrome associated with pituitary hyperfunction, the major concerns are osteoporosis and premature cessation of epiphyseal growth. Severe osteoporosis can be detected in dental radiographs. Orally, pigmentation on mucocutaneous surfaces may also be visualized. The oral pigmentation can be multifocal or diffuse and macular.

Pituitary tumors can be treated with surgery, radiation therapy, or drugs. These therapies have oral ramifications. With respect to surgery, an intraoral approach may be employed for transsphenoidal resection of pituitary tumors. There have been reported cases where this lead to severe gingival recession on the buccal surface of the maxillary anterior teeth. (Currently, a variety of techniques can be utilized for covering the root surfaces.) The severe gingival recession can lead to extreme sensitivity and the premature loss of those teeth.

With regards to radiation therapy, the modality used is typically external beam therapy. The dose varies depending on the protocol and range from 4,000 cGy to 5,500 cGy. Radiation fields include the superior border of the parotid gland and these patients may experience varying degrees of xerostomia (Dry mouth), altered taste sensation, and decreased smell capacity. These complications are typically mild and most resolve within months of completion of therapy. If the xerostomia be severe or prolonged, there is an increased risk of dental caries (cavities) and fungal infections. Patient comfort is facilitated by keeping the oral mucosa moist. This can be accomplished by the use of saliva substitutes or with a water bottle. Frequent follow-up dental examinations are recommended and the daily utilization of a fluoride gel in a customized carrier may be recommended. The daily application of fluoride gel, along with immaculate oral hygiene, is the most reliable method of prevention of post-irradiation dental caries. In regards to fungal infections it may occur with increased frequency in the post irradiation period. The most common locations are the corner of the mouth, and plain beneath dentures. This infection is easily treated with antifungal creams or powders and oral rinses.

Drugs used to treat these tumors may cause oral side effects. Many of the androgens, estrogens, and progestins, cause sore and tender gums. In severe cases, bleeding gums and gingival hyperplasia can be seen. A strict regimen of oral hygiene along with dental follow-up will minimize the severity of gingival inflammation and enlargement. Medications such as bromocriptine and pergolide may also lead to xerostomia. In prolonged xerostomia, as mentioned previously, there is an increased risk of dental caries and fungal infections. The same precautions should be taken as the aforementioned radiation induced xerostomia.

Other common side effects of medications include nausea and vomiting. In chronic cases, there is a risk of eroding the dentition. This is especially true on the palatal surfaces of the maxillary anteriors where the gastric acid is usually projected. As the enamel is eroded away, there is a risk of the dentition becoming sensitive and the exposed dentin is at a greater risk of developing dental caries. It is recommended that the patient thoroughly rinse his or her mouth soon after vomiting to reduce the prolonged gastric acid exposure to the tooth structure. The application of topical fluoride to the eroded dentition will also reduce the sensitivity and decrease the risk of caries.

In summary, the patients with a history of pituitary tumors are a special group of patients with many different medical needs. The dental team needs to be aware of the changes in the oral cavity that may occur in these patients. Combined with the physical presentations, one should be aware of the possible underlying medical condition and make appropriate referrals. Once a diagnosis is made, one must be aware of the oral presentations of the disease and potential side effects of the medical therapies. Working together with the endocrinologist, the dentist can help monitor and maintain the oral health of the patient.

The Role of Octreoscan® in Patients With Pituitary Tumors

W.W. de Herder, M.D., Department of Internal Medicine III and Clinical Endocrinology
University Hospital Dijkzigt, Rotterdam, The Netherlands

Introduction

Somatostatin is a protein-like substance (peptide), which generally exerts an inhibitory effect on a variety of hormone-producing (endocrine) glands. Somatostatin-producing cells are widely distributed throughout the human body. Many endocrine tumors arising from endocrine glands possess high numbers of so-called receptors (parking places) for the peptide somatostatin. Somatostatin can inhibit the increased hormonal production by these tumors by binding with somatostatin receptors. In some cases, binding of somatostatin to its receptor can also inhibit the growth of some of these tumors. Somatostatin itself is not suitable for medical therapy, because it needs to be directly administered into the bloodstream and it is rapidly degraded in the body, thereby losing its potency to inhibit excessive hormonal production. For this reason, "somatostatin analogs", like octreotide (Sandostatin®), have been developed. Because these substances exert their effect by binding to specific receptors, a radioactive, labeled somatostatin analog that can be safely administered to humans would be potentially suitable for the visualization by means of a gamma camera of tumors carrying somatostatin receptors in patients. This finally lead to the development of Octreoscan® for somatostatin receptor scanning (scintigraphy). A scan image created by binding of the radioactive labeled Octreoscan® to a tumor abundant in somatostatin receptors is by definition called a positive scan." On a negative scan image, no binding of radioactivity to the tumor is shown (for examples see the figures). Octreoscan® images always show uptake of radioactivity in the normal liver, spleen, kidneys, thyroid gland and mostly in the normal pituitary gland.

Hormonal studies obtained after the administration of somatostatin(analogs) to patients with tumors that are known to possess somatostatin receptors closely correlate with studies with cultured cells of these tumors after the administration of somatostatin(analogs) and results of Octreoscan®. This suggests that a positive Octreoscan® in a patient with a hormone-producing tumor, which possesses somatostatin receptors, predicts a therapeutical effect of a somatostatin analog on the hormonal hypersecretion by these tumors. Octreoscan® is also a useful tool in the diagnostic work-up of patients with hormone-producing tumors possessing somatostatin receptors, to localize the primary tumor, as well as metastatic spread.

What Is The Role of Octreoscan® in Patients with Pituitary Tumors?

- Most growth hormone (GH)-secreting pituitary adenomas possess somatostatin receptors. Octreotide therapy in patients with acromegaly results in:
- Symptomatic relief.
- A significant decrease of the mean GH levels in the blood.
- In approximately 60% of patients, normalization of insulin-like growth factor (IGF)-I levels in the blood.
- In approximately 50% of patients, slight, but significant decreases in pituitary tumor size.

However, most clinical studies do not show a good correlation between the of Octreoscan® and the GH response to a single subcutaneous dose of octreotide. In parallel with GH-secreting adenomas, most thyrotropin (TSH)-secreting pituitary adenomas also possess somatostatin receptors. Like in acromegaly, the clinical impact of Octreoscan® for patients with TSH-secreting adenomas seems limited: increased pituitary uptake of Octreoscan® generally may predict a good sensitivity of TSH secretion to the inhibitory effect of octreotide, but this can be more easily predicted on the basis of an acute octreotide test.

At present there is no established medical treatment for clinically nonfunctioning and gonadotropin-secreting pituitary adenomas (NFPA). The clinical distinction of these tumors from other diseases in the pituitary region may be difficult. About 40%-50% of NFPA possesses substantial amounts of somatostatin receptors. Generally, octreotide therapy in patients with NFPA does not result in significant tumor reduction. Significant improvement of visual field defects may be the result from other non-tumor-related effects of octreotide. Using Octreoscan®, increased pituitary uptake of radioactivity can be observed in approximately 60% of NFPA patients.

Prolactin (PRL)-secreting pituitary tumors are generally not sensitive to octreotide. Octreoscan® is expected to be of limited importance in the differential diagnosis of tumors in and around the pituitary region, because most meningiomas, low-grade astrocytomas, metastases from cancers (like breast cancer), hematological cancers (like Hodgkin and non-Hodgkin lymphomas) and inflammatory lesions can be visualized by means of Octreoscan®. Glioblastomas, craniopharyngiomas and other cysts are usually negative on Octreoscan®.

No suppressive effect of octreotide has been demonstrated in the majority of patients with untreated Cushing's disease, who have increased cortisol levels in the blood. In contrast, in patients with Nelson's syndrome, who are only on cortisol replacement therapy, long-term inhibition of excessive small corticotropin (ACTH) secretion by somatostatin and octreotide has been demonstrated. In some cases, stabilization of tumor growth and restoration of visual field defects accompanied this. Octreoscan® is usually negative in patients with small ACTH-secreting pituitary tumors, but can be positive in patients with large ACTH-secreting macroadenomas, like in Nelson's syndrome. However, Octreoscan® is an important technique for the identification of endocrine tumors that are not of pituitary origin that secrete ACTH ectopically.

In conclusion, Octreoscan® has only limited value for the diagnosis of disorders in or around the pituitary region. However, it is an important diagnostic tool for the diagnosis and staging of patients with other (neuro-)endocrine disorders. A good example of this is the detection and staging of endocrine pancreatic tumors in patients with familial multiple endocrine neoplasia (MEN)-I syndrome.

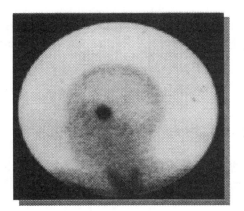 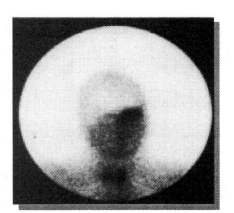

Legend to the figures; Octreoscan images of two patients:
The left patient has an enlarged pituitary gland, caused by a GH-secreting pituitary tumor. The head is rotated to the right. There is high uptake of the radioactivity in the tumor. Also, the thyroid gland in the neck is shown. The right patient has a so-called inner ridge meningioma in the pituitary region. The head is face forward. There is high uptake of the radioactivity in the tumor. Also, the thyroid gland in the neck is shown.

The Role of Octreoscan in Patients

41

Heredity and the Pituitary Tumor

Robert F. Gagel, M.D., Chief, Section of Endocrinology, Professor of Medicine
University of Texas MD Anderson Cancer Center

A question that patients frequently ask is "Why have I developed a pituitary tumor?" A second is "Could I pass this pituitary tumor on to my children?" In most cases, the answers to these questions are not straightforward. However, research is beginning to provide answers to some of these questions.

There is increasing evidence that small changes in DNA, the chemical structure which directs development and function of human beings, may be responsible for some pituitary tumors. Each of us has two complete copies of all of the DNA needed for life. We inherit one copy from one parent and another from the other. Together, these DNA copies serve as a blueprint for development of specific parts of the human body, such as the pituitary gland. There are approximately three billion bases of DNA. The DNA is further subdivided into structural units, called genes, which are responsible for telling a cell to perform a specific function. There is increasing evidence that small changes in the DNA structure of a gene can cause a major disturbance of cell growth and development; a collection of cells growing at an increased rate can cause a tumor. Figure 1 shows schematically how a mistake in a single cell could result in accelerated growth of that cell type resulting in a tumor.

How Does One Acquire A Defect in DNA Which Causes a Tumor?

Each of us starts life as a single fertilized egg. The egg divides very rapidly to create two, four, eight, sixteen, etc. cells. As a cell divides, it is necessary to copy all of the DNA in the cell (three billion bases) and to pass it to the new cell. To accomplish this task the cell has developed a very sophisticated copying mechanism, but there are occasional errors. For example, if you were asked to copy 1,000 numbers, it is likely that an error or two would creep into the transcribing process. Although the cell has developed a sophisticated mechanism to proof the copy and detect major errors, some slip through the editing process. If one of these errors occurs in a very important gene which controls cell function or growth, then the cell may begin to divide at an increased rate.

A second mechanism for acquiring a genetic abnormality is to inherit it from a parent. If one of your parents has a small error in a pituitary growth regulatory gene and this defect is present in eggs or sperm, there is a 50% possibility this defect could be passed to a child. A child who inherited this genetic abnormality would have a greater chance of developing a pituitary tumor.

Research over the past five years has identified two specific genetic abnormalities which causes pituitary tumors in families.

Acquired Abnormalities of DNA Which Cause Acromegaly

Acromegaly is caused by abnormal growth of the specific pituitary cell type which produces growth hormone. Research has discovered that approximately one-third to one-half of these pituitary tumors have an abnormality of a specific gene, called gsp, which regulates cell growth and hormone production. The abnormality in the gsp gene is very small and changes only one building block of the roughly three billion which comprise all of the DNA in the cell. Unfortunately, this change occurs in a critical portion of the gsp gene and results in increased pituitary cell growth and hormone (growth hormone) production. Over time, the increased rate of cell growth can cause a sizable pituitary tumor. The information about the gsp abnormality is relatively new and no specific treatments have been developed to counter the abnormal gene activity. However, an understanding of the cause of pituitary tumor development suggests that it may be possible at some future date to reverse this abnormality. Indeed, one of the actions of octreotide (Sandostatin), a drug commonly used to treat acromegaly (see Pituitary Network Newsletter, September 1994), may be to suppress or bypass the function of this particular gene. It seems likely that this information will lead to new pituitary tumor treatment strategies in the future.

Inherited Pituitary Tumors

A small number of pituitary tumors develop as a result of the inheritance of a specific gene from a parent. A family history is an important part of treatment of a pituitary tumor. Are there individuals in the family who have had a pituitary tumor? Sometimes it may be difficult to determine whether a relative had a pituitary tumor because it may be called a "brain tumor." Review of the specific medical records for the affected patient may be necessary to be certain of a diagnosis.

In a condition called multiple endocrine neoplasia, type 1 (MEN 1) there is the association of pituitary tumors, tumors of the parathyroid glands (glands which control the level of calcium in the blood), and cells in the pancreas which produce insulin and other hormones. The predisposition to develop a pituitary tumor in these families is inherited directly from an affected parent. Each child has a 50/50 chance of inheriting the gene causing this disorder from an affected parent. For example, if an affected parent marries and has eight children, it is likely that four of these children will inherit the predisposition to develop a pituitary tumor. It is important to understand that inheriting the gene is a matter of chance — either a child does or does not inherit the abnormal copy of the gene.

Approximately 10 years ago a Swedish group localized the gene which causes MEN 1 to the eleventh chromosome (there are a total of 23 chromosomes in each cell) and recently a group at the National Institutes of Health identified the causative gene, named menin. The gene functions as a brake for pituitary cell growth. Over 90% of families with MEN 1 have a DNA change which results in inactivation of this gene which leads to increased cell growth and tumor formation (Figure 2).

It is now possible by relatively simple genetic tests to determine the specific DNA change. This work is so new, however, that the test is not yet commercially available and is only available in research laboratories. If you have access to the worldwide web, information about the future commercial availability of the test can be found at: http://endocrine.mdacc.tmc.edu (see genetic testing section). In a family with an identified mutation or DNA change, it is possible to predict with 100% certainty whether a child is affected.

It seems certain that other abnormalities of the DNA will be identified in the future. These discoveries will certainly lead to a greater understanding of how pituitary tumors develop and, if experience with other tumors is any indication, will lead to strategies for prevention and treatment. Stay tuned!

References

1   Melmed S: Pituitary Neoplasia. Endocrinol Metab Clin North America 1994;23:81-92.
2   Gagel RF: Multiple Endocrine Neoplasia, in: Wilson JD, Foster DW (ed): Williams Textbook of Endocrinology. Philadelphia, W.B. Saunders Company, 1992, 1537-1553.
3   Chandrasekharappa SC, Guru SC, Manickam P, et al., Positional cloning of the gene for multiple endocrine neoplasia-type 1. Science 1997; 276:404-7.
4   Lemmens I, Vandeven WJM, Kas K, et al. Identification of the Multiple Endocrine Neoplasia type 1 (MEN 1) Gene. Human Molecular Genetics 1997; 6:1177-1183,Figure Legends:

Heredity and the Pituitary Gland (sidebar)

An acquired DNA change in a single cell causes more rapid growth and development of a pituitary tumor

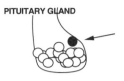

PITUITARY GLAND

DNA change in *gsp* gene causes a single cell to grow and divide at a more rapid rate.

The cell with the DNA change divides more rapidly than normal cells, resulting in a greater number of cells.

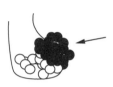

Continued growth results in the development of a pituitary tumor-additional changes in the DNA may occur which cause more rapid development of a tumor.

Figure 1. Schematic diagram showing how an activating mutation can lead to cell growth and pituitary tumor formation.

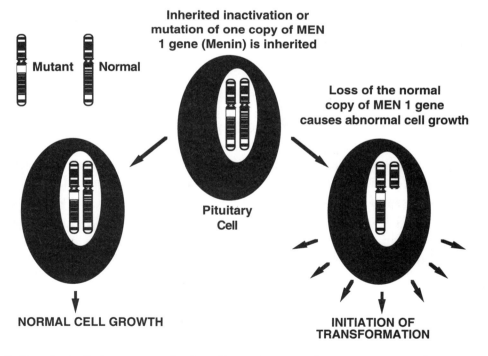

Mutant   Normal

Inherited inactivation or mutation of one copy of MEN 1 gene (Menin) is inherited

Loss of the normal copy of MEN 1 gene causes abnormal cell growth

Pituitary Cell

NORMAL CELL GROWTH

INITIATION OF TRANSFORMATION

Figure 2. Paradoxically loss or inactivation of genetic material can cause tumor formation. Loss or inactivation of both copies of the menin gene, located on chromosome 11q (shown shaded in white), leads to tumor formation. A cell with one mutant and one normal copy of this gene grows normally.

A Discussion Of Multiple Endocrine Neoplasia-Type I

*E. A. Koller, M.D., J. M. Treese., K. M. M. Shakir, M.D., Department of Internal Medicine,
Section of Endocrinology, National Naval Medical Center, Bethesda, Maryland*

If I have a pituitary tumor, is there a chance that I could get other tumors?

If I have a pituitary tumor, is there a chance that other family members could get pituitary tumors?

The answers depend on what type of pituitary tumor you had and whether the syndrome of Multiple Endocrine Neoplasia I (MEN I), Multiple Endocrine Adenomas-Type I, or Wermer's Syndrome, runs in your family.

Multiple Endocrine Neoplasia is a genetic (inherited) disorder in which several endocrine systems may be affected: the parathyroid glands, the anterior pituitary, the adrenal gland, and the pancreatic islet cells. It occurs in approximately 2 of 50,000 persons. Although some patients present with multiple endocrine glands affected at one time, the more typical scenario is for the patient to have one type of endocrine gland affected and then have other types of endocrine affected in subsequent years. Patients seldom present with disease prior to the age of ten. More than 90% of adults with MEN I will present by age 50. (Refer to the diagram.)

Hyperparathyroidism is the most common, and usually the earliest, disorder seen. 75% or more of MEN I patients develop hyperparathyroidism. Several of the 2-6 parathyroid glands are over-active resulting elevated parathyroid hormone (PTH) and calcium levels. Patients may present with these biochemical findings or with significant clinical disease such as kidney stones or bone loss. (Note: All familial (inherited) hyper-calcemia is not due to MEN I).

50% or more of MEN I patients develop pituitary lesions. There are several types of tumors (generally non-malignant) which may occur in the anterior pituitary. Some tumors may produce more than one type of hormone. Some tumors may be biochemically "silent" because they do not produce complete or functional hormone, but may still cause symptoms (headache or reduction in visual fields) and be detected by CAT (computed axial tomagraphy) scan or MRI (magnetic resonance imaging). The most common type of functional pituitary tumor for MEN I patients is the prolactinoma. With prolactinomas, there is over-production of the hormone, prolactin. This may cause galactorrhea (milk discharge) in non-postpartum women.

Prolactimonas may result in abnormal menses and infertility in women and erectile dysfunction and infertility in men. Other tumors may result in excess growth hormone production. Excess growth hormone causes gigantism if it occurs before a child/adolescent has completed puberty. It also causes acromegaly with its coarsening of facial features, bony overgrowth, enlargement of internal organs, and excess perspiration. Tumors that cause Cushing's Disease produce excess adrenocorticotropin hormone (ACTH) and/or melanocyte-stimulating hormone (MSH). Patients may present with new-onset central obesity, easy bruising, glucose intolerance, and dusky skin color. Much less common are tumors which produce thyroid-stimulating hormone (TSH), which could result in hyperthyroidism (a state of excess thryoid hormone secretion). Theoretically it is also possible for pituitary tumors to produce gonadotropins, follicle-stimulating hormone and leutinizing hormone, leading to aberrant feminization or masculinization.

More than 75% of patients have pancreatic islet cell tumors. These tumors tend to be in multiple locations. Some tumors may produce more than one hormone, but usually these tumors secrete no hormone or only one hormone. Although tumors may be malignant 30% of the time, they tend to spread slowly. The most common functional type of pancreatic tumor in MEN-I is a gastrinoma. Symptomatic patients present with peptic ulcer disease and/or diarrhea. Asymptomatic patients may need provocative (stimulatory) testing to identify abnormal hormonal responses. At least one third of pancreatic tumors are insulinomas. Excess insulin may cause hypoglycemia (low blood sugar) manifest by headache, confusion, seizures, or loss of consciousness. Much less frequently, pancreatic islet cell tumors can secrete the functional hormones; ACTH, glucagon, PTH, and vasoactive intestinal peptide. Pancreatic islet cell tumors can also secrete hormones like pancreatic polypeptide which do not cause identifiable clinical syndromes, ie., symptom complex.

There may be abnormal growth in the adrenal glands, but most of the time, no active hormone is released. Patients may also present with carcinoid tumors, most frequently in the lungs or in the intestines. The serotonin that they typically produce may cause flushing, trouble breathing, and diarrhea. Such carcinoids have also been reported to secrete ACTH. Lastly, lipomas (fatty tumors) may also occur at a higher rate in MEN-I families.

MEN I is transmitted through family members as an autosomal dominant trait; that is to say, there is a 50% chance that a child will inherit the disorder from an affected parent. Only one parent needs to carry the genetic material for the disease. A child of either gender may develop the disease. The disorder may have incomplete penetrance. In other words, some family members who carry the genetic material for MEN I may not be as affected as other members, and it is unclear as to why this is so. It has also been estimated that 50% of new cases of MEN I are sporadic, ie. the result of new mutations. The gene locus responsible for this disorder was recently identified at the National Institutes of Health. There are least 12 mutations throughout the gene located on the "q" arm of chromosome 11. It is thought that the protein normally produced by this gene, "menin," suppresses tumors, so when the protein is missing or defective, tumors can arise. It is possible that commercial genetic tests, such as those which have been developed for screening of family members with a related disorder, MEN II, will become available.

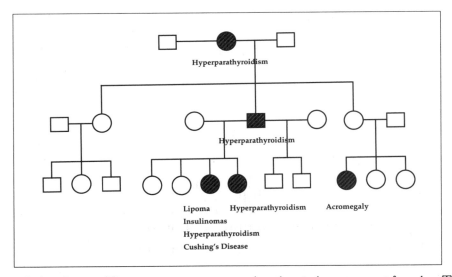

Fig. 1 A sample family tree. The squares represent males; the circles represent females. The first row is the first generation. The subseqent rows are later generations. Marriages are indicated by a connecting bar. Brother and sisters are indicated by connecting overhead bars. Family members with conditions that can be suspicious for MEN I are indicated by the shading.

" The starting point of all achievement is desire. Keep this constantly in mind. Weak desire brings weak results, just as a small amount of fire makes a small amount of heat."

Napoleon Hill

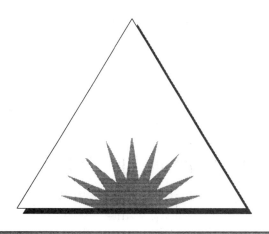

Ten Tools for Recovery

Charles B. Wilson, M.D., Professor, Department of Neurosurgery
University of California, San Francisco Medical Center

Editor's note: The following article is excerpted from the closing address of the Third Biennial Brain Tumor Conference which was delivered by Dr. Charles Wilson, Professor at the Department of Neurosurgery at the University of California, San Francisco, and a leading pioneer in the field of brain tumor research. Dr. Wilson's talk was entitled "Science Isn't Enough."

When you or someone close to you has a diagnosis of a brain tumor there are three immediate effects. One is practical—how will this affect your life? The second is physical—you may have some after-effect from the tumor or its treatment. And the third, on which I will dwell, is psychological.

Science has tried to discover the mechanisms for the powerful effects that our emotions have on our health, and it's given rise to terms such as psychoneuroendocrine effects and psychoneuroimmune effects.

I'm often asked, "Does stress cause cancer?" Who among us is not subjected to stress in some form? This is based on something called an immune surveillance hypothesis. And the hypothesis very simply is this: Every single day, something we breathe or eat carries in it something that may cause a cell to mutate and become a cancer cell. But we have this healthy immune system and that particular cell is destroyed and it never becomes a cancer. It's unlikely that stress directly causes cancer, but I'm convinced that it can unmask or certainly accelerate the appearance of cancer—and this comes from a hard core scientist who a few short years ago believed it was nonsense.

I believe also that stress can play a role both in progression of a disease and recurrence of a tumor. Stress can become very powerful—it is that emotion which leads to world class performance. But it has to be harnessed so that it can be a positive power and not something that has an erosive consequence.

I'd like to give you ten very specific things that you can do...not instead of conventional medicine, but in addition to it. And the theme of this is that there are certain things you can't control—you can't control that you have a tumor, you can't control where it is. But there are things you can control. So, rather than be dismayed and depressed over those things that you can't control, you focus on things over which you do have some control, and I can assure you that in these things I will recommend there is real power.

Seek Psychological Help.

On the front page of today's San Francisco Examiner is a headline: "It's Mind And Matter," and it's a story about sports psychology. These are world class elite athletes who often scoffed at the idea of needing any kind of psychological help, but you'd have to be pretty out of it not to recognize that sports psychology is a big thing. The Oakland A's, for instance, have a full-time sports psychologist. So there has to be a power within psychologically examining ourselves...who we are...our fears...our strengths...that helps us in dealing with our lives and whatever life may have brought us. But, I think more important from your standpoint, is that this type of examination can empower you in a way that has been shown many times to increase your chance of survival and have a profound effect on longevity.

By this (seeking psychological help) I mean learning coping skills and how to manage stress, whether by meditation or by some breathing exercise—but something you can be taught to do that gives you some sense of having control over what's happening.

Socialize, Socialize, Socialize.
Socialize with your friends, with your family. If you are socially isolated with cancer of the breast, your mortality is twice as high as those who are not socially isolated—a fairly impressive statistic.

If a patient has at least one confidant, a person to whom they can tell everything...the bad and the ugly...the fears...someone with whom they can absolutely spill everything, their chances of surviving over any given period of time is approximately doubled. And there are those who say a pet can have the same effect.

Join a Support Group.
Find some place where you can go to express your worries, your concerns—some place where you can laugh, and can bond with people who happened to end up in the same boat that you find yourself in.

Learn About Your Disease.
Initially it may be very stressful. You read about brain tumors, you see a picture of a scan, you can picture your own scan, you may get tight in the throat or feel sick in the stomach. But once you have learned something about your disease you become a partner in the team of people who will determine your future—that is your treatment and your management. Over time, learning about your disease improves your ability to cope.

Grieve.
Elizabeth Kubler Ross says you've got to grieve. It's a terrible thing that's happened. Your family grieves, you grieve, and it's okay, it's natural; but you've got to do that and then get on with life.

Face Your Own Mortality and Cope with Dying.
As I whizzed by my 60th birthday—and I'm looking forward in a few months to my 65th—in a way I came in touch, finally, with my own mortality. I realized that life is finite. Life can be beautiful, but it is certainly not forever. A part of the end of life is dying and it's okay to think about it; it's okay to wonder about it; and it's okay to be a little afraid about it—but it isn't okay not to think about it.

Try to Learn Something About Imaging.
I used to think this was not important, but I'm now persuaded that for some people (maybe not for you and certainly not for all) it can be very powerful. There are many ways of doing it. For instance, in San Francisco, Dr. Martin Rossman has introduced interactive guided imagery, which is just one form.

Decide to Develop Some New Interest or Some New Activity.
Despite all that's happened, decide that you're going to develop some new interest or some new activity. Maybe you've always wanted to go down to Glide Memorial Church in San Francisco and become a volunteer. Maybe you've always said "I'd like to take a class in Greek mythology," or maybe you'd like to learn jazz saxophone, write a book, learn to paint. Do something that's different, that's compelling, and that will give you a sense of new accomplishment.

Exercise and Eat Properly.
You may say, "I have a weak arm or a weak leg," or "I'm on Decadron and don't have much energy." Well, if you want to be inspired, just look in some day on the Special Olympics, or watch a wheelchair marathon. Exercise gives you a sense of discipline, gives you a sense of

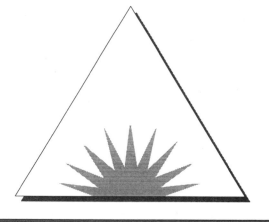

Ten Tools for Recovery

control, it makes you feel better. Psychiatrists learned long ago that probably exercise for depression is more effective than the couch.

And eat properly. You should be healthy. Just because you have a brain tumor does not mean that the body that happens to be harboring this tumor should be allowed to go along without maintenance and improvement. Vitamins will help.

Get in Touch With Some Higher Being.
It can be many forms and it can be many spirits. It will give you a strength and will give you a peace. Physicians are now learning that when religion matters to a patient, they should take that seriously.

The mind can be a powerful determinant in healing and recovery. Believe that you can beat this disease against all odds. Focus on those things in your life that you can control. But above all, put our trust in a higher spirit, because the strength that you can find in a spiritual experience has power beyond your imagination.

It's a beautiful day. It's the first day in the rest of your life, and I hope that my God and your God will bless you all.

"It's not whether you get knocked down. It's whether you get up again."

Charitable Air Medical Transport System in Place

This article was sent by Edward Boyer, President/CEO of Mercy Medical Airlift (MMA). He is concerned that "most people don't know that there are thousands of pilots and aircraft... ready, willing and able to provide free medical air transportation for ambulatory outpatients." MMA's purpose and long-range goal is to insure that no patients are denied access to distant specialized diagnosis, treatment or rehabilitation for lack of means of medical air transport.

Multiple sources of charitable air medical transportation are now available to most anybody in the U.S. There is no guarantee that every need will be met, but there are dedicated people working to help meet every need.

There are two national charitable programs that should be known by every medical organization, every health care worker and every family with a rare disorder patient. These are:

1. The National Patient Air Transport HOTLINE (NPATH) – (800) 296-1217. This one-of-a-kind unique hotline makes referrals to all known appropriate charitable, charitably-assisted and special patient discount commercial services based on an evaluation of the patient's medical condition, type of transportation required and departure/destination location. Patient referrals are made to over 45 different sources of air medical transport help.

2. The "special lift" air medical transport program operation in conjunction with NPATH HOTLINE. Sponsors of large-scale disease research or experimental treatment programs can take advantage of this program which will manage and coordinate the air medical transportation aspect of the special project – arranging to move large numbers of patients to and from special research or treatment facilities, one at a time, as required – via charitable means – nationwide.

At the present time a "Child-Lift 1" program is serving a special double-blind drug testing program for Congenital Lactic Acidosis. A "Child-Lift 2" program is transporting patients with Sturge-Weber Syndrome. Both of these programs are serving the Clinical Research Center of the University of Florida. A third very large nationwide "special-lift" program is currently being negotiated.

Both of these charitable air medical transport programs are operated by Mercy Medical Airlift, a non-profit charity specializing in developing, assisting and coordinating charitable public benefit air medical transport programs.

The HOTLINE can be reached at (800) 296-1217. To discuss possible future "special lift" programs call MMA at (800) 296-1911. MMA offices are in Manassas, Virginia but it services are nationwide. MMA operates the above described programs in support of the Air Care Alliance and works in full cooperation with, and supports all known public benefit volunteer flying organization, airline patients and other related patient air medical transport programs.

The Nurse's Role: Medical Management
The Endocrine Nurse's Society

The pituitary gland secretes six major hormones. They are: growth hormone, ACTH, prolactin, TSH, FSH, and LH. Pituitary dysfunction can occur when too much of any of these hormones is secreted or when too little of these hormones is secreted. As a patient you may have to take hormone replacement medications if you have a disease in which too little of a hormone is secreted, or you may have to take medications to control excess secretion of hormones if you have a disease that causes too much of a hormone being secreted. Your physician will diagnose your condition and prescribe the appropriate medications for you to take for your disease. The nurse will work with you to ensure that the medications that have been prescribed provide the optimum effect on your disease.

The nurse will first review with you the medications that you are to take. She will review with you the medication schedule that you will need to follow. You need to know the number of times that you need to take the medication, and the times of the day that this needs to be done. Be sure to share with your nurse any problems that you may encounter with taking your medications. For example, if you have a work situation or schedule that is rigid, there may need to be adjustments in the times of the day that you take your medications.

It is also important, for you the patient, to know about expected effects that the medication should have on the symptoms of your disease and your body. For example, if you have acromegaly which is caused by an excessive secretion of growth hormone, you might be given octreotide acetate. The medication is designed to decrease the secretion of growth hormone which should result in decrease in bone overgrowth and decreased facial puffiness. You might also experience an increase in your energy level.

The medications that have been prescribed for you are designed to act on your disease to either decrease excessive secretion of hormones or replace hormones that you are not secreting and that are necessary for health and a sense of well being. However, medications often have side effects that can indicate a problem with your continuing to take the medication. Therefore, the nurse will explain to you any side effects or untoward effects that have been noted to occur with the medication that you are taking. To build on the example in the previous paragraph, octreotide acetate has been noted to cause gallstone formation in some patients. This is important for you to know if you are taking that medication.

Not all medications will be taken by mouth. There are some medications that may be prescribed for you that you will need to administer to yourself by injection. If that is the situation with you, the nurse will teach you and a family member if possible to administer your medication by injection. This may take several learning sessions, and it is important for you to become comfortable with giving yourself an injection. Once you have learned the technique for self injection, you may want to review this on several occasions with the nurse to be sure that you are continuing to use the correct techniques.

Now that you have received your medications, know how and when to take them, you need to monitor the effect that the medications have on your body. It is best to keep a written record of these effects to share with your physician and nurse at each visit. This will assist them to recognize any unexpected effects that medication may be having on your body, and to evaluate the effectiveness of the medication in controlling your disease and its symptoms.

Patients with pituitary dysfunction often experience depression and psychological changes as

Pituitary Patient Resource Guide

a result of their disease. Pituitary dysfunction is difficult to diagnose despite the many tools available to the physician, and you, the patient, may become frustrated and experience a great deal of stress in the process of diagnosing your illness. Your family may also experience this as they see the changes that may occur during the course of your illness. The patient with pituitary dysfunction needs support and assistance to cope with his illness in an effective manner. The nurse can play a vital role in providing support to you and your family during this very difficult time.

Once your diagnosis has been made, the nurse can plan a vital role in assisting you to understand the changes that are occurring in your body as a result of your disease. It is important for you to understand the disease process: its cause and the treatment choices that are available to you. If at all possible, your family or significant other should be involved in the discussions involving diagnosis and treatment of your illness.

Each time that you visit the physician and the nurse, it is important to share your feelings and concerns about what you are experiencing. If you are having difficulties at work and seem unable to accomplish your work each day, you need to share this information with the nurse. Your energy level is important to discuss with your nurse. This may increase or decrease depending upon the disease that you have. For example, in Cushing's syndrome which may be caused by an excess of ACTH secretion, your energy level may increase, and you may find that you cannot concentrate. Students who have this excessive secretion of ACTH and cortisol, find that their grades go down as a result of the inability to concentrate.

Radiation therapy may be prescribed to treat your illness if it is caused by a pituitary tumor that is secreting excessive amounts on one of the pituitary hormones. Radiation therapy can be prescribed for acromegaly which is a disease caused by a tumor secreting an excess of growth hormone, and Cushing's disease which is caused by an excess of ACTH. You may or may not have had pituitary surgery prior to the initiation of radiation therapy. Radiation therapy is prescribed by a physician specializing in the field of radiation. The therapy itself is administered by a radiation therapist. Special planning is required prior to the initiation of the therapy. In a process called stimulation, you will be asked to lie very still on a table while the therapist uses a special x-ray machine to define the place on your head where the treatment will be aimed. The therapist will put special marks on your body which are not to be washed off during the treatment.

There may be some side effects to radiation therapy. Most often these include fatigue, skin changes, and loss of appetite. It is important to get plenty of rest during this time. Many patients, however, do maintain a regular work schedule with extra rest periods taken during off hours. At this time, it is important to maintain good nutrition despite the fact that you may not feel like eating. The nurse can work with you or refer you to a nutritionist who can assist you in maintaining adequate nutrition. It is important to keep your physician and nurse informed of your progress during the time that you are undergoing radiation therapy. They can assist you in managing the side effects that may occur during the treatment.

References

1. Romero JH: Hyperfunction and hypofunction in the anterior pituitary. Nursing Clinics of North American 31:769-777.
2. Radiation Therapy and You: A guide to self-help during treatment. National Cancer Institute. National Institutes of Health. Public Health Service. U.S. Department of Health and Human Services. Publication Number: 95-2227.1993.

Second Edition

A Creed For Those Who Have Suffered

I asked God for strength, that I might achieve.
I was made weak, that I might learn humbly to obey...
I asked for health, that I might do great things.
I was given infirmity, that I might do better things...
I asked for riches, that I might be happy.
I was given poverty, that I might be wise...
I asked for power, that I might have the praise of men.
I was given weakness, that I might feel the need of God...
I asked for all things, that I might enjoy life.
I was given life, that I might enjoy all things...
I got nothing I asked for — but everything I had hoped for.
Almost despite myself, my unspoken prayers were answered.
I am, among men, most richly blessed!

Roy Campanella

Section II

Specific Disorders

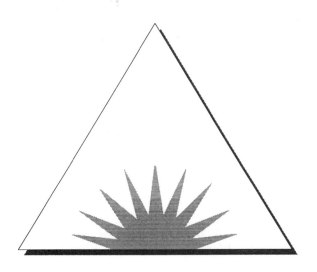

Second Edition

Cushing's Syndrome
National Institute of Diabetes and Digestive and Kidney Diseases

Cushing's syndrome is a hormonal disorder caused by prolonged exposure of the body's tissues to high levels of the hormone cortisol. Sometimes called "hypercortisolism," it is relatively rare and most commonly affects adults aged 20 to 50. An estimated 10-15 of every million people are affected each year.

What are the Symptoms?
Symptoms vary, but most people have upper body obesity, rounded face, increased fat around the neck, and thinning arms and legs. Children tend to be obese with slowed growth rates.

Other symptoms appear in the skin, which becomes fragile and thin. It bruises easily and heals poorly. Purplish pink stretch marks may appear on the abdomen, thighs, buttocks, arms and breasts. The bones are weakened, and routine activities such as bending, lifting or rising from a chair may lead to backaches, rib and spinal column fractures.

Most people have severe fatigue, weak muscles, high blood pressure and high blood sugar. Irritability, anxiety and depression are common.

Women usually have excess hair growth on their faces, necks, chests, abdomens, and thighs. Their menstrual periods may become irregular or stop. Men have decreased fertility with diminished or absent desire for sex.

What Causes Cushing's Syndrome?
Cushing's syndrome occurs when the body's tissues are exposed to excessive levels of cortisol for long periods of time. Many people suffer the symptoms of Cushing's syndrome because they take glucocorticoid hormones such as prednisone for asthma, rheumatoid arthritis, lupus or other inflammatory diseases.

Others develop Cushing's syndrome because of overproduction of cortisol by the body. Normally, the production of cortisol follows a precise chain of events. First, the hypothalamus, a part of the brain which is about the size of a small sugar cube, sends corticotropin releasing hormone (CRH) to the pituitary gland. CRH causes the pituitary to secrete ACTH (adrenocorticotropin), a hormone that stimulates the adrenal glands. When the adrenals, which are located just above the kidneys, receive the ACTH, they respond by releasing cortisol into the bloodstream.

Cortisol performs vital tasks in the body. It helps maintain blood pressure and cardiovascular function, reduces the immune system's inflammatory response, balances the effects of insulin in breaking down sugar for energy, and regulates the metabolism of proteins, carbohydrates, and fats. One of cortisol's most important jobs is to help the body respond to stress. For this reason, women in their last 3 months of pregnancy and highly trained athletes normally have high levels of the hormone. People suffering from depression, alcoholism, malnutrition and panic disorders also have increased cortisol levels when the amount of cortisol in the blood is adequate, the hypothalamus and pituitary release less CRH and ACTH. This ensures that the amount of cortisol released by the adrenal glands is precisely balanced to meet the body's daily needs. However, if something goes wrong with the adrenals or their regulating switches in the pituitary gland or the hypothalamus, cortisol production can go awry.

Pituitary Adenomas
Pituitary adenomas cause most cases of Cushing's syndrome. They are benign, or non-cancerous, tumors of the pituitary gland which secrete increased amounts of ACTH. Most patients have a single adenoma. This form of the syndrome, known as "Cushing's disease" affects women five times more frequently than men.

Ectopic ACTH Syndrome
Some benign or malignant (cancerous) tumors that arise outside the pituitary can produce ACTH. This condition is known as ectopic ACTH syndrome. Lung tumors cause over 50

percent of these cases. Men are affected 3 times more frequently than women. The most common forms of ACTH-producing tumors are oat cell, or small cell lung cancer, which accounts for about 25 percent of all lung cancer cases, and carcinoid tumors. Other less common types of tumors that can produce ACTH are thymomas, pancreatic islet cell tumors, and medullary carcinomas of the thyroid.

Adrenal Tumors

Sometimes, an abnormality of the adrenal glands, most often an adrenal tumor, causes Cushing's syndrome. The average age of onset is about 40 years. Most of these cases involve non-cancerous tumors of adrenal tissue, called adrenal adenomas, which release excess cortisol into the blood. Adrenocortical carcinomas, or adrenal cancers, are the least common cause of Cushing's syndrome. Cancer cells secrete excess levels of several adrenal cortical hormones, including cortisol and adrenal androgens. Adrenocortical carcinomas usually cause very high hormone levels and rapid development of symptoms.

Familial Cushing's Syndrome

Most cases of Cushing's syndrome are not inherited. Rarely, however, some individuals have special causes of Cushing's syndrome due to an inherited tendency to develop tumors of one or more endocrine glands. In Primary Pigmented Micronodular Adrenal Disease (PPMAD), children or young adults develop small cortisol-producing tumors of the adrenal glands. In Multiple Endocrine Neoplasia Type I (MEN I), hormone secreting tumors of the parathyroid glands, pancreas and pituitary occur. Cushing's syndrome in MEN I may be due to pituitary, ectopic or adrenal tumors.

How is Cushing's Syndrome Diagnosed?

Diagnosis is based on a review of the patient's medical history, physical examination and laboratory tests. Often x-ray exams of the adrenal or pituitary glands are useful for locating tumors. These tests help to determine if excess levels of cortisol are present and why.

24-Hour Urinary Free Cortisol Level

This is the most specific diagnostic test. The patient's urine is collected over a 24-hour period and tested for the amount of cortisol. Levels higher than 50-100 micrograms a day for an adult suggest Cushing's syndrome. The normal upper limit varies in different laboratories, depending on which measurement technique is used.

Once Cushing's syndrome has been diagnosed, other tests are used to find the exact location of the abnormality that leads to excess cortisol production. The choice of test depends, in part, on the preference of the endocrinologist or the center where the test is performed.

Dexamethasone Suppression Test

This test helps to distinguish patients with excess production of ACTH due to pituitary adenomas from those with ectopic ACTH-producing tumors. Patients are given dexamethasone, a synthetic gluco-corticoid, by mouth every 6 hours for 4 days. For the first 2 days, low doses of dexamethasone are given, and for the last 2 days, higher doses are given. Twenty-four hour urine collections are made before dexamethasone is administered and on each day of the test. Since cortisol and other glucocorticoids signal the pituitary to lower secretion of ACTH, the normal response after taking dexamethasone is a drop in blood and urine cortisol levels. Different responses of cortisol to dexamethasone are obtained depending on whether the cause of Cushing's syndrome is a pituitary adenoma or an ectopic ACTH-producing tumor.

The dexamethasone suppression test can produce false-positive results in patients with depression, alcohol abuse, high estrogen levels, acute illness, and stress. Conversely, drugs such as phenytoin and phenobarbital may cause false-negative results in response to dexamethasone suppression. For this reason, patients are usually advised by their physicians to stop taking these drugs at least one week before the test.

CRH Stimulation Test

This test helps to distinguish between patients with pituitary adenomas and those with ectopic ACTH syndrome or cortisol-secreting adrenal tumors. Patients are given an injection of CRH, the corticotropin-releasing hormone which causes the pituitary to secrete ACTH. Patients with pituitary adenomas usually experience a rise in blood levels of ACTH and cortisol. This response is rarely seen in patients with ectopic ACTH syndrome and practically never in patients with cortisol-secreting adrenal tumors.

Direct Visualization of the Endocrine Glands (Radiologic Imaging)

Imaging tests reveal the size and shape of the pituitary and adrenal glands and help determine if a tumor is present. The most common are the CT (computerized tomography) scan and MRI (magnetic resonance imaging). A CT scan produces a series of x-ray pictures giving a cross-sectional image of a body part. MRI also produces images of the internal organs of the body but without exposing the patient to ionizing radiation.

Imaging procedures are used to find a tumor after a diagnosis has been established. Imaging is not used to make the diagnosis of Cushing's syndrome because benign tumors, sometimes called "incidentalomas", are commonly found in the pituitary and adrenal glands. These tumors do not produce hormones detrimental to health and are not removed unless blood tests show they are a cause of symptoms or they are unusually large. Conversely, pituitary tumors are not detected by imaging in almost 50 percent of patients who ultimately require pituitary surgery for Cushing's syndrome.

Petrosal Sinus Sampling

This test is not always required, but in many cases, it is the best way to separate pituitary from ectopic causes of Cushing's syndrome. Samples of blood are drawn from the petrosal sinuses, veins which drain the pituitary, by introducing catheters through a vein in the upper thigh/groin region, with local anesthesia and mild sedation. X-rays are used to confirm the correct position of the catheters. Often CRH, the hormone which causes the pituitary to secrete ACTH, is given during this test to improve diagnostic accuracy. Levels of ACTH in the petrosal sinuses are measured and compared with ACTH levels in a forearm vein. ACTH levels higher in the petrosal sinuses than in the forearm vein indicate the presence of a pituitary adenoma; similar levels suggest ectopic ACTH syndrome.

The Dexamethasone-CRH Test

Some individuals have high cortisol levels, but do not develop the progressive effects of Cushing's syndrome, such as muscle weakness, fractures and thinning of the skin. These individuals may have pseudo Cushing's syndrome, which was originally described in people who were depressed or drank excess alcohol, but is now known to be more common. Pseudo Cushing's does not have the same long-term effects on health as Cushing's syndrome and does not require treatment directed at the endocrine glands. Although observation over months to years will distinguish Pseudo-Cushing's from Cushing's, the dexamethasone-CRH test was developed to distinguish between the conditions rapidly, so that Cushing's patients can receive prompt treatment. This test combines the dexamethasone suppression and the CRH stimulation tests. Elevations of cortisol during this test suggest Cushing's syndrome.

Some patients may have sustained high cortisol levels without the effects of Cushing's syndrome. These high cortisol levels may be compensating for the body's resistance to cortisol's effects. This rare syndrome of cortisol resistance is a genetic condition that causes hypertension and chronic androgen excess.

Sometimes other conditions may be associated with many of the symptoms of Cushing's syndrome. These include polycystic ovarian syndrome, which may cause menstrual disturbances, weight gain from adolescence, excess hair growth and sometimes impaired insulin action and diabetes. Commonly, weight gain, high blood pressure and abnormal levels of cholesterol and triglycerides in the blood are associated with resistance to insulin action and diabetes; this has been described as the "Metabolic Syndrome-X." Patients with these disorders do not have abnormally elevated cortisol levels.

How is Cushing's Syndrom Treated?

Treatment depends on the specific reason for cortisol excess and may include surgery, radiation, chemotherapy or the use of cortisol-inhibiting drugs. If the cause is long-term use of glucocorticoid hormones to treat another disorder, the doctor will gradually reduce the dosage to the lowest dose adequate for control of that disorder. Once control is established, the daily dose of glucocorticoid hormones may be doubled and given on alternate days to lessen side effects.

Pituitary Adenomas

Several therapies are available to treat the ACTH-secreting pituitary adenomas of Cushing's disease. The most widely used treatment is surgical removal of the tumor, known as transsphenoidal adenomectomy. Using a special microscope and very fine instruments, the surgeon approaches the pituitary gland through a nostril or an opening made below the upper lip. Because this is an extremely delicate procedure, patients are often referred to centers specializing in this type of surgery. The success, or cure, rate of this procedure is over 80 percent when performed by a surgeon with extensive experience. If surgery fails, or only produces a temporary cure, surgery can be repeated, often with good results. After curative pituitary surgery, the production of ACTH drops two levels below normal. This is a natural, but temporary, drop in ACTH production, and patients are given a synthetic form of cortisol (such as hydrocortisone or prednisone). Most patients can stop this replacement therapy in less than a year. For patients in whom transsphenoidal surgery has failed or who are not suitable candidates for surgery, radiotherapy is another possible treatment. Radiation to the pituitary gland is given over a 6-week period, with improvement occurring in 40%—50% percent of adults and up to 80 percent of children. It may take several months or years before patients feel better from radiation treatment alone. However, the combination of radiation and the drug mitotane (Lysodren) can help speed recovery. Mitotane suppresses cortisol production and lowers plasma patients. Other drugs used alone or in combination to control the production of excess cortisol are aminoglutethimide, metyrapone, trilostane and ketoconazole. Each has its own side effects that doctors consider when prescribing therapy for individual patients.

Ectopic ACTH Syndrome

To cure the overproduction of cortisol caused by ectopic ACTH syndrome, it is necessary to eliminate all of the cancerous tissue that is secreting ACTH. The choice of cancer treatment — surgery, radiotherapy, chemotherapy, immunotherapy, or a combination of these treatments — depends on the type of cancer and how far it has spread. Since ACTH-secreting tumors (for example, small cell lung cancer) may be very small or widespread at the time of diagnosis, cortisol-inhibiting drugs, like mitotane, are an important part of treatment. In some cases, if pituitary surgery is not successful, surgical removal of the adrenal glands (bilateral adrenalectomy) may take the place of drug therapy.

Adrenal Tumors

Surgery is the mainstay of treatment for benign as well as cancerous tumors of the adrenal glands. In Primary Pigmented Micronodular Adrenal Disease and the familial Carney's complex, surgical removal of the adrenal glands is required.

What Research is Being Done on Cushing's Syndrome

The National Institutes of Health (NIH) is the biomedical research component of the Federal Government. It is one of the health agencies of the Public Health Service, which is part of the U.S. Department of Health and Human Services. Several components of the NIH conduct and support research on Cushing's syndrome and other disorders of the endocrine system, including the National Institute of Diabetes and Digestive and Kidney Diseases (NIDDK), the National Institute of Child Health and Human Development (NICHD), the National Institute of Neurological Disorders and Stroke (NINDS), and the National Cancer Institute (NCI).

NIH-supported scientists are conducting intensive research into the normal and abnormal function of the major endocrine glands and the many hormones of the endocrine system. Identification of the corticotropin releasing hormone (CRH), which instructs the pituitary gland to release ACTH, enabled researchers to develop the CRH stimulation test, which is increasingly being used to identify the cause of Cushing's syndrome.

Improved techniques for measuring ACTH permit distinction of ACTH-dependent forms of Cushing's syndrome from adrenal tumors. NIH studies have shown that petrosal sinus sampling is a very accurate test to diagnose the cause of Cushing's syndrome in those who have excess ACTH production. The recently described dexamethasone suppression-CRH test is able to differentiate most cases of Cushing's from Pseudo Cushing's.

As a result of this research, doctors are much better able to diagnose Cushing's syndrome and distinguish among the causes of this disorder. Since accurate diagnosis is still a problem for some patients, new tests are under study to further refine the diagnostic process.

Many studies are underway to understand the causes of formation of benign endocrine tumors, such as those which cause most cases of Cushing's syndrome. In a few pituitary adenomas, specific gene defects have been identified and may provide important clues to understanding tumor formation. Endocrine factors may also play a role. There is increasing evidence that tumor formation is a multi-step process. Understanding the basis of Cushing's syndrome will yield new approaches to therapy.

NIH supports research related to Cushing's syndrome at medical centers throughout the United States. Scientists are also treating patients with Cushing's syndrome at the NIH Warren Grant Magnuson Clinical Center in Bethesda, Maryland. Physicians who are interested in referring a patient may contact Dr. George P. Chrousos, Developmental Endocrinology Branch, NICHD, Building 10, Room 10N262, Bethesda, Maryland 20892, telephone (301)496-4686.

Where Can I Find More Information?

The following materials can be found in medical libraries, many college and university libraries, and through interlibrary loan in most public libraries.

1. Cooper, Paul R. "Contemporary Diagnosis and Management of Pituitary Adenomas,"
Park Ridge, Illinois: American Associatior of Neurological Surgeons, 1991.
2. DeGroot, Leslie J., ed., et al. "Cushing's Syndrome," Endocrinology. Vol. 2,
Philadelphia: W. B. Saunders Company, 1995. 1741-1769.
3. Isselbacher, Kurt J., ed., et al. "Cushing's Syndrome Etiology," *Harrison 's Principles of Internal Medicine.* Vol. 2, No. 13, New York: McGraw-Hill Book Company, 1994 1960-1965.
4. Orth, David N., Kovacs, W.J., DeBold, C.R., "The Adrenal Cortex; Hyperfunction, Glucocorticoids; Hypercortisolism (Cushing's Syndrome)", Williams *Textbook of Endocrinology.* Ed. 8, Philadelphia: W.B. Saunders, 1992. 536-562.
5. Conn, R.B., Gomez, T., Chrousos, G.P, "Current Diagnosis," No. 8, Philadelphia:
W.B. Saunders 1991, 868-872.
6. NCI Research Report: Cancer of the Lung Prepared by the Office of Cancer Communications, National Cancer Institute, NIH Publication No. 93-526.

What Other Resources Are Available?

Cushing's Support and Research Foundation, Inc.
65 East India Row 22B, Boston, Massachusetts 02110
(617) 723-3824 or (617) 723-3674
Louise L. Pace, Founder and President

Pituitary Tumor Network Association
16350 Ventura Boulevard, Suite 231
Encino, CA 91436
(805)499-2262 Fax: (805)499-1523
Robert Knutzen, Chairman

Acromegaly

Shereen Ezzat, M.D., FRCP(C), FACP, University of Toronto,
Wellesley Hospital, Toronto, Canada

Introduction

Acromegaly was first described as a unique new entity by Marie in 1886. It was not until 1909 that Cushing and Davidaff suspected that the pituitary may be the cause of this condition. Neurosurgical access to the pituitary with removal of tumors of that gland resulting in reversal of acromegalic features, further supported the role of the pituitary in acromegaly, It is now well recognized that pituitary growth hormone (GH) is regulated in part by dual signals from other parts of the brain. This article will review the recent advances in the understanding of the causes, diagnosis and management of acromegaly.

Prevalence (How Common Is This Condition?)

While pituitary adenomas have been documented in up to 25% of adult humans on autopsy examination, GH-secreting adenomas likely represent less than 1% of this total number. In a comprehensive survey of a relatively stable population of 3.1 million in the Newcastle region, 164 patients with acromegaly were identified over an 11-year period. This information suggests an annual incidence of 3 per million with a prevalence of about 40-60 per million. Thus far there have been no studies conducted to examine the incidence and prevalence of acromegaly in North America. Most experts in the field believe that North American figures are in the same order of magnitude as those from European studies. However, since the clinical diagnosis of acromegaly is frequently missed, its frequency is probably underestimated.

Etiology (What Causes Acromegaly?)

The clinical features of acromegaly arise from prolonged, sustained excessive secretion of growth hormone (GH) and its target hormone, insulin-like growth factor I (IGF-1, also known as somatomedin-C). Computed tomography (CT) and magnetic resonance imaging (MRI) of the pituitary allow excellent visualization of the source of this GH excess. In addition, advances in hormone identification techniques have resulted in more specific characterization of the various pituitary tumor cell types responsible for this condition. Each of the GH-producing tumor subtypes can now be correlated with a different pattern of tumor growth and clinical features. A precise tissue diagnosis of the subtype of GH pituitary tumor may be of great value in predicting the clinical course.

Primary pituitary tumors account for the majority of cases of acromegaly. These arise from the GH-secreting cells (somatotrophs), and appear densely or sparsely granulated with GH-containing granules under electron microscopy. The densely granulated tumors grow more rapidly and are often associated with striking clinical presentation over many years. These are seen more commonly in younger patients. The sparsely granulated form, however, usually grows to invade adjacent sites within the brain (towards the optic apparatus), sideways (to invade the eye movement nerves within a structure called cavernous sinuses) or downward extension (to erode through the sphenoid sinuses). GH producing cells can also make prolactin. One quarter of GH-secreting pituitary tumors are associated with hyperprolactinemia, that is clinical evidence of prolactin excess.

The cause of pituitary adenomas remains unknown. Most pituitary tumors arise de novo and are not genetically inherited. Most of the evidence suggests that an acquired defect disrupts the chemical pathways that govern cell growth and hormone secretion in the pituitary. These defects can be traced back to specific genes within the pituitary. It appears that multiple

Acromegaly

disruptions or alterations are necessary to result in unrestrained cell growth and tumor formation. Recently the gene responsible for a heritable form of disease called multiple endocrine neoplasia type I (MEN-I) was identified. Patients born with a defective copy of this gene are at risk of developing tumors in the pituitary, parathyroid glands, and the pancreas. When they acquire a defect in their other copy of that gene (MEN-I gene) they develop a tumor. Identification of this gene will now facilitate screening of family members with suspected MEN syndromes. Furthermore, by scanning different regions of the gene in a pituitary tumor, we may possibly be able to distinguish heritable forms of pituitary tumors from those that represent isolated or sporadic cases. Clearly many such factors that can potentially lead to abnormal growth of pituitary cells will require further investigation and correlation with patients' clinical backgrounds so that more firm and practical conclusions can be made.

Over the last few years several reports have described patients with acromegaly and non-pituitary tumors involving the pancreas, lung, breast and ovary. Growth hormone excess with its associated features (excessive sweating, fatigue, acral enlargement, etc.) subsequently resolved after successful surgical removal of these tumors. While some of these tumors appear to be capable of producing and secreting GH outside the pituitary, the majority of these non-pituitary tumors secrete GH-releasing hormone (GHRH) which can be measured in the blood to confirm the diagnosis. The pituitary gland in patients with ectopic GHRH secretion becomes hyperplastic and may be enlarged on CT or MRI imaging. This is an additional reason underscoring the need for precise histologic examination of all "pituitary tumors" removed from patients suffering from acromegaly.

Clinical Presentation (How Do People Present With This Condition?)
The clinical features associated with acromegaly include the effects of GH oversecretion, followed by the compressive effects of an expanding pituitary mass. Younger patients generally present with more aggressive disease. While coarsening of facial features may seem obvious in retrospect, only 10% of patients with active acromegaly consult a physician for that complaint. Excessive sweating, interruption of menstrual periods, impotence, diabetes and skin tags are early common features of the disorder. It is also not uncommon for patients to present with seemingly unrelated complaints such as sleep apnea, jaw malocclusion, arthritis, or colonic polyps. Adenomatous polyps of the colon appear to be associated with skin tags and may become a significant cause of morbidity and mortality in aging patients with acromegaly.

Diagnosis (How is this condition diagnosed?)
The diagnosis of acromegaly is confirmed by demonstrating excessive, autonomous secretion of GH. Isolated, random sampling of blood GH is inadequate in establishing the diagnosis as GH secretion is pulsatile and can vary widely from minute to minute. GHRH (growth hormone-releasing hormone) stimulates GH production and release, while SS (somatostatin) inhibits its release. SS secretion is also episodic and is increased during tasting, sleep and obesity. Thus, blood GH levels may spontaneously reach 5 times "the normal range" in healthy individuals, while patients with active acromegaly may have GH levels within the "normal range." The demonstration of lack of GH suppression to <2 mg/L following the ingestion of 75 grams of glucose confirms the diagnosis of acromegaly.

While bodily growth in adults is primarily under the influence of GH, its effects are largely mediated through insulin-like growth factor I (IGF-1), previously known also as somatomedin-C. This growth factor is produced in most tissues, and also acts locally to regulate cellular growth and differentiation. Circulating IGF-1, however, is derived mostly from the liver under the influence of GH. Thus, blood levels are elevated in most patients with active acromegaly. Poorly controlled diabetes mellitus results in impaired liver production of IGF-1. Similarly, blood IGF-l levels decline moderately in normal aging individuals, and during starvation. IGF-l levels also increase during normal pregnancy reaching 2-3 times non-pregnant values. With this exception, an elevated age-adjusted IGF-1 level confirms the diagnosis of acromegaly. Furthermore, since blood levels of IGF-1 do not fluctuate as rapidly as GH, serial IGF-1 levels represent a practical and reliable alternative for measuring disease activity.

Following the biochemical confirmation of acromegaly, CT or MR-imaging should be used to localize the site of excess hormone production. In the absence of a definite pituitary tumor, an ectopic tumor source of GHRH or GH in the chest, abdomen,or pelvis is usually considered. Ectopic acromegaly can be diagnosed by measuring GHRH in the blood along with CT scanning of the suspected region of the body.

Treatment (What Are The Treatment Options?)
The aims of treatment in acromegaly are to achieve a biochemical remission of the GH excess along with its associated complications and to relieve the comprehensive effects of a growing pituitary mass. The options for management include medical therapy, surgery, and irradiation of the pituitary.

Transsphenoidal Surgery
Selective transsphenoidal removal of pituitary adenomas rapidly decompresses large tumors and reduces GH levels. Facial features and soft tissue swelling improve within days after surgery. Predictors of a successful surgical outcome include a pre-operative GH level of < 40 mg/L and a pituitary tumor <10 mm in diameter. The incidence of complications and success rate are related to the experience of the neurosurgeon with this procedure. In a worldwide review of 1200 patients with acromegaly, only 60% had GH levels below 5 mg/L immediately post-operatively. Many patients with early responses often relapse biochemically several years post-operatively, reflecting incomplete tumor removal especially when the tumor has invaded adjacent structures. Random individual blood GH levels are insufficient evidence for a biochemical cure. Reversal of the initial biochemical criteria used to make the diagnosis of acromegaly are necessary before the patient can be declared to be in remission.

Medications
Two agents are presently available for use in acromegaly. Bromocriptine (Parlodel) is a "dopamine agonist" which lowers GH secretion in some patients with GH-secreting pituitary adenomas. Generally, doses of up to 20 mg daily are necessary to achieve a reduction in GH. Side effects include gastrointestinal upset, light headedness on standing, and nasal congestion. Biochemical remission and tumor shrinkage are seen only 10%—15% of patients with acromegaly. Interestingly, patients report improvement in their symptoms despite persistently elevated GH and IGF-Ievels. The availability of bromocriptine in oral form, however, makes it an attractive first line primary drug or as part of an adjunctive treatment regimen for acromegaly. Other dopamine agonists such as CV 205-502, however, may prove to be more effective than bromocriptine in treating patients with acromegaly.

Octreotide (Sandostatin) is a potent synthetic analogue of the natural hypothalamic hormone somatostatin (SS). It is administered subcutaneously (like insulin) and lowers GH secretion within 1 hr. Its effects may be sustained for up to 8-12 hrs. A minimum of 8-hourly dosing (3 injections daily) of 100 mg is necessary, with the occasional patient requiring up to 1500 mg/day. Long term effectiveness of octreotide has been demonstrated in several studies. Clinical response is also favorable. Headaches in particular respond promptly within minutes of drug administration. Octreotide has also been successfully used in patients with ectopic GHRH-secreting tumors.

The major side effects related to the chronic use of octreotide are related to its inhibitory effects on gastrointestinal and pancreatic function. A third of patients experience loose bowel movements with biochemical evidence of mild malabsorption. In addition, gallstones, due to impaired action of pancreatic hormone secretion, has been reported in approximately 10% of patients. Although serum insulin levels fall during early treatment, diabetes is a very rare complication. In fact, we have noted reduced insulin requirements and improved sugar control in acromegalic patients with diabetes mellitus who are treated with octreotide.

A longer acting form of octreotide (Sandostatin-LAR) which is injected intramuscularly every 3 weeks is currently under development. Fewer fluctuations in GH levels have been described in patients using this form of Sandostatin than its regular subcutaneous form. It is anticipated that many patients who are now using Sandostatin will have the opportunity to switch to the LAR form. Hopefully availability in North America will be as soon as mid 1998.

Radiotherapy
Both conventional and heavy-particle beam irradiation have been used as primary and adjunctive treatments for acromegaly. Unfortunately, a response is not seen for 2-5 years during which time the patient is exposed to the harmful metabolic effects of GH excess. Reduction in pituitary function occurs insidiously in half of patients within 10 years of treatment. Neurologic complications such as visual loss, weakness, and memory impairment have rarely been reported. This modality of therapy is usually reserved for those patients who have failed surgical and medical therapy.

Summary And Recommendations
Acromegaly is a serious pituitary disorder inasmuch as it can be associated with significant long-term complications including increased morbidity and mortality. The insidious nature of its onset often eludes its diagnosis, leaving patients with a chronic debilitating condition that is sometimes difficult to treat. Heightened suspicion for subtle features of presentation should result in early biochemical and radiographic confirmation of the disease. Treatment should be individualized depending on the patient's age, associated risk factors, and radiographic evidence of tumor extension. Particularly in the absence of local invasion, patients should first undergo selective transsphenoidal resection of their pituitary adenomas by an experienced neurosurgeon. Long-term follow-up is critical in identifying relapses, at which point additional medical therapy should be instituted.

An initial trial of a dopamine agonist (such as Parlodel) is warranted due to its ease of administration in patients with unfavorable surgical outcome. Injectable octreotide (Sandostatin) is another medical a alternative. Long term therapy will be necessary, as withdrawal of any agent is associated with return of GH excess and tumor re-expansion. Every effort should be made to lower GH Levels to the point where they are suppressed after glucose administration to less than 2 mg/L along with normalization of blood IGF-1 levels.

Finally, radiotherapy should be reserved as a third option due to its slow onset of action and associated serious side effects.

Suggested Readings
1   Ezzat S, Forster MJ, Berchtold P, Redelmeier DA, Harris AG. Acromegaly: Clinical and biochemical features in 500 patients. Medicine (Baltimore) 1994;73:233.
2   Colao A, Ferone D, Marzullo P, et al. Effect of different dopaminergic agents in the treatment of acromegaly. J. Clin. Endocrinol. Metab. 1997;82:518.
3   Ezzat S, Snyder PJ, Young WF, et al. Octreotide treatment of acromegaly: A randomized multicenter study. Ann. Intern. Med. 1992;117;711.
4   Flogstad AK, Halse J. Grass P, et al. A comparison of octreotide, bromocriptine, or a combination of both drugs in acromegaly. J. Clin. Endocrinol. Metab. 1994;79;451
5   Ezzat S. Living with acromegaly. Endocrinol. Metab. Clin. North Am. 992;21:753.

A Layman's Quick Checklist for the Acromegalic

Morton A. Hirschberg

Symptoms

Introduction

Acromegalics undergo physical and psychological changes from the onset of their disease. An acromegalic may experience a few or many of the symptoms listed. During the course of the disease additional symptoms, some of a more severe nature, may develop. Finally, this document is written from the perspective of a mature acromegalic.

Physical Changes

Before puberty excessive growth to extreme height. After puberty, inappropriate growth. Growth can be of the fingers, hands, feet, jaw, eye ridges, and head. Soft tissue growth can be both external, such as the pads of the fingers or swelling of the feet, or internal with virtually every internal organ being enlarged. Fingers can become fat so rings do not fit, the feet large and wide so that shoes do not fit, and the head larger so that hats do not fit. Growth of the jaw may lead to separations or big gaps between the teeth. The tongue may grow and become very wide.

Due to the slow development of physical changes, this insidious disease may take many years before a correct diagnosis is made. Complications among those having the disease for any length of time arise from cardiovascular problems (i.e. enlarged heart and attending blood supply system) or colon cancer. These two are the leading causes of death among acromegalics.

Physical Symptoms

- Headaches (from mild to severe).

- Black and blue marks of the sole and/or instep of the feet.

- Deepening of the voice.

- Eye ridges thicken and eyes look deep set (look like a cave man).

- Skin discoloration or darkening.

- Fatigue (unusual tiredness or loss of energy).

- Hirsutism or hair growth on arms, legs, shoulders, chest and back.

- Saliva gland enlargement.

- Abnormal menstrual cycle in women.

- Numbness and/or weakness of the hands.

- Arthritis and/or related symptoms (pain in the joints).

- Kidney stones.

- Bone spurs or bony growths on the spine.

- Carpal tunnel syndrome. Caused by growth of hands without corresponding connective tissue growth (the tendons do not grow).

- Lower lip grows.

- Drooling while either awake or asleep (see also sleep apnea).

- Feet grow and/or swell (may not be bilateral).

- Colon polyps (the colon may also get longer).

- Reduced sexual drive and possible impotence.

- Lower testosterone level in males.

- Nose grows.

- Osteoporosis.

- Loss (weakening) of cognitive abilities and/or memory lapses.

- Skin odor.

Physical Symptoms

- Skin tags or other growths.

- Sleep apnea. Irregular breathing and breathing stoppages while asleep.

- Thickening and toughening of the skin.

- Sudden and excessive sweating and hot flashes.

- Thyroid gland swelling and/or other thyroid problems.

- Snoring (see also sleep apnea).

- Thickening of head or jaw (may not be
- bilateral or uniform).

- Teeth separation or other facial deformities.

- Tingling, burning sensations or pain in the extremities (worse when tired - that old crazy bone feeling, only continuous).

- Vision impairment and/or blindness.

ics.

Psychological Changes

Psychological changes are not well studied among acromegalics or well reported. This may be especially true of prepubescent acromegalics. Nonetheless, this is an important aspect of the

Psychological Changes

- Loss (weakening) of cognitive abilities and/or memory lapses.

- Mania (but no depression. All that growth hormone gives one a constant high).

- Megalomania (feeling of great power and invincibility).

- Rage (fits of almost uncontrollable temper - with remorse afterward ...oh that wonderful growth hormone!)

disease, and the following symptoms or personality changes may occur.

Tests

Introduction

A growth hormone blood test can pretty much determine whether or not one is an Acromegalic. X-rays, Magnetic Resonance Imagery (MRI), and colonoscopy testing may follow. No mention is made of an angiogram and unless there is a surgical error this test is not normally administered. Angiograms are not discussed here except to say that they are not risk free. Complications arise in 3%—5% of the patients tested.

Blood Testing.

Risks: really none, but an Acromegalic may be poked several times before a vein is penetrated due to tough, thick skin and veins. Glucose blood testing may also be performed where blood is drawn every half hour after a short (12 hours or so) fasting period. Risks: really none, but the blood may clot during glucose testing requiring multiple pokes. A good phlebotomist is a great asset. Telling some phlebotomists you are an Acromegalic and have tough skin may make them nervous. Don't let yourself be poked more than three times by anyone.

Colonoscopy.

Acromegalics develop colon polyps and an order of magnitude greater frequency than the normal population. Five percent of the normal population develops polyps while 55% of Acromegalics do (based on one study). A rectal examination itself cannot determine the presence of polyps. Risks: bleeding, pain, and perforation of the colon. The latter does occur with a 1%–3% frequency while bleeding and pain may be more frequent. There is also the associated risk of the general anesthetic. The alternatives to a colonoscopy, while perhaps less risky, present far less diagnostic value. These are: (1) Ingesting barium and having x-rays. Risks: virtually none, but may not indicate the absence of polyps, especially if there are cloudy areas on the x-ray, and, (2) Partial scoping. Risks: as with full scoping, however, no anesthetic is administered. This is not the most fun in the world. Results may not be definitive and if polyps are found a complete scoping will be required anyway. Tell the doctor performing the colonoplain scopy you are Acromegalic. Tell him your colon may be long. That will help him. Bottom line (no pun intended), a full scoping seems to be the best option from any viewpoint (again, no pun intended).

Magnetic Resonance Imagery (MRI)
Brain scans with and without contrast (Gadolinium) to completely confirm the diagnosis and determine the size and position of the tumor. Arterial blood flow can also be obtained when the contrast material (Gadolinium) is injected. Risks: without the contrast, none. With it, allergic reactions are possible but rare. If you are claustrophobic, take a walk around the machine. You will see it is hollow and you can see through it. It is not like a cigar wrapper. There are also machines which are completely open but the results are better with the more confining machine. Have them play music for you. I like the ear plugs and no music. Just like riding in a helicopter.

X-ray
Even before an MRI, x-rays of the hands and feet can show bone growth as well as soft tissue growth. Risks: those usually associated with x-ray; In general, virtually none.

Remedies

Introduction
There are three basic remedies for treatment of Acromegaly: drug therapy, radiation, and surgery. Complete normalization, generously speaking, occurs in between 55%–80% of Acromegalics. This means that various combinations of remedies, even all three, may be required. Each is now discussed separately.

Drug Therapy.
There are two major drugs used to treat Acromegaly: bromocriptine (Parlodel) and octreotide acetate (Sandostatin). Neither of these drugs will kill the tumor, although there might be some reduction in size. They are used strictly to control the disease by reducing the growth hormone until it is in the normal range. If they can be tolerated and are effective, a life long regimen may be in order. Drug therapy is perhaps the least intrusive remedy for Acromegaly.

Bromocriptine (Parlodel) is taken orally. Side effects include stomach problems such as nausea. Dosage is increased incrementally to establish tolerance and effectiveness. The drug is usually taken at meal times to reduce unwanted gastronomic side effects.

Octreotide acetate (Sandostatin) is taken by injection. There is a wide range of possible side effects including stomach problems. Nausea, loose stools and gas (flatulence) are among them. Asymptomatic gall stones is perhaps the most serious of the possible side effects and occurs in 30%–50% of those taking the drug. Dosage is increased incrementally to both establish tolerance and determine effectiveness. Daily injections of 1-3 shots may be required. A time spacing of the drug is suggested to keep the growth hormone level uniform throughout the day. More about octreotide may be found on the PTNA web site. Octreotide is a relatively expensive drug.

Radiation
There are two forms of radiation therapy: conventional radiation and Gamma knife (stereotactic radiosurgery).

Conventional Radiation. Daily treatments over a four to six week period (20-30 treatment sessions). Conventional radiation is not as well focused as is the Gamma knife. Side effects include: hair loss, burning, temporary and permanent memory loss, and a litany of glandular problems brought on by pituitary damage. Side effects may occur long after treatment and could result in requiring life long drug therapies as a corrective measure.

Successful results may take effect from several months to 10 years after treatment. This remedy, then, would most likely be used in conjunction with surgery and/or drug therapies.

Gamma Knife (Stereotactic Radiosurgery). Multiple emanations of cobalt 60 are administered in one treatment sitting. While the beams are focused and are low level, there are Risks: Side effects are as above. Not everyone is a suitable candidate for Gamma knife. This remedy is not effective if the tumor is too large.

Successful results may take effect from several months to several years after treatment. This remedy then would most likely be used in conjunction with surgery and/or drug therapies.

Of the two, Gamma knife would be my first choice.

Surgery
There are two forms of surgery available: frontal craniotomy and transphenoidal.

Frontal craniotomy. This form of surgery, which involves opening the skull and moving the brain to expose the pituitary area, is rarely done anymore. Risks: high. Side effects run a huge gamut including stroke.

Transphenoidal. This has become the surgical procedure of choice. Risk: usually less than 1% exhibit complications. Of course, there is a risk with any general anesthetic. Effects can be that many symptoms such as headaches still persist. In addition, it may not be possible to excise the entire tumor, leaving growth hormone levels high. This procedure is performed by going through incisions made in the nose and behind the upper lip. No visible scars show and pain is just about nil. If surgery is repeated, risks jump to a 5% complication rate. It may still be necessary to have drug or radiation therapy after a successful surgery.

All things considered, transphenoidal surgery has to be considered the best remedial alternative for continued health and longevity, especially with the prospect that drug and radiation therapies will not be required. Anything over 50% seems like great odds!

Epilogue
Finally, once an acromegalic, always an acromegalic. Testing and monitoring must be performed on a regular basis.

Sleep Apnea and Acromegaly

Ken Ho M.D., Ron Grunstein M.D., Garvan Institute of Medical Research, St Vincent's Hospital (KH)
& Dept of Respiratory Medicine, Royal Prince Alfred Hospital (RG), Sydney, Australia

"Everyone laughs about my snoring" is a very common complaint among patients with acromegaly. Snoring is no laughing matter. It may be a signal that something is seriously wrong with breathing during sleep. It may mean that the upper part of the air passage to your lungs is narrowed. More importantly it is often an indication of the presence of sleep apnea. Apnea is a Greek word meaning "want to breathe" and in medical terminology it means an interruption to breathing during sleep. As a result, patients may not get enough oxygen and suffer from poor quality sleep. It is now known that snoring and sleep apnea are manifestations of different degrees of the same problem with snoring being a mild, and apnea being a severe form of obstructed breathing.

How Common is Sleep Apnea in Acromegaly?

Sleep apnea is very common in acromegaly. In our study of 53 acromegalic patients, 51 (96%) snored heavily during sleep while 43 (80%) suffered from sleep apnea. Eight of the last 10 patients diagnosed with acromegaly at our institutions were discovered because of sleep apnea. Sleep apnea affects approximately 1 in 20 middle aged men in the general population. Thus sleep apnea is 15-20 times as common in acromegaly.

What Causes Sleep Apnea in Acromegaly?

Acromegaly causes growth of body tissues and retention of fluid. The tongue is often enlarged and there is swelling of soft tissue around the throat causing narrowing of the upper airway. During sleep, the muscles of the tongue and of the soft palate relax and sag. This leads to constriction of the airway which is already narrowed, thus making breathing labored and noisy. Collapse of the airway wall blocks breathing entirely, causing obstructive sleep apnea. When breathing periodically stops, snoring is broken by pauses. As pressure to breathe builds, the muscles of the abdomen and chest work harder, which temporarily interrupts sleep. This in turn activates the muscles of the throat to "uncork" the airway. The effort is akin to slurping a drink through a floppy wet straw. A listener hears deep gasps as breathing starts. With each gasp, the sleeper awakens, but so briefly and incompletely so that sleep is continuously interrupted throughout the night.

There is a second type of apnea called central sleep apnea. In this form of sleep apnea, mechanical obstruction to airflow is not the problem. The cause lies in the part of the brain that controls breathing during sleep. The brain appears to "forget" to send the necessary instructions to the breathing muscles. Eventually falling levels of oxygen in blood sound an alarm in the brain, causing the sleeper to awake and start breathing. Our studies show that up to one third of acromegalic patients with sleep apnea suffer from this form of apnea. Interestingly, most of the patients with central apnea also suffer from obstructive apnea, that is, both forms of sleep apnea are present in the same patient.

Why is Sleep Apnea Important?

Disturbed sleep produces profound daytime sleepiness that often disrupts work and personal life. People with sleep apnea fall asleep at inappropriate times; at work or behind the wheel of a car. Recent studies show that sleep apnea sufferers have 2 to 5 times as many automobile accidents as the general population. People with sleep apnea may have trouble concentrating and become unusually forgetful. They may seem uncharacteristically irritable, anxious or depressed. These problems may appear suddenly or emerge over many years. The person may not notice these problems or may minimize their severity. Often family members, employers or co-workers first recognize a pattern change in mood or behaviour that may prompt a visit to the doctor. Sleep apnea also increases the risk of developing high blood pressure, heart attacks and strokes.

Does Sleep Apnea Improve with Treatment of Acromegaly?
Successful treatment of acromegaly significantly improves sleep apnea. Some patients may be completely cured of sleep apnea while others experience a marked degree of improvement, or a milder degree of sleep apnea. This means that acromegalic patients should be re-evaluated in a sleep laboratory to determine whether further treatment is necessary. There may be many reasons why sleep apnea may persist after treatment for acromegaly. It may be that treatment itself was not curative so that the patient may be left with a mild degree of acromegaly. Given that sleep apnea affects up to 5% of the adult population, the patient may have an underlying predisposition to developing sleep apnea independent of acromegaly. Other factors that predispose to sleep apnea include obesity and the use of alcohol and sleeping pills.

How do I Know I May Have Sleep Apnea?
You may be told that snoring is so loud that it can be heard rooms away, even by neighbors. A particular pattern of snoring interrupted by pauses, then gasps, reveals that breathing stops intermittently during sleep. You may have noticed problems of daytime sleepiness, forgetfulness, irritability or some difficulty concentrating.

How is Sleep Apnea Diagnosed?
When you see your local physician, he may wish to talk to your bed partner or other members of your household about your sleep and waking behavior. The ultimate diagnoses depends on investigations that can be performed at a Sleep Evaluation Center. The Sleep Physician will evaluate your problems and will ask you to spend a night or two in the Sleep Evaluation Laboratory to monitor many aspects of your sleep. This includes recording brainwaves, muscle activity, leg and arm movements, heart rhythm as well as the level of oxygen in your blood.

Treatment of sleep apnea in acromegaly is very much dependent on effective treatment of acromegaly itself. The patient can be helped significantly even if residual apnea persists after treatment of acromegaly. Patients who are overweight should go on a weight reduction diet and should be encouraged to limit alcohol intake and avoid taking sleeping pills. There is no effective medication for sleep apnea. A standard and effective treatment for obstructive sleep apnea, irrespective of cause, is Continuous Positive Airway Pressure (CPAP, pronounced 'see-pap') Therapy.

This involves wearing a mask over the nose during sleep. Pressure from an air compressor forces ordinary room air through the nasal passages and into the airway under gentle pressure, thereby splinting the airway open and allowing unobstructed passage of air and uninterrupted sleep. CPAP is used primarily for obstructive apnea. CPAP machines can be rented on a trial basis or purchased after a sleep study has been performed to determine the correct pressure setting.

In summary, sleep apnea is a common complication of acromegaly and may be the presenting problem in many patients with undiagnosed acromegaly. If untreated, sleep apnea impairs physical and mental performance. In general, successful treatment of acromegaly is accompanied by improvement of sleep apnea although this may not disappear completely even if a patient is completely cured of the disease.

Suggested Reading:

Grunstein R, Ho KY, Sullivan CE. Sleep apnea in acromegaly. Ann Intern Med 1991; 115: 527-532.

Grunstein R, Ho KY, Sullivan CE. Effect of octreotide, a somatostatin analog, on sleep apnea in patients with acromegaly. Ann Intern Med 1994; 121: 478-483.

Pascualy RA, Soest SW. Snoring and sleep apea: A personal and family guide to diagnosis and treatment. New York, Demos Vermande, 1996.

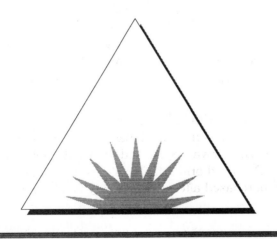

"If you are constantly looking back, chances are pretty good you'll fall into a hole ahead."

Colorectal Cancer and Acromegaly

Carey B. Strom, M.D., Assistant Professor of Clinical Medicine
UCLA School of Medicine, Los Angeles, California

Colorectal cancer represents 22% of the deaths in the United States each year, second only to heart disease. Gastrointestinal cancer represents 23% of the deaths from cancer each year; colorectal cancer is the highest among gastrointestinal cancers in terms of incidence and mortality. There are 150,000 new cases of colorectal cancer per year and 60,000 deaths as a result of this disease per year. One's lifetime risk of developing colorectal cancer is up to 6%. The mortality rate has been decreasing despite increasing incidence.

It is widely accepted that benign colorectal polyps, if not removed, can gradually develop into cancer over many years. The incidence increases with age. The estimated prevalence of polyps in asymptomatic people over the age of 50 is up to 30%. The estimated prevalence of polyps in acromegalies is up to 35%. Other risk factors for the development of colorectal polyps and cancer include diet, inheritance, familial occurrence, ulcerative colitis, Crohn's disease and personal history of colorectal polyps or cancer. There have been many studies that have shown that a high fat, low fiber diet increases the incidence and recurrence of polyps. There is also some evidence that fish, chicken, vitamin A and a high carbohydrate diet may be somewhat protective.

Acromegaly results from unrestrained secretion of growth hormone and insulin-like growth factor 1 (IGF-1) and usually occurs as a result of a pituitary adenoma. Both growth hormone and IGF-1 have been shown to stimulate proliferation of normal cells and tumor cells in the test tube. In addition, growth hormone inhibitory peptide, somatostatin, have been shown to inhibit the growth of human colonic tumors in mice. Dr. Shereen Ezzat, myself and Dr. Shlomo Melmed reported in the May issue of the Annals of Internal Medicine from 1991, that acromegalics have a 35% incidence of colonic polyps as compared to 30% in the normal population.

There has also been an association between skin tags and colon polyps in patients with acromegaly. It has also been shown that skin tags are a cutaneous marker for colon polyps independent of the presence of acromegaly.

Colorectal polyps have been identified with increasing frequency in the recent years as a result of the introduction of screening with tests of stool for occult (hidden) blood, flexible sigmoidoscopy, colonoscopy and a barium enema. It is widely held theory that adenomatous (benign but potentially malignant) polyps are precursors of colorectal cancer and, thus, the removal may decrease the incidence in mortality from colorectal cancer. There have been five controlled trials involving over 300,000 patients to illustrate the benefit of colorectal screening. The studies found that there is a substantial improvement in the terms of the stage at which the cancer is detected for those patients who have a diagnosis made as a result of screening, as opposed to patients who have a diagnosis made as a result of symptoms.

The earlier the cancer is detected, the better the chance of survival. The screening tests that we use in clinical practice include a digital rectal examination that can detect up to 10% of colorectal polyps or cancers, stool for occult blood which can detect colorectal cancer in approximately 50% of adults without symptoms, flexible sigmoidoscopy which can detect up to 60% of colorectal polyps and/or cancer and colonoscopy. (The difference between the flexible sigmoidoscopy and colonoscopy is the depth of penetration of the scope into the colon).

Colonoscopy detects 95% to 100% of all colorectal polyps and cancers. One is also able to biopsy and potentially remove polyps with this procedure. The polyps that tend to be more dangerous and subsequently go on to turn into cancer include polyps that are larger than 1 cm and those which have high grade dysplasia (a pathologic diagnosis). If one is found to have colorectal polyps on a sigmoidoscopy exam, it is generally recommended that a colonoscopy be performed to remove those polyps and to check the rest of the colon for polyps. It is felt that up to 40% of patients that have polyps within the reach of the sigmoidoscope may have more polyps higher up in the colon. After the colonoscopy is performed and the polyps are removed, it is recommended that patients have periodic screening with recurrent colonoscopy in the future.

The national polyp study also compared the effectiveness of colonoscopy vs. barium enema. The study showed that barium enema could only detect 30% of small polyps (less than 0.5 cm) and 50% of the medium to large polyps that were detected by colonoscopy.

The past decade of studies have given better awareness to the role of genetics in colorectal cancer, the so-called familial colorectal cancer syndrome. Although it is known that Lynch syndrome and familial adenomatous polyposis account for 6% of new cases reported each year, it is felt that familial occurrences do account for a large number of sporadic cases. As mentioned before, the lifetime risk for colorectal cancer in the general population is probably 5% to 6%; however, with a family history of colorectal cancer in one first degree relative, that risk increases to 20%, and with two first degree relatives having colorectal cancer, the risk can increase to 30%.

Even if one family member has only one benign polyp, the risk of contracting colorectal cancer increases for the whole family. Ulcerative colitis that has been long standing, increases one's risk twentyfold for the development of colorectal cancer. Crohn's disease also has a 2% to 3% increased risk over the general population for colorectal cancer. If a person has a personal history of colorectal cancer or polyps, there is up to a 40% recurrence of these tumors; therefore, patients need close follow-up.

It is recommended that persons over the age of 45 have stool for occult blood annually and flexible sigmoidoscopy every three to five years.

It is also recommended that if patients are found to have blood in the stool and/or polyps at sigmoidoscopy, a colonoscopy be performed to remove the polyps that were seen previously and also to examine the rest of the colon. It is also recommended that if a patient has a family history of colon polyps and/or colon cancer, that patient should have a colonoscopy. If a patient has a history of ulcerative colitis and/ or Crohn's disease, they may also benefit from colonoscopy. Acromegalics should also have the colon examined because of the higher incidence of colorectal polyps and possibly cancer.

Through appropriate screening methods, probability of contracting colorectal cancer will be reduced to 30% and the probability of dying from it will be reduced to 50%.

Forthcoming developments in colorectal cancer and its relation to benign polyps, such as abnormalties sighted in chromosome 5, 7, 17 and 18, may form the basis for future genetic screening. I think that it is important to try and prevent this development of colorectal polyps and cancer by dietary manipulation, as well as by appropriate screening measures.

Prolactinomas

Michael O. Thorner M.D., D.Sc., FRCP, Professor of Medicine, University of Virginia,
Health Sciences Center, Charlottesville, Virginia

What is a Prolactinoma?

A prolactinoma is a tumor in the pituitary gland which secretes a hormone called prolactin. Pituitary tumors are clinically evident in about 14 people in 100,000. However in postmortem studies about 1 in 20 subjects have a small prolactinoma. This tumor is in over 99% of cases benign. It is the most common type of pituitary tumor. Prolactin is the milk hormone and levels of this hormone in the blood rise during pregnancy to stimulate and prepare the breast for lactation. After delivery of the baby the prolactin levels will fall unless breast feeding takes place. However if the baby is allowed to suckle then the mother's prolactin will rise in response to the suckling to maintain milk production.

What is the Cause of Prolactinomas?

While research continues to unravel the mechanisms of disordered cell growth in the pituitary, the cause of pituitary tumors remains unknown. Most pituitary tumors are sporadic in nature and are not genetically transmitted from parents to offspring.

Where is the Pituitary Gland?

The pituitary gland sits virtually in the middle of the head. The pituitary gland sits in a bony box (sella turcica (saddle). The eye nerves sit right above the pituitary gland. If a pituitary tumor expands the size of the pituitary it may give rise to local symptoms such as headache or visual disturbance. The visual disturbance is due to pressure on the eye nerves. Tumors may over secrete a hormone. Prolactinomas over secrete prolactin giving rise to elevated levels of prolactin in the blood (hyperprolactinemia). Disturbances of other pituitary functions may also arise.

What is the Importance of Hyperprolactinemia?

Women who develop hyperprolactinemia usually notice that they have a change in the pattern of their menstrual cycles. They may lose their periods altogether (amenorrhea), their periods may become irregular or their periods may become very heavy (menorrhagia). They may notice that the breasts secrete milk inappropriately (galactorrhea). In addition they often notice a reduction in their sex drive (libido) which may be associated with pain on intercourse due to vaginal dryness.

Men with hyperprolactinemia may develop hypogonadism and galactorrhea. However the onset is very insidious and since men do not have any objective measure to observe (like periods in women) they often deny that they have a problem. In this situation their partner is usually a more objective assessor of their sexual performance. Thus most men only present very late in the course of their disease with symptoms of the large tumor; they usually complain of headaches and/or visual disturbances. After they are treated, they then recognize that their sexual function was abnormal.

What is the Differential Diagnosis?

Elevated levels of prolactin can occur from multiple different causes. The most frequent cause is the taking of medications which act by blocking the effects of dopamine at the pituitary or depleting dopamine stores in the brain. These include major tranquilizers such as trifluoperazine (Stelazine) and haloperidol (Haldolt and metoclopramide (Reglan). Less frequently, drugs such as alpha methyldopa, and reserpine may elevate prolactin levels. Another cause of hyperprolactinemia is any disease within the pituitary fossa which may interfere with the delivery of dopamine from hypothalamus to the prolactin secreting cells. Thus, non functioning tumors and actively secreting tumors (causing acromegaly and Cushing's Syndrome) may also cause mild hyperprolactinemia. The way these are distinguished is usually by the degree of elevation of prolactin and the size of the tumor as visualized on MRI scan or CT scan. Breast manipulation and stimulation as well as chest wall injury may cause hyperprolactinemia by reflex stimulation. However prolactin elevation from this cause is usually modest.

How is Prolactinoma Treated?

The first line of treatment for a prolactinoma is medical rather that surgical. Approximately 80% of patients may expect their prolactin levels to be restored to normal with return of normal gonadal function. The size of pituitary tumor will also be reduced by medical treatment.

Medical treatment consists of the prescription of a dopamine agonist drug. The first effective dopamine agonist drug for this condition was bromocriptine. It is the first line of treatment. It is critical that treatment is initiated slowly, since this will prevent the development of side effects. Thus, many authorities recommend that treatment is initiated with a quarter of a 2.5 mg tablet taken on going to bed in the evening together with a glass of milk and a cookie. In this way the absorption of the drug from the gut is slowed and no side effects usually develop. The dose is increased every three days to one quarter of a tablet with breakfast and on retiring, and then increased to half a tablet at night and a quarter with breakfast. The dose is then increased to half a tablet twice a day; then one tablet at night and half with breakfast and finally one tablet twice a day A serum prolectin is checked when the patient is on one tablet twice a day. If it is not normal a third tablet is added at lunch time by first taking half a tablet and then if this is well tolerated the dose is increased to a full tablet.

Other regimens of bromocriptine administration are used by physicians. But the one listed above is the one least likely to cause side effects. Bromocriptine is the only dopamine agonist which is approved for the treatment of hyperprolactinemia and for the treatment of infertility associated with it. Cabergoline, an orally active long-acting dopamine agonist, has recently been approved by the Food and Drug Administration for hyperprolactinemia. It has the advantage of only needing to be taken once or twice per week and some patients who are unable to tolerate Bromocriptine or other dopamine agonists are better able to tolerate this drug. However, it is considerably more expensive. Pergolide, another dopamine agonist, is available in the United States. It is not approved for this indication. The dose usually needed to treat hyperprolactinemia is either 50 micrograms once a day, or 100 micrograms once a day.

The most common side effects are nausea and vomiting and dizziness particularly on standing up. These usually do not occur if the therapy is initiated as described above. If they do occur the patient should back off to the previous dose which was not associated with side effects. It is important to recognize that tolerance to side effects occurs even though the prolactin lowering effects are preserved. This means that over time the side effects will disappear even though the patient continues to take the medication.

Is Surgery Ever Warranted for Prolactinoma?

If medical therapy cannot be tolerated or if it is unsuccessful then surgery should be considered. If medical therapy has been continued for a year and the prolactin levels are still elevated, and gonadal function has not been restored, then medical therapy can be considered to have failed. It may be considered to be partially successful if prolactin levels are lowered by >80% even though levels are still elevated. In this situation medical therapy should be continued possibly with the addition of surgery or radiation therapy. Similarly, if the size of the pituitary tumor on MRI has not reduced in size within a year, or has increased in size, this also can be considered as failure of medical therapy.

The results of surgery are very dependent on the skill and experience of the neurosurgeon. If the serum prolactin is less than 250 ng/ml in the best centers there is an 80% chance of normalization of the serum prolactin. The higher the prolactin the lower the chance of normalization of the serum prolactin by surgery. Depending on the size of the tumor and completeness of surgical resection, studies show that 20%–50% of subjects will experience a recurrence of hyperprolactinemia. When this occurs, it is usually within 5 years from the time of surgery. However following removal of a large portion of the tumor it may be possible to normalize the serum prolactin by medical therapy, while this may have not been possible prior to surgery.

How Does a Patient Choose an Appropriate Neurosurgeon?

It is important for the patient to discuss with the surgeon the number of operations to remove pituitary tumors that he/she has performed and what the expected results are in his hands and in the major centers. The best results come from surgeons who have completed many hundreds or thousands of such operations.

What Evaluation of Pituitary Function is Necessary?

The anterior pituitary gland produces a variety of hormones which affect many different endocrine functions. These include ACTH, or corticotropin, which stimulates the adrenal glands to produce cortisol; thyrotropin, which stimulates the thyroid gland to produce thyroid hormone; the gonadotropins LH and FSH, which stimulate the ovaries to regulate ovulation and the testes in men to regulate spermatogenesis and testosterone production. In addition, prolactin and growth hormone are produced by the pituitary gland to regulate lactation and growth, respectively. These pituitary functions are usually normal in patients who have a prolactinoma. These can be evaluated by a simple blood test which measures not only the hormone which is produced from the pituitary, but that which is produced by the target gland in response; for example, TSH is measured as well as serum thyroxin or free thyroid hormone levels.

How Can the Pituitary Tumor be Visualized?

The pituitary and pituitary tumors can be visualized by one of two techniques, either Computer Assisted Tomography (CAT Scan) or by Magnetic Resonance Imaging. Magnetic Resonance Imaging, or MRI, is the preferential method for identifying pituitary tumors. This test should be performed in any patient who is suspected of having a pituitary tumor. If a pituitary tumor is found, and is then either followed or treated medically or surgically, it is probably advisable to repeat the scan at one year. Many physicians repeat the scan annually, while others repeat the scan based on clinical symptoms and signs. Another practice is to double the interval between scans, so that after the first year, it may be another two years before the scan is repeated, and then four years, etc. in the asymptomatic patient.

What is the Relationship of Prolactinomas to Pregnancy and Oral Contraceptives?

If the woman has a microprolactinoma, then there is no reason that she cannot conceive and have a normal pregnancy after successful medical therapy. The risk of swelling of the pituitary, giving rise to symptoms from hypopituitarism or compression of vital structures is less than one percent. In patients than one percent. In patients with macroadenomas, the risk is greater, and some people consider it as high as twenty-five percent. The important issue is that the patient should be carefully evaluated prior to becoming pregnant, and should have an MRI scan and plotting of objective visual fields. During pregnancy, if there is no swelling of the pituitary, pregnancy should be uneventful, but the patient should consult their endocrinologist if they should develop symptoms,

What is the Risk of Osteoporosis In Hyperprolactinemia?

Hyperprolactinemia does not cause osteoporosis unless hypogonadism is also present. All patients who are hypogonadal have an increased risk of development of osteoporosis. The usual recommendation is that the patient should be treated for the hyperprolactinemia so that gonadal function is restored to normal. In addition, they should take the appropriate amount of calcium (1 gm calcium gluconate or carbonate), exercise, and other general preventative measures used in prevention of osteoporosis. particularly headache, nausea, vomiting, excessive thirst or urination or extreme lethargy. Most endocrinologists see patients at two-monthly intervals through the pregnancy. If a patient has completed a successful pregnancy, the chance for completing further successful pregnancies is extremely high. As soon as a patient is pregnant, it is usually advised that she stop taking Bromocriptine or dopamine agonist drug, and this is only re-started if the patient develops symptoms from expansion of the tumor during pregnancy.

Oral contraceptives were at one time considered to be involved in the development of hyperprolactinemia. However, this has since been proven to be untrue, and therefore patients who have hyperprolactinemia who have been treated with bromocriptine or other dopamine agonists may also take an oral contraceptive for contraceptive purposes. Similarly, post-menopausal estrogen replacement is quite safe to take in patients with prolactinoma, providing that the prolactinoma is treated with medical therapy or surgery.

"The path of no risk is
the biggest risk
of all."

Indications for Treatment of Microprolactinomas: An Update

Anne Klibanski, M.D., Chief, Neuroendocrine Unit,
Massachusetts General Hospital, Harvard University

Although the presence of a macroprolactinoma (greater than or equal to 1 cm) obligates therapy, treatment of patients with idiopathic hyperprolactinemia or microprolactinomas remains controversial. Infertility or clinically significant galactorrhea have long been recognized as standard indications for treatment of hyperprolactinemia. Infertility may be associated with amenorrhea or anovulatory cycles. However, infertility also may be due to subtle ovulatory disorders including luteal phase dysfunction which may be more difficult to diagnose. Also, hyperprolactinemia may be intermittent in nature, and several prolactin levels may be needed to establish the diagnosis. Intermittent hyperprolactinemia associated with infertility may also occur exclusively in the periovulatory phase of the menstrual cycle. A subset of women are thought to be more sensitive to the rising levels of estrogen associated with the ovulatory phase of the cycle, and hyperprolactinemia occurring during this time period may lead to infertility. Therefore, even mild prolactin elevations in infertile women warrant therapy.

Other indications for treatment include signs and symptoms of androgen excess or headaches. Hyperprolactinemia is known to be associated with androgen excess in a subset of patients, and elevations in serum testosterone, free testosterone and DHEAS have been reported. Prolactin may have a direct stimulatory effect on adrenal androgen production. In women with documented hyperprolactinemia together with mild signs of androgen excess, treatment of hyperprolactinemia with dopamine agonist therapy typically results in normalization of serum androgens. Although headaches do occur in patients with prolactin-secreting macroadenomas, there is as well an association between hyperprolactinemia and headaches, even in patients with microadenomas or normal head scans. Therefore, in patients with hyperprolactinemia and headaches, particularly if the onset of headaches coincides with menstrual irregularity or symptoms potentially attributable to hyperprolactinemia, a trial of dopamine agonist therapy may be warranted.plain A more controversial point is whether women with microprolactinomas or idiopathic hyperprolactinemia without these indications for therapy should be treated, or whether they should be followed with observation alone. Two major points to be considered in this regard are the effects of follow-up without treatment on tumor size, and the metabolic consequences of hypogonadism and estrogen deficiency.

Tumor Size in Untreated Hyperprolactinemia

In a number of retrospective and prospective studies, patients with idiopathic hyperprolactinemia or microprolactinomas have been found to have a zero to 22% incidence of tumor progression. In a retrospective series of 25 patients reported from the NIH, one patient (4%) had tumor growth. The most comprehensive prospective series was reported by Schlechte et al. in which thirty women with hyperprolactinemia who were not treated were evaluated at yearly intervals for three to seven years. Of the 27 women who had serial x-ray evaluations, two had evidence of tumor progression, and four, with initially normal radiographic studies, developed radiographic evidence of a pituitary tumor. None of these patients developed a macroadenoma or pituitary hypofunction associated with these radiographic changes. On the basis of both retrospective and prospective data, it has been documented that the majority of patients with idiopathic hyperprolactinemia or microprolactinomas do not have evidence of tumor progression. Therefore, medical therapy based on tumor size is considered primarily in those women who have clear-cut evidence of tumor enlargement on an MRI scan, or who have the new appearance of a microadenoma with previously normal MRI scans. It is critical to emphasize that patients who do not receive therapy must be monitored carefully with serial prolactin levels and MRI scans.

Osteopenia in Hyperprolactinemia

Hypogonadism frequently accompanies hyperprolactinemia and is often manifested clinically by amenorrhea and/or other ovulatory disorders. Because mean serum estradiol levels in amenorrheic hyperprolactinemic women are typically low and comparable to the early follicular phase estradiol levels seen in normal women, hyperprolactinemic ammenorrheic women have an absolute or relative estrogen deficiency state. Such women lack the rise in serum estradiol levels typically seen in the mid-follicular, ovulatory and luteal phase of the cycle. The long-term metabolic consequences of amenorrhea and its associated estrogen deficiency in young women have been the *Osteopenia in Hyperprolactinemia*: Hypogonadism frequently accompanies hyperprolactinemia and is often manifested clinically by amenorrhea and/or other ovulatory disorders. Because mean serum estradiol levels in amenorrheic hyperprolactinemic women are typically low and comparable to the early follicular phase estradiol levels seen in normal women, hyperprolactinemic amenorrheic women have an absolute or relative estrogen deficiency state. Such women lack the rise in serum estradiol levels typically seen in the mid-follicular, ovulatory and luteal phase of the cycle. The long-term metabolic consequences of amenorrhea and its associated estrogen deficiency in young women have been the subject of a number of studies. Osteopenia has been found to affect both cortical and trabecular bone compartments and progressive cortical trabecular bone loss has been demonstrated in untreated patients. In a cross-sectional study of women treated for hyperprolactinemia with transsphenoidal surgery, spinal bone mineral content was 15% higher in women who had post-operative restoration of menses. These data suggested that restoration of normal gonadal function with treatment of hyperprolactinemia might have a beneficial effect on bone loss. In a study conducted at the MGH by Biller et al, trabecular bone density by CT was investigated prospectively in 52 hyperprolactinemic women with a mean follow-up interval of 1.8 years. Of the 39 women with a history of amenorrhea, 49% had a spinal bone density of more than 1 SD below normal. Because a decrease of 1 SD of bone mineral density is associated with a marked increase in fracture incidence, these data indicate that hyperprolactinemic women are at increased fracture risk before they enter menopause. Of the group of women who remained amenorrheic during the entire study, there was a significant decrease in mean trabecular bone density. In those patients who were followed after restoration of menses by treatment of hyperprolactinemia, there was an increase in bone density in only a subset of patients. Of note, women with oligoamenorrhea had a trabecular bone density which was midway between the hyperprolactinemic women and the normal controls. Therefore, chronic amenorrhea and its associated estrogen deficiency leads to progressive osteopenia in such women. Data from published studies indicate that, as in other hypogonadal states, the trabecular bone compartment may be first affected by hyperprolactinemic amenorrhea and may be less likely to show improvement following restoration of normal function. These data estrogen deficiency may have a permanent decline in bone density which may persist until the menopause. It is also important to note that hyperprolactinemic women who have regular menstrual periods do not have evidence of osteopenia. Therefore, prolactin has not been shown to have an independent, deleterious effect on bone density, and osteopenia is only an important consideration in those women who have associated menstrual disturbances.

Conclusions

For those patients not desiring fertility, and who show neither clinically significant galactorrhea, symptoms of androgen excess, nor headaches, the two most important indications for medical therapy are tumor size and hypogonadism. Women who have hyperprolactinemia with a normal MRI scan, or a microadenoma, can be followed with serum prolactin levels and head scans. Treatment is required if there is a significant increase in tumor size, development of amenorrhea, or other clinical indications.

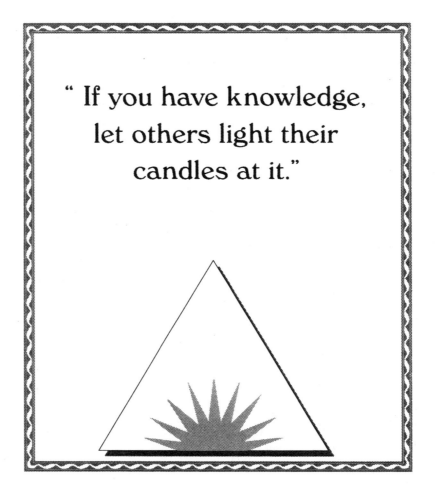

" If you have knowledge, let others light their candles at it."

TSH-Secreting Pituitary Tumors

Francoise Brucker-Davis, M.D., Visiting Associate, NIDDK Molecular and Cellular Endocrinology Branch, National Institutes of Health, Bethesda, Maryland

If you, or a member of your family, have been diagnosed with a TSH pituitary tumor, this paper will summarize the main points necessary to understand this disease and its treatment.

Definition

A TSH (Thyroid-Stimulating Hormone) pituitary tumor arises from one of the TSH secreting cells localized in the anterior pituitary. This tumor secretes an excess of TSH (sometimes even more active than the normal TSH) and often also alpha-subunit (one of the two components of TSH). The cells secreting the other pituitary hormones usually have a normal function; however, in some cases, the tumor can secrete one or more other hormones (active or not).

Frequency

TSH pituitary tumors are rare; they represent about 2% of all pituitary tumors.

Cause

Right now, the cause is unknown; no familial predisposition has been found. Scientists work hard to identify the factors called oncogenes that transform a normal cell into a tumorous cell. In the future, when these factors are identified, we hope that specific treatment will be able to target the oncogenes, and reverse the tumoral transformation.

Pathology

The tumors are overwhelmingly benign adenomas (very few will have a malignant transformation, with the possibility of distant metastases, like in any cancer).

Natural Evolution

Even if the pathology of the tumor is benign, we know that the local evolution can be very aggressive, with extension toward the optic chiasm (crossing of both optic nerves), with the potential risk of sight impairment or even blindness, or toward other important brain structures. There is not much room around the pituitary gland, so it is understandable that if the tumor keeps on growing, there can be serious consequences.

Size

The exact size is better evaluated by the surgeon: if the tumor is less than 1 cm, it is a micro-adenoma; if it is more than 1 cm, it is a macro-adenoma. The smaller tumors are less likely to be invasive or complicated and are more often cured by surgery alone. Unfortunately, diagnosis is often made at the stage of macro-adenoma.

Symptoms

The symptoms occur insideously, and it sometimes takes years before you realize that there is something wrong.

- **Symptoms related to the secretion of excess TSH:** TSH is the hormone that drives the thyroid gland; an excess of TSH will result in excessive production of thyroid hormones, called hyperthyroidism. The main symptoms are: palpitations, fast heart beats, tiredness, increased frequency of bowel movements, weight loss, nervousness, heat intolerance, excess sweating, irregular periods in women.

- **Symptoms related to the tumor itself (shared by all other pituitary tumors):** Headaches, visual defects (serious complication of a big tumor with upward extension).

• **Other:** If another hormone is secreted at the same time, you can experience other symptoms of hormonal imbalance: for example, in the case of secretion of GH (growth hormone), symptoms of acromegaly.

Diagnosis

Your endocrinologist will coordinate your work-up in order to confirm the diagnosis, eliminate other causes of hyperthyroidism and inappropriate secretion of TSH and have a good idea of the extension and sometimes complications of your tumor. The extent of the work-up depends on the center where you will be evaluated and treated. Research centers will run more sophisticated tests that are not mandatory for the diagnosis but will help to better understand TSH-pituitary tumors and eventually find a more specific treatment. The minimal work-up should include:

Hormonal Work-up

• Level of TSH and alpha subunit in the basal situation and usually after stimulation by TRH (TRH-TSH Releasing Hormone is the hormone that drives the secretion of TSH by the pituitary).
• Level of thyroid hormones.
• Level of the other pituitary hormones to check if their secretion is increased (if the tumor secretes more than one hormone) or impaired (a big tumor can compress and compromise the function of the adjacent normal pituitary).
• It is important to know it before surgery.
• Visualization of the tumor by MRI or CT-scan of the pituitary. This will provide information on the size and extension of the tumor.
• Visual fields, to check if there is any sight impairment.

Treatment

TSH-pituitary tumors are rare and can be locally aggressive in their evolution. After thorough evaluation, you need to be treated and followed by a specialized team that is experienced in dealing with TSH-pituitary tumors (remember, all pituitary tumors are not alike): Besides your endocrinologist, the team should include outstanding neurosurgeon and radiation therapy specialist. The three main tools for treatment are:

1. Surgery

Surgery is the treatment of choice. The procedure is called transsphenoidal surgery. The surgeon will try to remove selectively the adenoma, sparing the normal pituitary. In the case of well-encapsulated tumors, a cure is possible with surgery alone, mainly in the case of micro-adenoma. However, only prolonged follow-up will confirm the cure. In the case of an invasive tumor, the surgeon can remove as much as is safely possible, thus improving the efficacy of subsequent external radiation and/or octreotide treatments. The procedure is minimally traumatic with a low risk of complications in expert hands: a leak of cerebral fluid with its risk of infection (meningitis), damage of the normal pituitary or a transient water imbalance (diabetes insipidus or the opposite, retention of water) are possible.

2. External Radiation

If the surgeon knows that there are tumorous cells left (invasive tumor) or in the case of recurrence after surgery, external radiation is necessary. The radiation destroys residual tumor; however, the effect is slow and some patients will need medication (octreotide), while awaiting the full effect of radiation. Unfortunately, normal pituitary cells also are sensitive to radiation, meaning that normal pituitary function can be compromised in the following years. Another good reason to have continuing endocrine follow-up is so that replacement hormones can be introduced when necessary. If you have not yet completed your family, it is important for you to know that radiation will progressively decrease your fertility, and the possible therapeutic options should be discussed. Lastly, in the long run, some patients may develop memory problems as a consequence of this irradiation.

Medical Treatment

The majority of TSH pituitary tumors are sensitive to an analog of somatostatin (octreotide). This drug has recently been approved by the FDA for acromegaly, but not yet for TSH-pituitary tumors; as such, it may only be administered by certain research centers. It is the drug of choice if surgery and/or external radiation are not curative. This drug is palliative and cannot cure the disease, but it can decrease the secretion of TSH and stop the growth of the tumor. At high doses, a shrinking of the tumor may occasionally occur. Octreotide is given by subcutaneous injections, two to three times a day. Possible side effects include stomach problems with diarrhea (which usually improve after a few injections) and gallbladder stones.

Hormonal replacement is sometimes necessary, if pituitary function is impaired. Anti-thyroid medications (PTU or Tapazole) or destruction of the thyroid by radioactive iodine usually have **no place** in the treatement of TSH-pituitary tumors because TSH levels go up when thyroid hormones decrease and tumor growth may be stimulated.

Follow-up

A long follow-up is necessary, even when surgery seems to have been curative. Here again, because of the aggressiveness and rare nature of the tumor, it should only be managed by an experienced team. Your endocrinologist will look for signs of recurrence, and also screen for possible complications of your treatment (i.e: pituitary insufficiency after external radiation, gall bladder stones on octreotide).

Reviews should be more frequent at the beginning and then on a yearly basis when you are stable. Again, it should include blood work (hormonal evaluation), MRI or CT scan of the pituitary and visual fields testing, plus an ultrasound of the gallbladder to screen for stones, if you are on octreotide.

Suggested Reading

1. B.D. Weintraub, PA. Petrick, N. Gesundheit and E.R. Oldfield. TSH-secreting pituitary adenoma. *In Frontiers in Thyroidology*, 1986, vol. 1, 7 1-77, Ed. G. Medeiros-Neto and E. Gaitan (Plenum publishing corporation)
2. N. Gesundheit, P. Petrick, M. Nissim et al. TSH-secreting pituitary adenomas: clinical and biochemical heterogeneity: case reports and follow-up of nine patients. *Annals of Internal Medicine* 1989; 111: 827-835
3. Ph. Chanson, B.D. Weintraub and A. Harris. Octreotide therapy for TSH-secreting pituitary adenomas: a follow-up of *52* patients. *Annals of Internal Medicine* 1993;

Clinically Nonfunctioning Pituitary Adenomas: Characterization And Therapy

Laurence Katznelson, M.D., Instructor in Medicine
Neuroendocrine Unit, Massachusetts General Hospital, Harvard Medical School

The majority of patients with pituitary adenomas present with signs and symptoms reflecting excess hormone production. Approximately 25%–30% of patients with pituitary tumors do not have classical hypersecretory syndromes, such as acromegaly or Cushing's disease. These tumors are referred to as clinically nonfunctioning adenomas, because patients may appear otherwise normal. Patients may present with headaches, visual loss, fatigue, weight gain, lethargy, or, in women, change in menstrual status due to local compression from the tumor. The vast majority of these tumors are benign. Recent progress in our ability to characterize and treat these tumors will be discussed here.

Clinical Manifestations

Because of the lack of clinical manifestations of anterior pituitary hormone excess, tumors may grow to a large size before they are diagnosed. The tumors are often first detected when patients present to an ophthalmologist for evaluation of visual changes and visual field deficits are found. Growth of the tumor into the cavernous sinuses may lead to cranial nerve palsies, resulting in abnormal control of facial and ocular movements. Patients may also describe chronic or worsening headaches. These tumors may also be detected incidentally during the evaluation of another problem. For example, it is not uncommon to discover a tumor incidentally during an evaluation in the emergency room for head trauma.

Partial or complete hypopituitarism (low pituitary hormone levels) is frequently demonstrated in patients with large clinically nonfunctioning tumors because of compression of the adjacent, normal pituitary gland. Secondary thyroid or adrenal insufficiency may be detected in 81% and 62% of patients, respectively. A mild degree of hyperprolactinemia is present in up to 80% of patients and is likely to be produced by the remaining, normal pituitary gland as a result of compression of the hypophyseal stalk by the tumor with loss of hypothalamic inhibitory signals. Symptoms of hypopituitarism include loss of appetite, weight loss, fatigue, decreased energy, joint pains, and dizziness. Clinically symptomatic diabetes insipidus (DI) is an uncommon finding at the time of initial presentation in patients with pituitary adenomas. DI refers clinical to the presence of significant urination and intractable thirst and results in excessive concentration of blood salts. One of the first clues for the presence of DI is new onset frequent urination at night. The presence of DI in association with a sellar (the sella turcica is the bony area that surrounds the pituitary gland) and/or suprasellar mass suggests that the lesion may not be a primary pituitary tumor.

Hypogonadism (sex hormone insufficiency) is detected in up to 96% of patients with pituitary macroadenomas (> 1 cm). Symptoms of hypogonadism in women include irregular or nonexistent menses and infertility, and, in men, inability to attain erections. In both sexes, complaints of lack of sexual drive are common. Hypogonadism is usually associated with inappropriately normal or decreased serum gonadotropin (LH and FSH, the pituitary hormones responsible for reproductive function) levels, indicating central hypogonadism. The cause of hypogonadism in this setting may be multifactorial. In addition to insufficiency of LH and FSH secretion due to tumor mass effect, patients with such tumors may also have sex hormone deficiency as a result of associated hyperprolactinemia. Surgical management of these tumors with resultant reduction in mass effect may result in reversal of the hypogonadism. However, the majority of patients with clinically nonfunctioning adenomas require gonadal steroid replacement.

Diagnostic and Clinical Issues

As stated above, people with this type of tumor often appear otherwise normal and present with complaints attributable to tumor size (headaches, change in vision), hormone deficiency (hypopituitarism), or may be diagnosed incidentally during an evaluation for another problem. It is crucial to evaluate the extent of tumor growth and involvement of local structures with radiographic imaging including an MRI scan. In addition, compression of the optic chiasm frequently occurs resulting in loss of peripheral vision including temporal field deficits that may lead to blindness. Therefore, visual field testing is a necessary component of the evaluation.

Because many patients with clinically nonfunctioning pituitary adenomas lack a specific serum hormone marker (as seen with acromegaly or Cushing's disease, for example), it may be difficult to distinguish these tumors from other intra- and suprasellar non-pituitary masses that may mimic pituitary adenomas in their clinical, endocrinologic, and radiographic presentation. The differential diagnosis of such lesions includes craniopharyngiomas, meningiomas, arachnoid cysts, granulomatous diseases, gliomas, metastatic tumors, and chordomas. The pre-operative diagnosis of pituitary adenomas has been facilitated by 1) use of serum markers, and 2) gonadotropin responses to TRH (thyroid hormone releasing hormone).

LH and FSH circulate as a dimer (combination) of a common alpha (a) and beta (b) subunits. The combination of these subunits is necessary for hormone function. In patients with these tumors, isolated a or b-subunit elevations may be detected. Demonstration of elevated serum levels of hormones and/or free subunit levels, typically a-subunit and FSH, may suggest the presence of a pituitary adenoma, indicating the utility of such tumor markers. It may be difficult to determine whether elevated LH/FSH levels reflect secretion by normal or neoplastic gonadotrophs. For example, LH and FSH levels are increased in patients with primary gonadal failure. This is particularly relevant in the evaluation of a post-menopausal woman with a sellar mass because menopause itself is associated with elevated gonadotropin levels. Therefore, when interpreting levels of serum markers, it is important to consider the clinical setting and to compare intact gonadotropin and free-subunit levels.

Patients with clinically nonfunctioning tumors may demonstrate unique gonadotropin responses following administration of TRH (thyroid hormone releasing hormone: controls thyroid hormone production). In up to 40% of patients, administration of TRH results in stimulation of serum levels of gonadotropins and/or free subunits. These data suggest that TRH receptors, not found on normal gonadotroph membranes, are expressed on neoplastic gonadotroph cells. In a recent study, TRH tests elicited an exaggerated response of LHb subunit in 11 of 16 women with clinically nonfunctioning adenomas and normal basal serum LH and LHb levels. Therefore, a TRH test may be diagnostically useful in the evaluation of patients with intrasellar lesions.

Therapy

Initial therapy is directed toward reduction of tumor mass and management of acute or chronic neuro-ophthalmologic or neurologic symptoms. Optic chiasmal compression frequently results in visual field deficits, including bitemporal hemi- or quadrantanopsias. Cranial nerve palsies may result from extension of the adenoma, particularly if the tumor invades the cavernous sinus with compression of cranial nerves III, IV and VI. It is important to establish the extent of the tumor on an MRI scan and assess its potential to compress adjacent structures. Visual field deficits or other evidence of local compression will warrant urgent therapy, with surgery the initial therapy of choice.

A. Surgical Therapy

Surgical therapy in experienced hands is safe and often highly successful in tumor debulking. Surgery will lead to pathologic diagnosis important in differentiating primary pituitary disease from other sellar and extrasellar lesions.

The therapeutic approach is dependent upon whether the tumor is a macroadenoma (> 1cm) or a microadenoma (<1cm) by radiologic imaging. If an asymptomatic patient has a microadenoma, and a clinical diagnosis of a nonfunctioning adenoma has been made, then surgical excision is not recommended. Such lesions are often incidentally found after MRI scans for other reasons. Our approach is to repeat the scan at yearly intervals to determine whether there has been further growth. If an asymptomatic patient has a macroadenoma, but close to 1 cm, then the case may be argued for observation in a similar fashion.

Primary therapy for macroadenomas is neurosurgical debulking of the tumor mass. The timing of surgery depends on the presence of visual field deficits and neurologic symptoms, and immediate neurosurgery may be necessary to decompress the optic chiasm and cranial nerves to prevent irreversible damage. Transsphenoidal surgery results in improvement in visual field deficits in up to 90% of cases, with full recovery of vision achieved in approximately 63% of patients. There are limited data on the frequency of completeness of tumor removal, as many of the studies were done prior to the availability of modem sensitive radiological techniques. Given the low morbidity and mortality from this technique and the high frequency of successful outcomes, transsphenoidal surgery is the initial therapeutic choice. Probably the most important determinant of surgical outcome is the clinical skill and experience of the neurosurgeon.

Hypopituitarism may improve following tumor resection and reversal of functional deficiencies has been reported. Recovery of thyroid, adrenal, and gonadal function occur in up to 60% of cases. Therefore, unless hormone levels measured pre-operatively are very low or patients are clinically symptomatic, replacement therapy of thyroid and gonadal deficiency is withheld until post-operative evaluation several weeks following surgery. Adrenal insufficiency should be replaced with appropriate glucocorticoid therapy pending re-evaluation.

Growth hormone function, as determined by provacative testing including ITT or arginine infusion, is deficient in almost all subjects pre-operatively. GH deficiency in patients with pituitary macroadenomas is usually not reversible. There is much interest in the use of growth hormone replacement therapy in this population.

B. Adjuvant Therapy

Radiation Therapy

Patients with significant residual tumor following transsphenoidal surgery or those with recurrent adenoma may benefit from adjuvant radiation therapy. The decision to administer postoperative radiotherapy should depend upon the size of the residual tumor and the importance of preserving pituitary function. We recommend post-surgical follow-up MRI scans at six month intervals during the first year, one year intervals for five years, and two year intervals thereafter if there is no clinical evidence of recurrence and visual fields remain stable. If there is evidence of tumor growth, then radiation therapy is instituted promptly, or repeat transsphenoidal surgery is considered. Conventional radiation therapy is administered through a wide beam to the tumor area through multiple ports to deliver 45 Gy (4500 rads) at 1.8 Gy (180 rads) per day as the usual dose. Other techniques that administer radiation in a more focused manner include proton beam radiation, gamma knife radiation, and radiation with a stereotactic linear accelerator.

Patients receiving radiotherapy should undergo serial evaluation of pituitary hormone function because radiation may result in partial or complete hypopituitarism. Adrenal, thyroid and gonadal insufficiency develop in two-thirds of patients over 5 years following radiation therapy. These data demonstrate that anterior pituitary hormonal deficiencies are common following radiotherapy and emphasize the necessity of careful, serial monitoring of hormonal function during the five to ten years following radiotherapy.

Endocrine Therapy

Recent studies have investigated the exciting possibility of adjuvant medical therapy for patients with clinically nonfunctioning pituitary tumors. Medical therapy is based on the assumption that suppression of hormone secretion may be accompanied by reduction in tumor size. Investigations with the somatostatin analog, octreotide, and the dopamine agonist, bromocriptine, have shown promise for use of adjuvant medical therapy.

Somatostatin Analog

Somatostatin is a peptide (protein) that plays an inhibitory role in the normal regulation of multiple systems, including the pancreas, gastrointestinal hormone secretion and peristalsis, and in the central nervous system. Recently, somatostatin analogs have been investigated in the management of pituitary tumors. Studies have demonstrated efficacy of somatostatin analogs in the management of acromegaly. In this system, somatostatin reduces secretion of GH leading to medical remission. Somatostatin analogs have greater clinical utility than native somatostatin because of the longer half-life following subcutaneous administration. The somatostatin analog octreotide (Sandostatin) has been used widely in the management of somatotroph adenomas.

The development of therapeutic strategies for clinically nonfunctioning adenomas has been based on the assumption that suppression of gonadotropin biosynthesis and release may lead to a decrease in hormone secretion and tumor size. Data supporting the use of somatostatin and its analogs to regulate hormone secretion by clinically nonfunctioning adenomas is derived from studies detecting somatostatin receptors in such tumors. High affinity somatostatin receptors (proteins that have the capacity to take up somatostatin and its analogs) have been detected in up to 40% of glycoprotein hormone producing pituitary adenomas. The presence of somatostatin receptors on clinically nonfunctioning pituitary adenomas therefore suggests a role for somatostatin analogs in the therapy of patients with such tumors.

Several reports have demonstrated the utility of octreotide in the management of patients with clinically nonfunctioning pituitary adenomas. We studied six subjects with a-subunit secreting pituitary adenomas and demonstrated a significant decrease in serum alpha-subunit levels in 50%, and a dose-responsive decrease in tumor size in two. Improvement in visual field deficits were also noted in these patients. These data suggest that octreotide may result in clinical improvement in a small subset of patients. The variable response to octreotide may be a function of the density of somatostatin receptors. Therefore, a trial of octreotide may be reasonable in patients who have already undergone attempt at surgery and have significant residual disease.

Radiological imaging of somatostatin receptors has been performed clinically using radio-labeled octreotide. This technique represents a non-invasive, outpatient investigation that may be highly useful in detecting the presence of somatostatin receptors and therefore help identify which patients may optimally respond to octreotide therapy.

Bromocriptine

Bromocriptine (Parlodel), a dopamine-like agent, has been administered to patients with clinically nonfunctioning pituitary adenomas, with conflicting results. Dopamine receptor binding sites have been detected on such tumors suggesting a potential role for bromocriptine in reducing tumor size. Administration of bromocriptine may result in a decrease in serum gonadotropin and free-subunit levels in most patients. However, the effect on tumor size has been variable. There have been occasional reports of tumor regression in response to bromocriptine therapy with accompanying improvement in visual fields. However, the majority of subjects with clinically nonfunctioning pituitary adenomas do not show reduction in tumor size in response to bromocriptine.

In summary, recent laboratory and clinical investigations have led to advances in our ability to characterize and manage clinically nonfunctioning pituitary adenomas. The availability of more sensitive and specific glycoprotein hormone free-subunit assays may facilitate pre-operative characterization of these tumors.

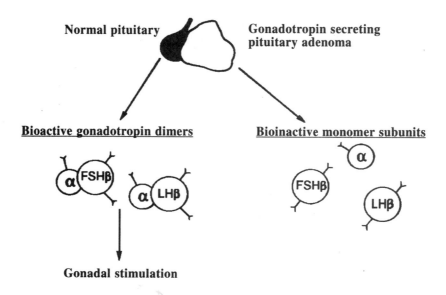

Legends:
Figure 1: Secretion of gonadotroph free-subunits by clinically nonfunctioning pituitary adenomas. The normal pituitary gland secretes intact LH and FSH which are bioactive at the level of the gonads. In contrast, clinically nonfunctioning pituitary adenomas secrete the free gonadotropin a and 3-subunits. These free subunits are bioinactive at the gonadal level.

References

1. Snyder PJ. Gonadotroph cell adenomas of the pituitary. Endocrine Rev. 1985;6:552-63.

2. Katznelson L, Alexander JM, Bikkal HA, Jameson JL, Hsu DW, Klibanski A. Imbalanced follicle-stimulating hormone beta-subunit hormone biosynthesis in human pituitary adenomas. J Clin Endocrinol Metab. *1992;74:1343-51.*

3. Kovacs K. Light and electron microscopic pathology of pituitary tumors: immunocytochemistry. In *Secretory Tumors of the Pituitary Gland.* Black PM, Zervas NT, Ridgway BC, Martin JB, eds. Raven Press, New York. 1985;365-76.

4. Daneshdoost L, Gennarelli TA, Bashey HM et al. Recognition of gonadotroph adenomas in women. N Engl J Med. 199 I;324:589-94.

5. Katznelson L, Alexander JM, Klibanski A. Clinical review 45: Clinically nonfunctioning pituitary adenomas. [Review] J Clin Endocrinol Metab. 1993;76(5): 1089-94.

7. Klibanski A. Chronic somatostatin analog administration in patients with alpha-subunit secreting pituitary tumors. J Clin Endocrinol Metab. 1992; *75(5):1318-25.*

Craniopharyngiomas and Rathke's Cleft Cysts

Keith E. Friend, M.D., Assistant Professor, Section of Endocrine Neoplasia
and Hormonal Disorders, University of Texas MD Anderson Cancer Center

Craniopharyngiomas are intracranial tumors that can occur at any age, but are most commonly found during childhood or adolescence; they account for about 10% of all central nervous system (CNS) tumors in these younger age groups. Craniopharyngiomas are usually not discovered until they impinge upon important structures around them. For this reason, although they are almost always benign tumors, they are frequently quite large when detected, ranging from an average of about one inch across to more than 4 inches.

The symptoms produced by a craniopharyngioma vary depending upon the tumor's location. If it compresses the pituitary stalk or involves the area of the pituitary gland itself, the tumor can cause partial or complete pituitary hormone deficiency. This frequently results in one or more of the following: growth failure, delayed puberty, loss of normal menstrual function or sexual desire, increased sensitivity to cold, fatigue, constipation, dry skin, nausea, low blood pressure, and depression. Pituitary stalk compression can also increase prolactin levels enough to cause a milky discharge from the breast.

If the craniopharyngioma involves the optic tracts, chiasm, or nerves, then visual disturbances can result. Involvement of the hypothalamus, an area at the base of the brain, may result in obesity, increased drowsiness (somnolence), temperature regulation abnormalities, or a water balance problem such as diabetes insipidus. A partial list of other common symptoms, arising for a variety of reasons, includes personality changes, headache, confusion, and vomiting.

The symptoms produced by craniopharyngiomas are, as the preceding list illustrates, quite diverse. The initial treatment for most people with craniopharyngiomas, however, is usually surgery. The goal of surgery is generally to completely remove the tumor while improving or at least preserving pituitary, visual and brain function. Depending upon the location of the tumor, the surgeon may choose to approach it one of several ways. If the tumor is primarily in the area of the pituitary, a transsphenoidal route (through the nose and sinuses), is often used, as is done with many pituitary adenomas. If the tumor is not in this region, the surgeon may choose to approach it using one of several types of craniotomy, a procedure in which an opening is made in the skull to allow access to the tumor.

In instances where the tumor cannot be completely removed, radiation treatment has been clearly demonstrated to increase the chance of survival. Radiation is also used as an initial therapy for some people with craniopharyngiomas. The goals of radiation treatment are similar to those of surgery, to destroy tumor while preserving or improving pituitary, visual and brain function, as well as to prevent regrowth. A variety of methods are available to administer radiation to the tumor, including conventional radiation therapy (requires several weeks of treatment) and methods such as gamma knife (single day). These procedures involve allowing the radiation to travel from a source outside the body, to the tumor inside. Occasionally, radioactive material is placed directly inside the tumor. Because hormone deficiencies can develop many years after radiation treatment, all individuals treated in this manner should have periodic evauations by an endocrinologist throughout their lifetimes, not just in the immediate period after surgery.

Craniopharyngiomas are thought to arise from the remains of a structure (Rathke's pouch), formed at the time, early in pregnancy, when a fetus' organs are developing. During this process, a small amount of tissue (Rathke's pouch) bulges or pouches out from the throat area and moves up to eventually become part of the pituitary gland. This accounts for the name given to this type of tumor (cranio=skull, pharynx=throat, oma= tumor). Most craniopharyngiomas are cystic (contain fluid) and many also contain some calcium deposits. This relatively unique type of appearance helps in their identification prior to the time of surgery.

Successful management of craniopharyngiomas often requires the involvement of several specialists (neurosurgery, radiation therapy, endocrinology). As people adjust to life after the initial treatment of the tumor, additional support services are also often required, and should be individually tailored to meet the specific needs of patients and their families. For example, some individuals need aid adapting to diminished vision, others require emotional or psychological assistance. By combining effective initial treatment, along with careful follow up, many people with craniopharyngiomas go on to live uncompromised or relatively uncompromised lives. This is not always the outcome, however, and this important fact should serve as a reminder that although significant improvement has been made in treating craniopharyngiomas, earlier detection and better therapeutic techniques still are required, and must remain a priority of both physicians and researchers.

Unlike craniopharyngiomas, Rathke's cleft cysts are not tumors, but instead are classified as developmental abnormalities. As the name implies, the cysts also arise from the developmental structure known as Rathke's pouch (cleft). Small Rathke's cleft cysts (less than 1/8 of an inch) are common and do not usually cause symptoms. When the cysts enlarge, however, they can interfere with pituitary function or impinge upon important structures such as the optic chiasm. For this reason, many of the symptoms produced by Rathke's cleft cysts are similar to those listed for craniopharyngiomas.

Treatment generally consists of surgically creating an opening or pouch (marsupialization) in the cyst, allowing the fluid inside the cyst to drain, thereby markedly decreasing its size. The majority of Rathke's cleft cysts treated this way do not recur. Attempts at complete removal of the cyst are generally not advisable because this increases the risk of surgical complication without improving benefits. Occasionally, cysts are not discovered until permanent damage has been done to the pituitary gland or optic chiasm. In these cases, surgical treatment will prevent further damage to these structures but will not correct that which has already occurred. With accurate diagnosis and careful management, however, people with Rathke's cleft cysts are usually treated quite successfully.

Section III

Treatments of Pituitary Disease

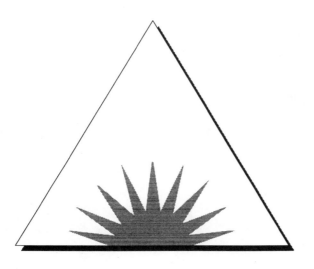

Second Edition

Medications for Pituitary Disease

Ariel L. Barkan, M.D., Pituitary and Neuroendocrine Center,
University of Michigan, Ann Arbor, Michigan

Patients with pituitary tumors often require medication therapy to suppress hormonal hyper-secretion, to replace the missing hormone(s) or to accomplish both tasks. It is absolutely imperative for the patient to participate actively in the choice of therapy and to comply with the treatment protocol.

An active discussion of the reasons for a particular treatment, the goals to be accomplished and the potential pitfalls is a necessary prerequisite for successful cooperation between a knowledgeable endocrinologist and an intelligent patient.

Replacement Therapy

The pituitary tumor itself or its treatment (surgery and/or radiation) can irreparably damage the proper function of the healthy pituitary cells. While surgical damage occurs right away (and thus is easy to detect), radiation causes delayed damage whose results may not be obvious for years. This requires a life-long follow-up to detect the earliest signs of the incipient pituitary failure.

Clinical pictures, as well as hormonal tests, play equally important roles and sophisticated stimulation test are sometimes needed. As a rule of thumb, there is a particular order in the disappearance of pituitary hormones. Growth hormone is the most sensitive one and vanishes first, followed by gonadotropins (LH and FSH), then ACTH and later TSH. In practice, however, the patient may develop a loss of only one hormone, or the order of disappearance may be broken with bizarre combinations and permutations.

Growth Hormone Deficiency

GH deficiency should definitely be treated in children to assure proper statural growth. This should be done only by a qualified pediatric endocrinologist. Currently, four preparations are available in the U.S.: Protropin® by Genentech, Genotropin® by Pharmacia & Upjohn, Humatrope® by Lilly, and Norditropin® by Novo-Nordisk. All are exceedingly expensive (approximately $20,000 per year) and require daily injections. Fortunately, other companies are poised to capture a slice of the market, and the price will inevitably fall. GH replacement for adult hypopituitary patients is officially approved by the FDA and should be covered by the insurance companies. Recent studies have suggested that adult hypopituitary patients may benefit from GH replacement in terms of normalization of bone density, muscle strength, general energy, etc. Whether GH replacement in adults can prevent cardiovascular complications and/or extend life span, is unknown. The conclusive studies are not yet available and there are some potential complications of GH therapy. This treatment has to be administered under close medical supervision by a qualified endocrinologist. The benefits of GH replacement in the elderly non-hypopituitary patients are uncertain and the side effects may be more severe in this group. This indication is not approved by the FDA. Apparently, GH can be bought for this purpose on the "black market" or through chains of the "for profit" establishments in Mexico, that advertise GH as a "Fountain of Youth" type innocuous drug. Talk to your endocrinologist before using it!

Gonadotropin Deficiency

In men, restoration of potency, and prevention of bone and muscle loss are accomplished by the intramuscular injections of Depot-Testosterone. The drug is given every 2-3 weeks,

200-300 mg. per injection. The existing oral preparations are totally ineffective and may cause liver damage. Testosterone skin patches and new oral androgens are under continuous development; ALZA Corporation has released its new Testoderm®, a scrotal patch, and Smith-Kline Beecham has released Androderm®, patches that can be worn on the arms, legs, back or abdomen. Transdermal testosterone replacement offers no physiological advantage vs. i.m. injections, is much more expensive and often causes skin irritation.

In women, estrogen in different forms (Estraderm® patches, Estrace®, and Premarin® or Ogen® tablets) are equally effective and the choice is dictated by the financial considerations and convenience (patches in some patients cause skin irritation, for example). If a woman has a uterus, periodic administration of progestagen (Provera® tablets) is needed. Fertility can be restored in both sexes by hCG/hMG therapy and should be done only by reproductive endocrinogists or gynecologists. In women, this should be closely monitored by ultrasound and estrogen measurements to avoid potentially severe (and occasionally fatal) complications. Treatment with clomiphene or GnRH pumps is usually ineffective in patients with pituitary damage.

ACTH Deficiency

This is by far the most important deficit to treat. Unrecognized or untreated, this condition may result in death during severe stressful illnesses (heart attack, pneumonia, etc.). Cortisone acetate (~37.5 mg/day), hydrocortisone (~25 mg/day) or prednisone (~7.5 mg/day) are usually given for life. During stressful illnesses (flu, for example) the dose should be doubled by the patient for the duration of acute disease. If an illness is accompanied by vomiting and/or diarrhea, the absorption of the oral drug may be impaired and this would require an injection. Contact your doctor immediately! Identification bracelets are mandatory: this is your best insurance policy in case you are brought to the hospital while unconscious.

TSH Deficiency

This results in hypofunction of the thyroid gland. Replacement therapy with levothyroxine is easy, reliable, cheap and 100% effective. Several good brand name preparations are available and all are equally effective: Synthroid®, Levoxyl®, and Levothroid® are practically interchangeable. Avoid generics; some are very unreliable. Also, steer away from older preparations such as desiccated thyroid, Proloid®, Ecthroid® or Thyrolar®.

Prolactin Deficiency

This of no practical importance in men. In women this will result in the inability to lactate (produce milk) but this is of little concern, since artificial baby foods are widely available.

Vasopressin Deficiency

Vasopressin deficiency causes diabetes insipidus. If mild, this may be left untreated as long as water is freely available. DDAVP is a synthetic hormone that is given by nasal sprays or tablets. The dose should be adjusted by your endocrinologist.

Overall, proper replacement therapy is highly effective and, while being a chore at the beginning, soon becomes routine and doesn't appreciably affect the quality of life.

Another group of medications (unfortunately very small) is directed toward suppression of persistent hormone hypersecretion. Bromocriptine (Parlodel®) is highly effective for suppression of prolactin hypersecretion and shrinks a large proportion of prolactin-secreting tumors. The latter may obviate pituitary surgery or radiation. The doses may range from 2.5 mg to more than 20 or 40 mg per day. Stopping the drug will almost inevitably result in re-expansion of the tumor and restoration of prolactin hypersecretion. Some patients cannot tolerate the drug because of nausea, abdominal pain or lightheadedness. In some women, these side effects may be ameliorated by the vaginal route of administration. Pergolide (Permax®) is not approved for treatment of hyperprolactinemia but is very effective. It may be an alternative for some patients who are intolerant to bromocriptine. Other medications are being developed and Parlodel-LAR®, an indictable form of bromocriptine (one injection per month) is undergoing trials.

Cabergoline (Dostinex®) has recently been approved for treatment of hyperprolactinemia (Pharmacia & Upjohn). It needs to be taken orally once or twice a week and may have less side effects than bromocriptine. The choice between different preparations is dictated by their efficacy and side effect profile in an individual patient as well as by the price.

Most importantly, remember that not every case of hyperprolactinemia results from a pituitary prolactinoma. All too often it is due to some other pituitary disease, medications, thyroid disease, renal failure or even chest wall damage. Every case of hyperprolactinemia should be investigated by a qualified endocrinologist before the final decision about treatment is made.

Bromocriptine is less effective for acromegaly. Even though the doses are usually higher, GH normalizes only in about 10% of patients and tumor shrinkage is rare. Nevertheless, for a responsive patient, this may be an excellent choice.

Octeotide® (Sandostatin) is highly effective in acromegaly. It normalizes GH secretion in ~60—80% of patients, and shrinks tumors measurably in a significant proportion of them. It is approved by the FDA, and the insurance companies will reimburse the cost at least partially. This is not an ideal medication: it requires 3—4 daily injections, it causes diarrhea and abdominal cramps, it may cause gallstones (a gall bladder surgery may be needed) and occasionally it may worsen the pre-existent diabetes. Only physicians thoroughly familiar with this drug should direct the treatment. A long-acting indictable preparation (once a month) is in the works. Octreotide is successfully used in some patients with TSH-producing pituitary tumors.

Lanreotide (Ipsen) is another somatostatin analogue that is available in Europe. It is as good as octreotide and a choice between the two will be decided solely by the price.

Unfortunately, there is no specific medication therapy for patients with LH/FSH secreting tumors or for ACTH-secreting tumors (Cushing's disease). In the latter, however, adrenal overproduction of cortisol may be chronically normalized by an anti-yeast medication, Keto-conazole.

Any patient diagnosed with pituitary disease or who is suspected to have one should be seen by an endocrinologist with expertise in this field. This will give the best chance for appropriate and speedy diagnosis, immediate therapy and successful long-term follow-up.

Hormonal Replacement Therapy For Hypopituitarism

David M. Cook, M.D., Oregon Health Sciences University

General Overview

Hypopituitarism is a general term which refers to any underfunction of the pituitary gland. This is a clinical definition used by endocrinologists and is interpreted to mean that one or more functions of the pituitary are deficient. The term includes both anterior and posterior pituitary gland secretions. Deficient pituitary gland function can result from damage to either the pituitary or the area just above the pituitary, the hypothalamus. The hypothalamus contains releasing and inhibitory hormones which control the pituitary, Since these hormones are necessary for normal pituitary function, damage to the hypothalamus can also result in deficient pituitary gland function, also referred to as hypopituitarism. Lastly there can be temporary decrease in pituitary function if there is prolonged exposure to an excess target gland hormone secretion. An example of this increase in negative feedback exposure to a target gland secretion would be Cushing's Disease. In Cushing's Disease excess ACTH secretion from a pituitary ACTH secreting pituitary tumor would, in turn, cause excessive cortisol secretion and suppression of the normal ACTH secreting cells of the anterior pituitary. Suppression would also occur at the hypothalamic level in the cells which produce the releasing hormone for ACTH referred to as CRH or corticotropin releasing hormone. If and when "feedback" suppression occurs, underfunction is temporary and will eventually return to normal.

Injury to the pituitary can occur from a variety of insults, including damage from a tumor, irradiation to the pituitary, trauma and abnormal iron storage (hemochromatosis) just to mention a few. With increasing damage there is a progressive decrease in function. There appears to be a predictable loss of hormonal function with increasing damage. There appears to be some hormones of the anterior pituitary which are lost with only minimal damage and those that resist damage until almost total pituitary function is lost. The progression from most vulnerable to least vulnerable is as follows; first is growth hormone (GH), next the gonadortopins LH and FSH, followed by TSH and finally the last to be lost, ACTH. Phrased another way, if ACTH is lost, predictably all other hormone functions are also lost. Those patients who have lost ACTH usually have lost all pituitary function and are referred to as suffering from panhypopituitarism or total pituitary underfunction.

Deficiency ACTH and Cortisol

Deficiency of ACTH resulting in cortisol deficiency is the most dangerous and life threatening of the hormonal deficiency syndromes. Loss of cortisol, the stress hormone, results in marked muscle weakness, nausea,vomiting and vascular collapse, i.e., low blood pressure and shock. This can occur as soon as four to five hours after surgical interruption of normal pituitary function. Replacement therapy of cortisol (also referred to as hydrocortisone) is difficult. Too much cortisol results in Cushing's syndrome and too little results in adrenal insufficiency. Unfortunately there are no laboratory tests to monitor cortisol therapy. The clinical endocrinologist must work with the patient to control successful replacement therapy. Weight gain, hypertension, edema and muscle weakness suggest too much cortisol. Weight loss, nausea and light headedness suggest too little. Since excessive cortisol is dangerous for normal bone structure, the least amount of cortisol per day is the major goal of therapy. The production rate of cortisol per day is in the range of 10 to 20 milligrams. When given orally some of the ingested cortisol is metabolized in the liver and lost to the general circulation. For this reason, oral doses needed for replacement therapy tend to be larger than production rates. Cortisol is normally secreted into the bloodstream more in the morning and virtually ceases during the night, In order to mimic this normal pattern a larger dose is usually given in the morning and less at night. Since cortisol is excitatory and can keep patients awake at night, the pm dose is usually given before dinner. If patients feel well with a single morning dose, this is even superior to twice daily dosing.

Cushing's syndrome can occur with levels or cortisol which are not excessive yet are constant without a low level during the night. For this reason, in addition to the disturbed sleep, cortisol is not given late at night. For similar reasons, cortisol preparations with long acting activity should be avoided. An example of a long acting preparation is dexamethasone. These preparations, by exerting their effects over a long period of time, can cause Cushing's syndrome.

Deficiency of TSH and Thyroid Hormone.

Deficiency of thyroid hormone causes a syndrome consisting of feeling cold, dry skin, constipation and muscle aching. This constellation of symptoms is very uncomfortable and is often the symptom complex which drives patients with pituitary disease to seek medical attention. In contrast to cortisol therapy, blood testing is available to monitor thyroid hormone therapy. Thyroid hormone disappears slowly from the bloodstream and only half disappears over a seven day period (Seven day half-life). Patients with pituitary damage of the TSH secreting anterior pituitary cells have low blood TSH levels which are normally an excellent guide to thyroid hormone therapy in patients with thyroid gland damage but not with pituitary damage. For this reason L-thyroxin values alone in blood act as a guide to chronic therapy. Values for thyroxin should be kept in the normal to high normal range during therapy. When initiating a dose of thyroid hormone or changing doses, a new steady-state level of thyroid is not achieved for a full two months. For this reason we do not suggest repeating thyroid mood tests for a full two months after changing or initiating a dose.

The usual replacement dose for thyroxin is 1.6ug per kilogram of body weight. Older individuals and those with heart disease should be started on much lower doses and the dose escalated slowly. Once a new steady state is reached there are a number to drugs which can change thyroid hormone requirements and they are listed below. Excessive thyroid hormone replacement causes hyperthyroidism which can cause heart beat irregularities and osteoporosis.

There is one clinical situation in which caution should be exercised in patients with pituitary disease receiving thyroid hormone therapy. In cases where there is combined thyroid and cortisol deficiency, if thyroid hormone is given without the cortisol, the increased metabolic rate resulting from the thyroid could accelerate the disposal rate of limited cortisol cortisol secretion and push the patient into adrenal (low cortisol) crisis. The principle here is that patients with pituitary disease beginning thyroxin therapy must be assessed for their ability to make ACTH and cortisol.

Deficiency of LH and FSH Causing Low Estrogen (Females) or Low Testosterone (Males).

Deficiency of estrogen and/or testosterone can cause a decrease in bone formation and osteoporosis. Estrogen can be given orally as conjugated estrogen's (Premarin) or as estradiol (estrace). Estrogen can also be given in patch form including patches applied twice weekly (estraderm) or once weekly (Climara). Patch forms are suggested in patients with elevated blood triglycerides since oral estrogens can aggravate hypertriglyceridemia in some patients. Regardless of estrogen preparation, unopposed estrogen is a risk factor for endometrial tumors in women who have not had a hysterectomy. Expressed another way all women taking estrogens who have a uterus must take progesterone. Progesterone may be taken in a small daily dose or in a larger dose for 12 days out of each calendar month. The former regimen is usually associated with less bleeding and is the preferred method by most women.

Testosterone therapy is delivered in injectable form or in patch form. Although there are oral preparations of male sex hormone they are not usually prescribed since they have the potential for liver toxicity. Injectable testosterone lasts about two weeks in most patients. Injections are given intramusculary and can be given by the patient after a period instruction. The injectable preparations are testosterone cypionate and testosterone enanthate. One is not suggested over the other. Both provide replacement therapy and are the least expensive way to give male sex hormone (testosterone). About half patients receiving injectable testosterone can feel the normal rise and fall of serum testosterone which occurs over the two week injectable sequence. Some have a sensation of a testosterone "rollercoaster" which can be uncomfortable. For these men, the patch forms of testosterone replacement which deliver testosterone over twenty four hours in a predictable fashion are suggested. There are two forms of patch testosterone include a scrotal patch and a skin patch. The skin patches are applied at night and the scrotal patch in the morning. One skin patch is insufficient and two need to be applied each day at night. The skin patch may cause skin irritation. If skin irritation occurs, application in different areas usually will suffice. The scrotal patch is applied in the morning. With the scrotal patch the scrotal skin must be shaved every two to three days. Similar to the skin patches, new scrotal patches are applied daily, this is necessary since the patches contain only enough hormone for a 24 hour period.

Antidiuretic Hormone Deficiency, Causing Diabetes Insipidus.
Patients with diabetes insipidus have increased thirst and urination. Replacement of antidiuretic hormone resolves these symptoms. Antidiuretic hormone action takes place at the kidney level, by stimulating the kidney to retain water. Insufficient antidiuretic hormone can cause dehydration and excess hormone water intoxication. The latter can be dangerous and must be anticipated and avoided by the patient and the clinical endocrinologist. Antidiuretic hormone is currently replaced by administration of DDAVP a synthetic analog (a compound with a slight change of the naturally occurring molecule to provide longer lasting effects). DDAVP can be given intranasally or by tablet. Most patients can do quite well with once daily dosing. We suggest this medication be given at night in order to avoid getting up at night to urinate. If patients watch their daily weight, they can avoid excessive water retention by omitting a dose if there is sudden retention of water.

Growth Hormone Deficiency
Since August 1996 there has been FDA approval of GH for GH deficient adults. Growth hormone is necessary in children for growth, but also appears necessary in adults to maintain body composition. Symptoms of GH deficiency in adults include fatigue, poor exercise performance and symptoms of social isolation. GH is only available in indictable form and must be given daily under the skin using insulin syringes. The dose should be determined by the clinical endocrinologist. This is one medication which is required by the company which supplies GH to be dispensed by a certified endocrinologist. GH is extremely expensive and should be given only to adults who have this deficiency established by the accepted diagnostic criteria.

Summary
Pituitary hormone therapy can be a challenge to the patient and physician. All the hormones involved have the potential for creating new problems if given in excessive or inadequate quantities. The "art" of replacement usually requires the expertise of a clinical endocrinologist who is familiar with pituitary physiology and pharmacology. With the recent availability of human growth hormone in replacement amounts for adults, patients may now be restored with all the possible hormone deficiencies that may result from pituitary damage.

Hormonal Replacement Therapy

" There are two times in
a man's life when he
should not speculate —
when he cannot afford it, and
when he can."

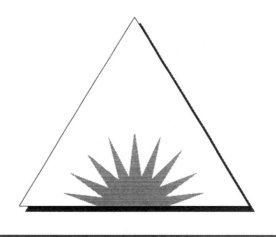

Growth Hormone Deficiency In Adults

Bengt-Ake Bengtsson, M.D., Ph.D., Associate Professor Head, Division of Endocrinology
Sahlgrenska University Hospital, Göteborg, Sweden

Growth hormone (GH) deficient children have been treated with GH since the late 1950s, and the effects of GH deficiency in childhood are well-known. They include short stature with normal body proportions, delayed bone maturation, excess adiposity, reduced lean body mass and fasting hypoglycemia. When the children have reached final height, treatment with GH has up to now been discontinued. Although it has been recognized for many years that GH is secreted in adult life, GH deficiency in adults has remained unrecognized in endocrine clinics the world over. Only recently have the grave consequences of GHD in adults been elucidated and with the advent of recombinant human GH, the supply of the hormone has increased, making it possible to explore the effects of treating adults.

The most common causes of GH deficiency in adults are pituitary and peripituitary tumors and their treatment. In the development of hypopituitarism, the loss of hormones follow a characteristic sequence. The secretion of GH appears to be the most sensitive and is the first to disappear, followed by the secretions of gonadotropins, thyroid-stimulating hormone and finally adrenocorticortrophin. Thus, almost all patients suffering from hypopituitarism also have GHD.

The somatotrope cells that secrete GH make up about 50% of the hormone-producing cells of the anterior pituitary. GH is secreted in a pulsatile manner and the secretion is regulated in a complex manner by hypothalamic peptides. GH secretion decreases with age and with higher body weight. The mechanism of the decline in GH secretion with increasing age is not known. GH has both direct and indirect effect on peripheral tissues. The indirect effects are mediated mainly by insulin-like growth factor I (IGF-1). Circulating IGF-l levels correlate to a greater or lesser degree with the GH status of the patient, with sometimes low plasma IGF- I concentrations in patients with GHD and high concentrations in patients with acromegaly.

GH has profound effects on body composition through its anabolic, lipolytic and antinatriuretic actions. GHD in adults is associated with characteristic changes in body composition such as increased body fat and decreased lean body mass and total body water. The increase in body fat is mainly located to abdominal regions. GH replacement therapy has been shown to have profound effects on body composition. Body fat, mainly abdominal, is reduced and lean body mass is increased. Within a half year of treatment, body composition has been found to be normalized. GHD of both childhood and adult onset has been associated with low bone mass, suggesting that GH is not only important for the accumulation of bone mass up to peak bone mass, but also for the maintenance of the adult skeleton. GH has been found to increase bone mass after one to two years of treatment.

Patients with hypopituitarism on routine replacement therapy have been found to have a doubled increased mortality in cardiovascular disorders such as cerebral stroke and myocardial infarction. Untreated, GHD might explain this premature death.

GHD has been associated with a number of cardiovascular risk factors such as low HDL and high LDL- cholesterol, increased concentrations of serum triglycerides and decreased fibrinolysis. Also, hypertension has been found to be more frequent in these patients, Treatment with GH induces favorable lipid changes such as an increase of HDL- and decrease of LDL- cholesterol concentrations. Furthermore, blood pressure has been found to decrease in response to treatment.

It was already observed many years ago that cardiac output decreased in response to hypophytsectomy. Recent studies have expanded our knowledge of cardiac performance in GHD. Thus, GHD is associated with reductions in maximum oxygen uptake, maximal heart rate, cardiac wall thickness, cardiac function and physical exercise capacity. Moreover muscle strength is being reduced. Treatment has been found to normalize cardiac performance, physical exercise capacity and muscle strength.

Patients with GHD often complain of fatigue, lack of concentration and memory difficulties. The fatigue reduces the working capacity, influences the professional career and impairs leisure activities. During recent years, instruments have been developed to assess "quality of life." By applying these instruments, the magnitude of problems associated with GHD in adults has been disclosed. Based on self-rating questionnaires, significant impairment of "quality of life" has been found in adult patients with GHD compared to matched healthy controls. The questionnaires disclosed significant differences in energy levels and emotional reaction, as well as social isolation, implying that these patients have reduced vitality, feel less energetic and have a depressed mood and a decreased sense of well-being. Furthermore, many patients are unable to work and have disability pensions.

From a clinical point of view, the improvement of "quality of life" is the most remarkable change that is observed among the patients in response to treatment with GH. There is especially an increase in the energy level and vitality. These effects are sometimes remarkable and could be observed within the first weeks of treatment. Recently, it has been shown that GH affects the neurotransmittors in the brain suggesting, that GH is of importance for brain function. Possibly these effects on the brain explain the improvement of "quality of life."

The approach to the diagnosis of adult GHD should include a high index of suspicion. Since these patients have, for the most part, hypothalamic-pituitary disease, the normal standard of care dictates that all hypothalamic-pituitary functions should be evaluated. This evaluation normally includes measurement of basal thyroid function tests, gonadotropins, gonadal steroids, prolactin, and cortisol as well as a test for hypothalamic-pituitary-adrenal reserve. The standard test which is used is the insulin tolerance test which also is the standard test for GH reserve. The measurement of serum IGF-1 may also be made but a normal IGF-1 does not exclude GHD in the adult.

GH replacement therapy is generally well tolerated, and side-effects can usually be avoided by starting with a low dose and increasing it slowly. The most common side-effects are related to fluid retention. These effects are dose-related, and respond to dose reduction.

In conclusion, evidence continues to accumulate that GH replacement therapy with GHD adults has substantial beneficial effects with improvement of body composition, skeletal mass, cardiovascular risk factors, cardiac function, exercise capacity and several aspects of "quality of life." The observed beneficial effects of GH treatment are of sufficient scale to justify considering this treatment as a routine replacement therapy in GHD adults. Recently, the regulatory authorities in Europe and in the USA approved this new indication for GH therapy.

Osteoporosis and Pituitary Disease

Anne Klibanski, M.D., Professor of Medicine, Harvard Medical School
Chief, Neuroendocrine Unit, Massachusetts General Hospital

Overview

Osteoporosis or loss of bone mineral is an important and often unrecognized long-term metabolic consequence of many pituitary disorders. In patients with osteoporosis, the normal balance between bone formation by cells called "osteoblasts" and bone resorption by the cells in bone called "osteoclasts" is disrupted. Osteoporosis is well known to be a major public health problem, Although there is a clear gender preference with women more affected than men, it is increasingly recognized that osteoporosis in men can also cause significant morbidity and mortality. The problem with osteoporosis is that it leads to progressive thinning of the bones which ultimately leads to fractures in any bone region but particularly in the spine, hip and wrist. Hip fractures in particular are associated with significant morbidity and mortality. Although it has been long recognized that women after the menopause will have bone loss as a consequence of their loss of normal hormonal function, particularly estrogen deficiency, thisplain problem has only recently been addressed in younger patients and in men as well. The most important factor is to understand that patients with pituitary disease are at increased risk for osteoporosis because of excess hormone secretion and/or hypopituitarism. Once this increased risk is recognized, patients should obtain appropriate screening to see whether this is a problem for them and then to decide with their physicians what the best therapeutic strategies are to prevent further long term problems.

Etiology

The etiology of osteoporosis in patients with pituitary disease is multifactorial. Patients who have evidence of pituitary tumors secreting too much ACTH (Cushing's disease) or hyperprolactinemia (prolactinomas) are at increased risk because of the effects of these high levels of hormones either directly or indirectly on bone mass. In the case of patients with Cushing's disease, the elevated levels of cortisol produced by the adrenal gland have a profound effect in interfering with normal bone metabolism, interfering with the normal absorption of calcium and vitamin D, and, having a direct effect on important growth factors that can stimulate normal bone development. The use of exogenous steroids for the treatment of many disorders is commonly known to be a risk factor for osteoporosis. Patients with Cushing's disease are at high risk for this development and should be screened appropriately. In addition, two other factors contribute to the bone loss scene in Cushing's disease. First, patients with Cushing's disease often have associated reproductive abnormalities such as amenorrhea and estrogen deficiency in women or testosterone deficiency in men. These hormone deficiency states will also lead to bone loss, Finally, growth hormone, which is important in maintaining normal bone health can also be decreased by the effects of cortisol in Cushing's disease. Patients with hyperprolactinemia have associated reproductive abnormalities as well. The amenorrhea and estrogen deficiency associated with an elevated prolactin present a clear risk factor for the development of osteoporosis. Similarly, men with hyperprolactinemia typically have low levels of the male hormone, testosterone. Testosterone deficiency is an important factor predisposing to bone loss and the development of osteoporosis in men. Similarly, although growth hormone is typically associated with a beneficial effect on bone, patients with acromegaly who have associated reproductive abnormalities may also develop osteopenia.

Hypopituitarism resulting from any pituitary lesion, radiation damage or other factors affecting normal pituitary function also leads to osteoporosis. As previously mentioned, hypogonadism is an important underlying factor which can lead to bone loss in patients with multiple underlying pituitary disorders, An important and recently recognized factor in bone is the contribution of growth hormone deficiency as an osteoporosis risk factor, Patients with growth hormone deficiency either acquired during childhood or adult life due to pituitary disease have been found to have a decreased bone mass. In addition, growth hormone administration has been shown to result in a small but significant improvement in bone mass in patients with growth hormone deficiency. Thyroid hormone also has an impact on bone mass and inappropriate replacement of thyroid hormone to patients with secondary hypothyroidism can also lead to increased bone loss.

Diagnosis

Osteoporosis, like hypertension and many other chronic disorders, has been called "silent" because at a point where it becomes clinically evident it has typically been long-standing and has already caused significant morbidity. The diagnosis of osteoporosis is often made because of clinical fractures, a decrease in height or the finding of diffuse loss of mineral on a routine x-ray. Unfortunately, by the time these events occur and are recognized, profound bone loss has often gone on for many years undetected. Therefore, patients who are at higher risk for the development of osteoporosis such as patients with pituitary disorders would be well advised to have a screening test done for this disease. The simplest and most widely available test is called a DEXA scan (dual energy x-ray absorptionery). These scans involve minimal radiation exposure, no injection or contrast agent. They can produce accurate, reproducible measurements of the bone density, of the spine, hip, wrist or other areas to determine whether there is significant evidence of bone demineralization present.

Evaluation

Once the diagnosis of osteoporosis is made, and evaluation must be done to identify the underlying and potentially reversible causes of its etiology. First, there are a number of systemic, metabolic and other underlying endocrine disorders which can lead to osteoporosis. Chronic renal disease, liver disease and other metabolic abnormalities can lead to decreased bone mineral content. Two additional endocrine etiologies other than those emphasized above, hyperparathyroidism (a disorder of the glands regulating calcium metabolism) and hyperthyroidism can also lead to calcium loss from bones and a decrease in bone mass. Alcoholism is a well known risk factor for osteoporosis. Undernutrition, dietary deficiencies of calcium, vitamin D and other important nutrients essential for maintaining bone health should also be excluded. Immobilization or a prolonged sedentary lifestyle can also contribute to osteoporosis as does the use of cigarettes. Medications can also lead to osteoporosis, often through effects of calcium and vitamin D. The antiseizure medication, Dilantin, is particularly notable in this regard. After a complete history and physical examination by your physician, a number of screening tests may be indicated as guided by these evaluations. Typically, calcium, phosphorous and albumin levels are drawn. An assessment of thyroid function is made and renal or liver function may be evaluated in the appropriate circumstance. Further evaluation is dependent on the individual findings by a physician's evaluation.

Therapy

A therapeutic approach to osteoporosis should incorporate four parallel strategies. First, in patient with clear-cut hormone deficiencies, replacement of hormone therapy such as estrogen and progesterone in women and testosterone in men should be strongly considered unless there are contraindications to their use, In the case of growth hormone deficiency, when documented, a consideration should also be given as to whether growth hormone treatment is a possible option in an individual patient. The establishment of a normal endocrine profile may also involve treating an unrecognized or still active pituitary condition such as Cushing's. As long as Cushing's' disease is active, or patients are taking amounts of glucocorticoid replacement that are higher than normal replacement, continued loss of bone remains a real and severe risk. Second, dietary intervention is important in maintaining normal nutrition, particularly in regard to the calcium and vitamin D components of a normal diet. Adult women and men with normal reproductive function should have at least 1000 mg or (1 gram) of elemental calcium in their diet each day. This is roughly equivalent to the amount of calcium in a quart of milk. If dietary consumption is inadequate, calcium can be supplemented through nonprescription calcium tablets in the form of calcium carbonate or calcium citrate. In a diet completely deficient of dairy products, particularly in patients without sun exposure, a multivitamin containing vitamin D should also be instituted. A third important component is reviewing with the patient's physician what other therapeutic options may exist. In patients who are unable to tolerate gonadal steroid replacement with estrogen or testosterone, or, in patients replaced with these hormone but who still have persistent osteoporosis because of nonreversible bone loss, thought should be give to the use of new treatment options available to all patients with osteoporosis. These included calcitonin, and a family of compounds known as bisphosphonates which specifically inhibit bone resorption, such as Fosamax. These medications, which are approved for the treatment of postmenopausal osteoporosis, should warrant serious consideration in the appropriae circumstance in a patient with osteoporosis due to other disorders as well. Finally, lifestyle alterations are an important component of any patient's treatment for osteoporosis. Exercise, particularly involving weight bearing bones can help maintain bone mass. Muscular strength and flexibility are also important in preventing falls, a major risk factor in clinical fractures, In patients with a history of alcoholism or cigarette smoking, serious discussions should involve the benefits of discontinuing these substances in terms of bone health as well as their other important health implications involving cardiac disease and malignancy. In elderly patients who may be prone to falls, studies have now shown that carefully reviewing the patient's living and walking area can decrease the number of falls and its associated morbidity .

Summary

Osteoporosis is a common, multifactorial disorder clearly associated with increased morbidity and mortality. It has only been recognized relatively recently that because of the complex hormone disorders which accompany pituitary disease, patients with this condition are at higher risk for the development of osteoporosis and fractures. Patients with pituitary disease should be evaluated for the possibility of osteoporosis. If identified, underlying hormonal and metabolic factors should be aggressively searched for and corrected as is appropriate for an individual patient. Bone health is a life-long process and the thinking that osteoporosis is only a disease of the elderly is completely untrue. As early as childhood and adolescence peak bone mass is developed and will be an important factor in bone strength throughout all of life. Adolescents with pituitary disease and associated hormone abnormalities may be at even greater risk for the development of osteoporosis because not only do they lose established bone, they also fail to achieve peak bone mass in their early life. Therefore, patients with pituitary disease of all ages should discuss osteoporosis with their physicians as part of their overall health concerns.

Surgical Management of Pituitary Tumors

Charles B. Wilson, M.D., D.Sc., M.S.H.A., Department of Neurological Surgery, University of California, San Francisco

The August, 1997 issue of the Journal of Clinical Endocrinology & Metabolism published this article by Charles B. Wilson, M.D., D.Sc., M.S.H.A. With permission of the author we are providing excerpts for your information.

The Procedure

Transsphenoidal surgery has become an operation with remarkably little morbidity and exceptionally low mortality rates. Hospital stays of 2 days are standard, and selectively patients are being discharged even earlier. Patients whose jobs are not physically demanding can usually return to work within 1 to 2 weeks after surgery. To be sure, complications, both minor and major, occur even in the most experienced hands. As one example postoperative loss of pituitary function, whether categorized as a side effect or a complication, is a serious concern in a patient of any age, but most critically in children and young adults. Considering the benign behavior of most pituitary adenomas, the preservation and possible improvement of anterior pituitary function assumes a priority equal to that of avoiding injury to critical parasellar structures.

I subscribe to the principle of specialized care, and if it makes sense for interested internists to acquire special knowledge and experience in endocrinology, it seems reasonable to apply the same rationale to specialization in pituitary surgery. Particularly in neurosurgery, practice makes perfect, and I advocate concentrating, rather than diffusing, surgical referrals -not in the sense of creating "centers." but by encouraging one of several neurosurgeons in larger communities to become the local expert in pituitary surgery. There is no question about it: such a plan for referrals for pituitary surgery can provide improved outcomes for your patients. Has managed care, including capitated care, complicated the referral process? Unquestionably it has, but I hardly need to remind you that inexpert pituitary surgery can be *very* expensive, in both the short term and the long term. Care of high quality is rarely costineffective, particularly in the care of children and patients with Cushing's disease.

Pathology

I am an advocate of immunostaining. At the University of California, San Francisco (UCSF) we do immunostaining routinely on all pituitary adenomas, even though it provides critically important information in only a minority of cases. Without immunostaining, for example, nodular corticotrophic hyperplasia might go undetected; and in the case of a large nonsecreting adenoma associated with hyperprolactinemia as a nonspecific effect of the compression and distortion of dopaminergic vascular pathways, the adenoma might be mistaken for a prolactin (PRL)-secreting adenoma and managed incorrectly. Only immunostaining differentiates an endocrine-inactive adenoma from a prolactinoma, each of which is managed quite differently.

Prolactin-Secreting Adenomas

The prolactinoma is the only pituitary adenoma for which medical management in the long term is fully satisfactory, and for that reason the proportion of patients with prolactinomas referred for surgical consultation varies widely in different geographic regions. I assume that the proportion of patients referred for surgical consideration in Northern California represents an approximation of general practice. The referred group in my practice includes patients who have unacceptable side effects caused by medication, patients with dopamine-insensitive adenomas, and those patients who, after becoming informed, for personal reasons select surgical over medical management.

In a significant proportion of patients referred to me for surgical consultation, I have advised medical over surgical management based on gender, age, and the probability of a surgical cure - 'cure' in the sense of long term freedom from recurrence.

In Table 1 are shown the indications I follow in recommending surgical removal of a microadenoma, and in Table 2 are shown the indications for removal of a macroadenoma. These indications for both small and large adenomas reflect my experience as well as my biases. Based on the basal PRL value and a high-resolution magnetic resonance image (MR), I can predict the likelihood of a surgical cure. If cure is not possible because of extrasellar spread, almost always on the basis of cavernous sinus invasion, surgery is not advised unless the patient fails to respond to medical management. When there is no likelihood of a surgical cure, surgery has the focused objective of reducing the adenoma's mass, either to reduce the production of PRL to a level that can be further reduced into a desirable range by a tolerated dose of a dopamine agonist or to relieve symptoms of compression and reduce the bulk of the adenoma before irradiation.

Dopamine agonists, such as Parlodel, inhibit tumor-cell replication in the great majority of prolactinomas, and for that reason patients known or proven to have residual or recurrent adenomas should be treated indefinitely with Parlodel. Often a dose as low as 1.25 mg, taken at bedtime, is sufficient to maintain or restore normal PRL levels and prevent tumor regrowth if the residual volume of adenoma is small or if the adenoma is highly dopamine-sensitive. In all cases involving incompletely removed or recurrent PRL-secreting tumors, long-term administration of a dopamine agonist is the first line of treatment. Irradiation is reserved for those few patients who have adenomas refractory to medical therapy and for the larger number of individuals who cannot tolerate the medication.

Growth Hormone-Secreting (Somatotrophic) Adenomas

For almost three decades, the preferred primary treatment for the patient with acromegaly has been surgery. In occasional cases of acromegaly, uncontrolled diabetes, hypertension, or congestive heart failure may counsel against anesthesia, and in such cases preoperative medical preparation, including somatostatin, may be advisable. Still, today - with the exception of such cases - the initial and usually definitive treatment for acromegaly is transsphenoidal surgery. As a general rule, younger patients have larger tumors and higher basal growth hormone (GH) values, whereas older patients with acromegaly are more likely to have smaller tumors and lower, or even normal, random GH values.

Following selective transsphenoidal adenomectomy, more than 80% of patients with acromegaly have a sustained remission. Until a long-acting somatostatin equivalent is available for general use, all incompletely removed adenomas should be treated postoperatively with radiation therapy. Although many months and even years may be required to restore normal GH production, irradiation affords a very high probability of eliminating further growth and, in time, restoring normal GH levels. I believe that patients with acromegaly have a special susceptibility to radiation-induced hypopituitarism, but this consequence of irradiation is less threatening than acromegaly to the patient's health.

Corticotrophic Adenomas (Cushing's Disease)

In the short term, Cushing's disease is the most serious and life-endangering condition caused by any pituitary adenoma; and for the surgeon, these tumors present the most difficult challenge of all pituitary adenomas. As I begin each operation for Cushing's disease, I have to assume that the operation will be difficult from beginning to end, and seldom am I pleasantly surprised by a truly "simple" case.

The patient with Cushing's disease has friable tissue, soft bone, and capillary fragility. Moreover, in many cases, obesity and other factors conspire to produce venous hypertension, a major complicating factor during the transsphenoidal exploration of a normal-size sella surrounded, literally, by a moat of turgid, confluent dural venous sinuses.

In adults with suspected Cushing's disease, unless MR imaging indicates a tumor larger than 5 mm in diameter, we proceed to preliminary sampling of the cavernous sinuses. This means that the majority of such patients - more than 75% - undergo venous sampling and concurrent cavernous sinus venography. The tumors of Cushing's disease are tiny, the typical adenoma having a diameter of considerably less than 5 mm. Their minute size, coupled with the generally accepted likelihood of a false-positive MR image in 15% of the normal population, argues convincingly for preoperative venous sampling in almost all cases.

Venous sampling is invaluable in surgical decision-making. It helps to determine which patients to operate on, how to conduct the intrasellar exploration, and what to do in the case of a negative exploration. I have several caveats. The cavernous sinuses, rather than the down-stream inferior petrosal sinuses, should be sampled bilaterally after the venographic anatomy is defined, and venograms of both cavernous sinuses should be obtained at the same time. If venous drainage from the sella is dominantly unilateral, then simultaneously obtained left-right values may not be reliable in indicating lateralization. A cavernous sinus venogram should be obtained because a filling defect in a cavernous sinus may disclose the presence of an intracavernous adenoma. A 2:1 or larger cephalic-to-peripheral ACTH gradient establishes the diagnosis of Cushings disease, and in our experience the additional testing with corticotrophin-releasing factor adds nothing to the value of samples taken from the cavernous sinus. If a patient with no anomalous venous drainage patterns exhibits a lateralizing ACTH gradient of 2:1 or greater, then removal of the appropriate half of the anterior pituitary gland will be curative in 80% of cases in which hemihypophysectomy is performed.

Cushing's disease is not a common disease - by one estimate, there are approximately 200 newly recognized cases annually. If left untreated, the disease is fatal. With no other tumor is the surgeon's experience more critical in determining outcome, and for this reason I suggest that inexperienced pituitary surgeons must gain experience with less complex tumor types, initially referring patients with Cushing's disease - particularly pediatric patients - to an experienced colleague. In my view, these rare and difficult cases should be concentrated in the capable hands of experienced pituitary surgeons throughout the United States. Requests for referral to an "out of plan" surgeon may be denied because of concern for cost, but a comparison of the long-term costs of a curative operation to those accrued from a failed first attempt creates a compelling argument for referral to an experienced surgeon for economic considerations alone - even without invoking the equally valid issue of appropriate patient care.

Endocrine Inactive Adenomas

In this category are adenomas that produce no clinically recognizable secretory product. At the time of diagnosis, the great majority of cases present with impaired vision and some expression of hypopituitarism, typically gonadotrophic insufficiency, with or without associated headache. Because of the increasingly prevalent use of high-resolution MR imaging, a new category of incidental and asymptomatic - presumed - pituitary adenomas requires the formulation of a new management algorithm, which I will consider separately.

For many years, my surgical objective in treating large endocrine-inactive adenomas was decompression of the optic nerves and chiasm with the assumption that irradiation was required afterwards to prevent regrowth. I did not attempt a total removal of large tumors - very possibly as a carryover from the established practice when these tumors were treated by craniotomy. However, as I gained experience and discovered that it was possible to achieve total removal of intrasellar macroadenomas while preserving compressed anterior lobe tissue, I changed the surgical objective from decompression to total removal. In the majority of large adenomas, a clean surgical plane separates the surface of the tumor from the compressed normal structures. By finding and developing this plane early in the process of removal, a surprisingly large proportion of large tumors can be removed completely. Subsequent follow up of these adenomas with serial MR images at 6-month intervals for the first 2 years and then yearly has shown a 5% rate of recurrence after 5 years. If tumors that invade the cavernous sinus are excluded, I believe that as many as 40% to 50% of endocrine-inactive adenomas can be cured by surgery alone, and for this reason the surgeon should go into the operation with complete removal, rather than decompression, as the goal. Loss of anterior pituitary function that existed before surgery has been an infrequent complication, and more often function that was lost preoperatively later returned spontaneously. To borrow from the lexicon of the olympics, the bar has been raised for pituitary surgeons.

Incidental (Coincidental) Pituitary Adenomas

Although I have kept no record of the number of patients with presumed incidental pituitary adenomas whom I have evaluated since the introduction of high-resolution MR images, I estimate that they constitute one out of five patients referred to me with the diagnosis of pituitary adenoma. Radiographically, some presumed adenomas are pure cysts rather than cystic adenomas, but if a cyst has attained a diameter of 1 cm, it should be managed in the same manner as an adenoma because both the pure cyst of this size and an adenoma, whether smaller or larger than 1 cm, have potential for further growth.

The defining features of a presumed incidental pituitary adenoma are these: (1) it is asymptomatic; (2) there is normal anterior pituitary function, including a normal GH response to provocative testing; (3) calcification is absent; and (4) the lesion is confined to the sella (Table 4). Of the anterior pituitary cell types, somatotrophs are the most vulnerable to compression, followed by gonadotrophs as a distant second. Although GH has a legitimate physiologic role throughout life, GH secretion is essential for the normal development of children. If GH secretion is normal, all other anterior pituitary functions are almost certainly normal as well. Because most craniopharyngiomas are calcified and because there is a compelling argument for early intervention, the presence of calcium should be excluded by CT scanning before the surgeon assumes that a mixed solid and cystic mass is an incidental adenoma.

What are the indications for surgical intervention? A decision to operate that is appropriate for an adolescent may be inappropriate for an elderly patient. Moreover, an adenoma that has doubled in size within 1 year, although still asymptomatic, should be viewed differently from an adenoma that has shown slight but unquestioned growth (expansion) over the course of 5 years. The listed indications for operation are only guidelines to be used in conjunction with clinical judgment. A pure cyst that, by its size, has qualified for inclusion with incidental adenomas has a likely potential for further growth; and in contrast to the common and innocuous small cysts seen so often in the pars intermedia, the cyst that is 1 cm or larger is, in my opinion, certain to have further expansion at some unpredictable rate of growth.

See tables on next page.

Surgical Management of Pituitary Tumors

Table 1	
Surgical indications for prolactin secreting microadenomas	
Personal choice	Primary amenorrhea
Intolerant of medication at an effective dose	Prolactin value of 200 mch/l
Desire for pregnancy	Male sex
Inadequate response (resistance) to medication	Extrasellar extension (suprasellar or intrasphenoid)

Table 2
Surgical indications for prolactin secreting macroadenomas
Personal choice (pattern of growth does not preclude surgical cure)

Unsuccessful trial of medication
    a. with potential for cure
    b. without potential for cure but bulk reduction advised to lower the effective dose of medication

Desire for pregnancy when a prior pregnancy was complicated by symptomatic expansion of tumor

Surgery for Pituitary Adenomas

Mark D. Krieger, M.D., William T. Couldwell, M.D., Ph.D., Martin H. Weiss, M.D.,
Department of Neurological Surgery, University of Southern California, Los Angeles, California

Pituitary adenomas are benign tumors which originate from any of the multiple cell types of the anterior pituitary gland. These tumors come to clinical attention when they result in signs and symptoms of an endocrinopathy (an over or underproduction of one or more of the hormones produced by the pituitary gland), or when they achieve sufficient size to produce mass effect (neurological symptoms resulting from compression of neighboring nervous system structures).

Diagnosis

Pituitary adenomas may present early in their growth if they result in an endocrinopathy. Even small adenomas may cause hormonal abnormalities, resulting in a variety of well defined clinical syndromes. Currently, these tumors are classified according to their hormone production, which determines the clinical syndrome (Table I). The most commonly overproduced hormone is prolactin, which results in the amenorrhea-galactorhea syndrome, and is frequently discovered during infertility workup. Growth hormone and corticotrophic hormone are seen with the next highest frequency, resulting in acromegaly or giganticism and Cushing's Disease, respectively. Overproduction of thyroid stimulating hormone and gonadotrophic hormone are seen with much lower frequency.

When pituitary tumors grow to a large size, they usually present with mass effect. This pattern is more typical of non-functioning pituitary adenomas (null cell adenomas), as functional tumors would be more likely to be detected at an earlier stage due to their associated hormonal abnormalities. However, functioning tumors may go undetected (or the patient may describe a vague complaint of feeling "not quite right," which may have been ignored by his primary physician) and present with mass effect. As these tumors grow, they protrude beyond the confines of the sella turcica (a bony structure which surrounds the pituitary gland). The optic chiasm, which lies directly above the sella turcica, is particularly susceptible to compression from the enlarging tumor. Compression of the chiasm results in a classical bitemporal hemianopsia (loss of the peripheral visual field of each eye). Large tumors may also result in headaches, and hypopituitarism from compression of the remaining pituitary gland. Null cell tumors are the most common category of pituitary tumors, presenting later in life than functioning tumors.

Management

The two major goals for the treatment of all pituitary tumors are: 1)relief of signs and symptoms attributable to mass effect (including visual loss), and 2) correction of associated endocrine abnormalities. It must be kept in mind that even non-secreting tumors may precipitate hypopituitarism (hormonal undersecretion). Thus, a full endocrinologic workup is always mandated.

Treatment requires a coordinated effort between a medical team (endocrinologists) and a surgical team (neurosurgeons) with cumulative experience in the management of these tumors. Contemporary imaging modalities, such as magnetic resonance imaging (MRI) or computerized tomography (CT), combined with the advent of radioimmunoassay techniques to measure miniscule pituitary hormone levels in the blood, have heralded a new era in the detection and management of pituitary adenomas, facilitating the diagnosis, surgical planning, and follow-up care of these patients. The quantification of the hormone levels is particularly important in providing a parameter to determine the response to treatment.

Medical (non-surgical) therapy is effective only in hypersecreting tumors. Tumors which secrete prolactin or growth hormone are susceptible to this form of management, and medication may be prescribed as a first line treatment. These patients may eventually require surgery, however, if the medication is ineffective or intolerable. No pharmacological therapy is available at this point in time for non-functioning tumors, or ACTH, TSH or gonadotrope secreting tumors. The primary mode of treatment for these tumors should therefore be considered surgical, with other options (radiation or observation) reserved for those patients in whom underlying medical conditions preclude surgery.

The Transsphenoidal Operation

If the neurosurgeon and the endocrinologist in conjunction agree that an operation is necessary, the usual procedure of choice is a transsphenoidal craniotomy. The transsphenoidal resection of pituitary tumors has a long history of development and refinement since first performed in 1907 by Schloffer, a rhinologist from Innsbruck, Austria. Prior to this time, only transcranial approaches to pituitary tumors had been attempted by the pioneers of our specialty. These earliest attempts at the turn of the century, however, resulted in a prohibitive mortality rate. Sir Victor Horsley, in a small series of ten cases, had two deaths. This rate would be unacceptable by modern standards, but was a significant improvement over the 50% to 80% mortality rates seen at the time. It should be recognized that this extraordinary incidence of mortality was generally accepted in the early efforts to develop the field of intracranial surgery.

As a consequence of these earlier experiences, attempts were made to modify the surgical techniques and the adjuvant management in an effort to make the surgical approach to the pituitary region a more reasonable option for both surgeon and patient. The technique of sphenoid sinus exposure (hence the term transsphenoidal) was developed by neurosurgeons such as Halstead and Cushing as a more focused approach to this region, with less collateral tissue injury. Cushing described a technique that combined a number of suggestions from previous authors, employing the sublabial incision (under the upper lip) used by most neurosurgeons today (Figure 1). Cushing also adopted the technique of submucous dissection of the nasal septum and employed the headlight to enable better visualization in the depths of the operative field. Utilizing the transnasal/transsphenoidal approach during the fifteen year period from 1910 to 1925, he operated on two hundred and thirty-one pituitary tumors with low morbidity and mortality. Tplain his represented the largest and most favorable experience of his generation.

This technique has greatly increased in popularity over the last 20 years as methods have continued to improve. This may also in part be attributed to the well recognized inadequacy of other approaches to this region, especially the subfrontal transcranial approach, for removal of the component of the tumor within the depths of the sella turcica. The transsphenoidal approach also has proven effectiveness in the treatment of visual disturbances from large adenomas. Our assessment of over 200 patients who presented with visual loss operated via the transnasal transsphenoidal route yielded evidence of improved vision in 81%, unchanged vision in 16%, and worsening vision in 3%. These results are similar to other large series, and certainly equal or exceed the results of large series of transcranial subfrontal explorations for visual loss. In addition, there exists clear documentation of the potential for improvement in pituitary function following transsphenoidal tumor resection with careful preservation of normal gland in cases with preexisting hypopituitarism. For smaller hormone secreting tumors, the efficacy of transsphenoidal surgery in selected patients has been well established, with some reports showin greater than 90% tumor control. In series including larger tumors, however, a more realistic 50-80% rate of tumor control is expected with surgery alone. Thus, the transsphenoidal approach's efficacy in treating small tumors situated deep in the sella and large tumors projecting above the sella establishes this as the approach of choice for the surgical management of most pituitary tumors, regardless of size (Figure 2).

Today, in the hands of an experienced surgeon, mortality of the transsphenoidal operation for pituitary tumors approaches zero. Operative morbidity (adverse outcome) includes transient, or, in some cases, permanent diabetes insipidus (DI), a dysfunction of the posterior lobe of the pituitary gland which results in frequent urination and may require medication to control. The incidence of this ranges from 1.8% permanent DI in one large series to a 17% incidence immediately postoperatively with large adenomas, most of which resolved with time. Leakage of cerebrospinal fluid occurs with an incidence of 1- 4.4% among different series, depending upon the size of the tumor and the follow-up time, but occurs disproportionately with larger tumors. Other complications are distinctly uncommon. As put forth by all pituitary neurosurgeons, complications amount to a relatively small percentage of the overall surgical experience, emphasizing the relative safety of the procedure. Most patients will leave the hospital after a stay of less than one week, with only minimal discomfort.

Though the above procedure is the primary choice for the majority of pituitary tumors, in some instances a transcranial approach may be recommended for a patient harboring a pituitary tumor. Such cases would include tumors with lateral extension out of the sella turcica, or with abnormal courses of the carotid arteries at the base of the skull which may pose a hazard to the transsphenoidal approach. Both of these circumstances may be anticipated by careful review of the preoperative MRI studies.

In summary, the coordinated efforts of the endocrinologist and neurosurgeon have greatly improved the quality of life for patients with pituitary adenomas. Should surgery be necessary, the transsphenoidal approach is usually undertaken, and is a safe and effective method for removing the vast majority of pituitary tumors.

Surgery for Pituitary Adenomas

Table 1.
Pituitary Adenoma Types and Their Incidence

Type	Incidence in Percentage
GH-cell adenoma	**15.1**
Densely granulated	7.1
Sparsely granulated	8.0
PRL-cell adenoma	**28.0**
Densely granulated	0.5
Sparsely granulated	27.5
ACTH-cell adenoma	**13.8**
Endocrinology active	8.1
Silent	5.7
TSH-adenoma	**0.6**
FSH/LH adenoma	**4.4**
Null Cell adenoma	**24.7**
Nonococytotic	17.4
Oncocytotic	7.3
Plurihormonal adenoma	**13.4**
GH-cell PRL-cell adenoma	5.2
Acidophol stem cell adenoma	2.5
Mammosomatotroph cell adenoma	1.4
Other	4.3
Total	**100.0**

GH = Growth hormone; PRL = Prolactin; ACTH = Corticotropin; TSH = Thyrotropin; FSH = Follicle-stimulating hormone; LH Luteinizing hormone.

From Kovacs K, Horvath E: Pathology of Pituitary Adenomas. In Collu R, Brown GM, Van Loon GR, eds., *Clinical Neuroendocrinology.* Blackwell Scientific Publication, Boston, 1998, with permission.

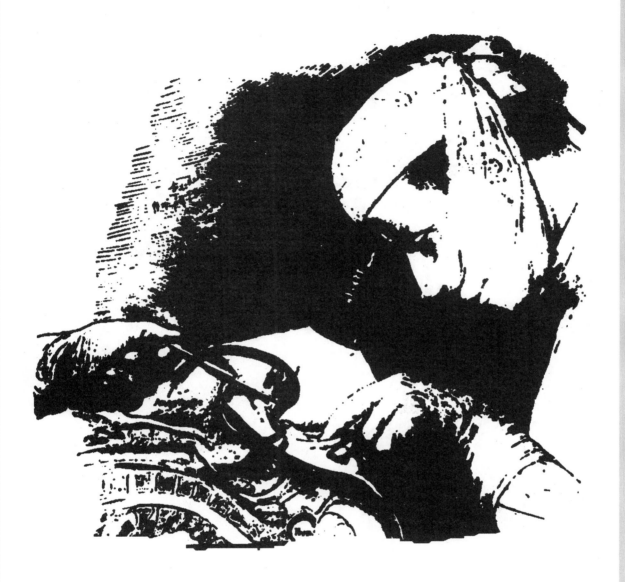

Figure 1. Cushing's adaptation of the transsphenoidal technique.
This 1912 drawing by the renowned medical illustrator Max Brödel shows the technique of transsphenoidal approach to the hypophysis. Note the sublabial incision adopted by Cushing at the time. (from Cushing H: The Weir Mitchel lecture: Surgical experiences with the pituitary disorders. JAMA 1914: LXIII: 1515 - 1525, with permission.)

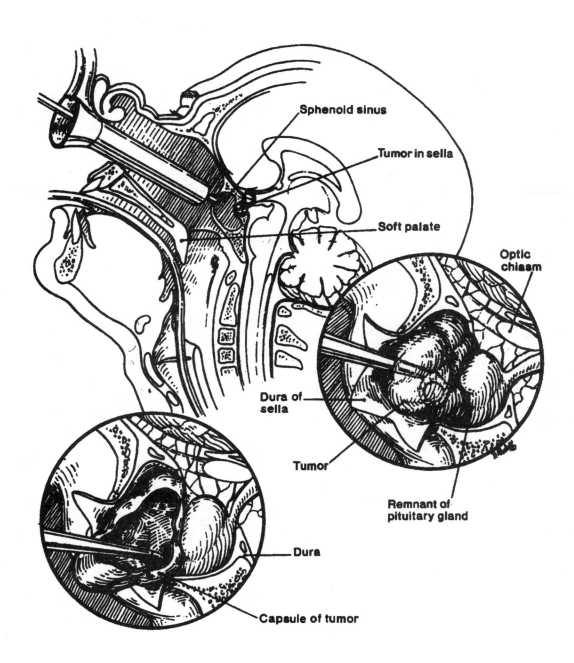

Figure 2. The transsphenoidal approach.
The transnasal transsphenoidal approach is preferred for access to the majority of pituitary adenomas.
It offers direct access to the tumor with no brain retraction and minimal morbidity. The current
popularity of the technique was facilitated by the advent of the operating microscope, better microsurgi-
cal instrumentation, and increased illumination.

Skull Base Approaches for Pituitary Tumors

Michael J. Link, M.D., John M. Tew, Jr., M.D.,
University of Cincinnati Medical Center and The Mayfield Clinic

Pituitary adenomas, although usually benign, may grow to considerable size and compress important neurologic and vascular structures at the skull base. When this occurs, surgery is indicated to decompress these structures, especially when vision is at risk. Decompression can usually be accomplished through a transsphenoidal approach as detailed in Figure 2. When the tumor to extend beyond the limits of the conventional transsphenoidal operation, a more extensive operation requiring a craniotomy combined with skull base approaches may be needed. We will review these approaches, their indications and results.

A knowledge of the anatomy of the pituitary region is important to understand the indications and expectations involved with surgery in this area (Figure 1). The pituitary gland sits in a bony saddle called the sella turcica near the center of the head. This position provides excellent protection for the pituitary gland however, any surgical approach will require a relatively "long reach" along the course of normal structures. Several skull base approaches, which have been devised to minimize the involvement of important structures, allow optimal exposure of the tumor so it can be effectively removed.

The sella turcica is located directly above the sphenoid sinus, a relationship that provides direct access to the pituitary gland via the nasal structures. On either side of the pituitary gland are the cavernous sinuses. Unlike the sphenoid sinus, which is an air filled, tissue-lined sinus that drains into the nose, the cavernous sinuses are actually a network of veins for the head and brain. Within the cavernous sinuses lie the carotid arteries, which are the main blood supply to the brain; and the third, fourth, and sixth cranial nerves, which control eye movement. The fifth cranial nerve, which provides facial and eye sensation, is in the outside wall of the cavernous sinus. All these structures and the veins of the cavernous sinuses are surrounded by the tough covering around the brain called the dura mater. The dura, making up the inside walls of the cavernous sinuses, separates these structures from the pituitary gland. Directly above the pituitary gland is the optic chiasm. The optic nerves, which are responsible for vision, leave the eyeballs and travel back to the optic chiasm where they partially cross before continuing to the back of the brain where vision is processed. Immediately above the optic-chiasm is the hypothalamus, an area of the brain involved in many important regulatory functions (e.g. appetite, wakefulness, release of pituitary hormones).

When pituitary tumors enlarge they can compress the above mentioned structures and cause significant neurologic deficits. The tumor may extend down into the sphenoid sinus and even erode the sphenoid bone causing headache, bleeding from the nose, or leakage of spinal fluid. As the tumor expands, it can invade the cavernous sinuses and surround the carotid arteries, causing double vision (third, fourth and sixth nerves) or facial pain (fifth nerve). If the tumor grows up it can compress the optic nerves and chiasm, resulting in a loss of vision. The outside visual field in each eye is usually affected first (tunnel vision); this can progress to complete blindness if left unchecked. If the tumor is large enough to affect the hypothalamus or even block the flow of spinal fluid through the brain, hydrocephalus can result.

The downward growth of the tumor, and to a limited degree the upward extent, can usually be addressed via the transsphenoidal operation. However, there is limited accessibility in the other directions. Therefore, a transcranial, skull base approach may be better suited to ensure effective tumor removal.

Subfrontal Approach

The most common approach to the pituitary region, after the transsphenoidal route, is the subfrontal approach. When tumors extend far above the sella turcica, this approach allows improved visualization of the optic nerves and chiasm and surrounding brain structures to ensure an adequate removal. The most common indication for this approach is progressive visual loss. Most patients have already undergone the transsphenoidal route in an attempt to decompress the optic chiasm from below before this operation is needed.

For the subfrontal approach a craniotomy is fashioned to remove the frontal bone to expose both frontal lobes of the brain to the level of the eyebrows (Figure 2). The frontal lobes are gently elevated and separated to allow a corridor to the pituitary region (Figure 3). Tumor is then removed from beneath and around the optic nerves and chiasm, and from surrounding brain and blood vessels (Figure 4). The bone overlying the sella turcica is removed with a high-speed drill to allow further tumor removal from the sella and sphenoid sinus (Figure 4). The risks of this approach include possible injury to the frontal lobes with resultant memory difficulties, seizures, or a loss of sense of smell. There is a also a risk of injury to the optic nerves and chiasm, pituitary stalk or the branches of the carotid arteries with resultant hemorrhage or stroke. Overall, the risk of a life-threatening complication is approximately 1%; the risk of other complications including spinal fluid leak or wound infection is not more than 5%. This approach does not allow access to the cavernous sinus but provides excellent decompression of the optic apparatus.

Transcavernous Approach

Pituitary tumors may invade one or both cavernous sinuses adjacent to the pituitary gland and may involve the frontal and/or temporal lobes of the brain. A frontotemporal craniotomy, with further removal of the bone surrounding the optic nerve and next to the cavernous sinus, can allow access to these types of tumors (Figure 5). For a long time surgery within the cavernous sinus was considered too risky because of concern about bleeding from the veins and injury to the delicate neurovascular structures within it. With improved knowledge of the surgical anatomy and new microsurgical techniques the cavernous sinus can be opened and the tumor removed. There remains a 20% chance of temporary or permanent injury to one of the cranial nerves and a 2% risk of injury to the carotid artery. While this approach allows excellent access to the cavernous sinus and region above the sella turcica, it is limited to only one side and does not provide access to the region below the pituitary.

LeFort Maxillotomy

Pituitary tumors will rarely grow through and around the sphenoid sinus being predominately in the sphenoid bone and below (the clivus). A LeFort maxillotomy, a more extensive approach from in front and below, can then be considered. The operation is similar to the transsphenoidal route with a much greater exposure of the skull base. This increased exposure is obtained by separating the bone containing the upper teeth from the cheek bones and nose (Figure 6). The operation is primarily performed through the back of the mouth (Figure 7). At the end of the surgery, the bones are reattached using small titanium plates and screws. Potential complications of this approach include meningitis, spinal fluid leak, trauma to the sixth cranial nerves (double vision), and malocclusion of the teeth.

Most pituitary tumors can be controlled with medication, transsphenoidal surgery, radiation, or a combination of these modalities. Various surgical approaches using conventional craniotomies with extended removal of skull base structures to provide access to the pituitary region can be employed to treat pituitary tumors that have not responded to, or are not suitable for, conventional treatment. Pituitary tumors, although benign, can invade critical nerves and blood vessels at the skull base, resulting in major neurologic deficits such as blindness, double vision, or hydrocephalus. When this occurs, surgery is indicated to remove the tumor from around these structures. We have reviewed the surgical approaches that can be used. The extent and direction of tumor growth determines the procedure. However, it must be emphasized that even with the extensive operations described, some pituitary tumors remain surgically incurable because of invasion of both cavernous sinuses and other important structures. As plain the knowledge of pituitary tumors grows so will the ability to gain effective treatment. Skull base approaches for direct surgical removal will likely continue to play an important role in that treatment.

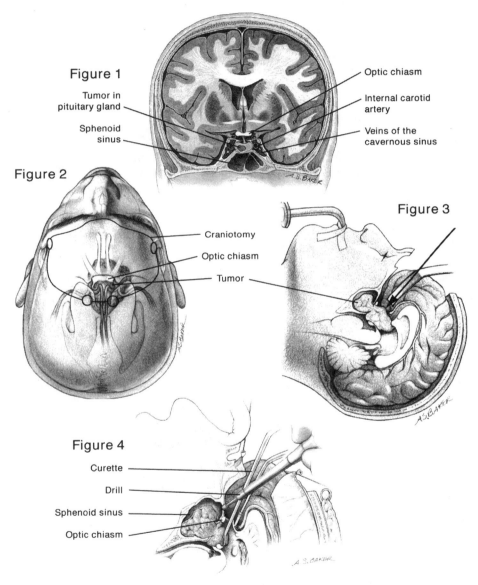

Figure 1: Coronal cross-section of the head at the level of the pituitary gland. (All figures reprinted with permission from Tew, J.M.,Jr, van Loveren, H.R., Keller, J.T.; Atlas of Operative Microneurosurgery, Volume II; W.B. Saunders, in press.)

Figure 2: Craniotomy outlined for subfrontal approach to large suprasellar pituitary tumor.

Figure 3: Sagittal cross-section shows the line-of-sight obtained with the subfrontal approach.

Figure 4: Removal of tumor and bone is depicted via the subfrontal approach.

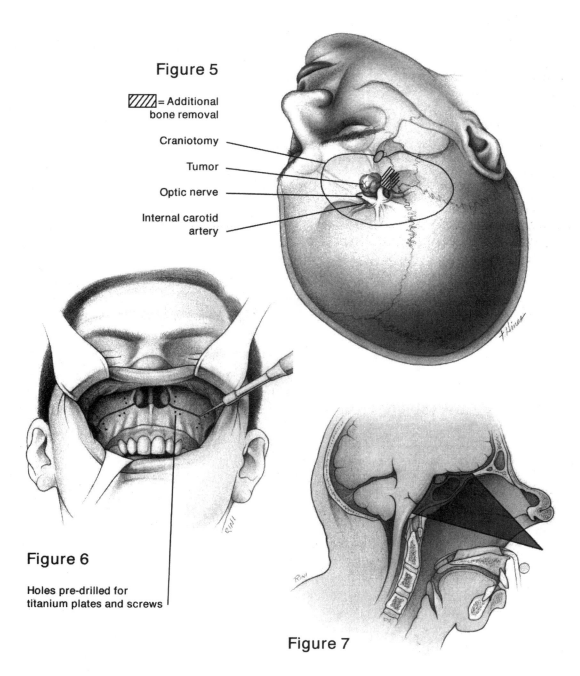

Figure 5

////// = Additional bone removal

Craniotomy

Tumor

Optic nerve

Internal carotid artery

Figure 6

Holes pre-drilled for titanium plates and screws

Figure 7

Figure Legends

Figure 5: Craniotomy outlined for the transcavernous approach. Additional bone removed at the skull base is depicted by cross-hatching. (All figures reprinted with permission from Tew, J.M.,Jr, van Loveren, H.R., Keller, J.T.; Atlas of Operative Microneurosurgery, Volume II; W.B. Saunders, in press.)

Figure 6: High-speed drill is used to separate the bone containing the upper teeth from the cheek bones and nose.

Figure 7: Depicts the wide area of exposure obtained with the Lefort maxillotomy.

The Role of Radiosurgery in the Treatment of Pituitary Tumors

Antonio A. F. De Salles, M.D., Ph.D., and Yvette Ficekova, M.D.
Division of Neuorosurgery, UCLA

Stereotactic radiosurgery is a technique used for the treatment of intracranial tumors that was developed to avoid the need for an open surgical removal. Radiosurgery is a combination of radiation therapy and stereotactic surgery. These two techniques, when performed together, provide a high concentration of radiation to the tumor, in such intensity, that the tumor is rendered sterile. When the tumor cells go on to divide, they die. The tumor decreases in size progressively, depending on the speed of reproduction of its cells. The process of tumor death and reabsorption may last from months to years. Scar tissue in the area of the tumor may be seen forever on MRI or CT.

Stereotactic surgery is a surgical technique designed to localize lesions inside of the skull with mathematical accuracy. This technique uses geometrical principles to direct probes, to guide sites of surgical incisions, and in the case of radiosurgery, to direct radiation beams to the intracranial lesion. Several forms of irradiation have been directed by stereotactic techniques. The particulate irradiation and the electromagnetic radiation are the most commonly used. Particulate radiation is made of nuclei of atoms accelerated by cyclotrons that were built in the forties for the development of the atomic bomb. Particulate energy has a special property called the Bragg peak. This allows calculations to make the beam stop at the tumor, thereby avoiding radiation of normal brain beyond the tumor. Recently, similar cyclotrons have been built for medical purposes. Few centers in the world have these cyclotrons because of the high cost of their construction and maintenance.

The electromagnetic energy, also called photon beam, is generated from the decay of the Cobalt-60 isotope, or artificially by collision of electrons accelerated to high speed to a plate of heavy metal. The collision releases photons which are generated and directed on high voltage linear accelerators. The energy generated by decay of Cobalt-60 or linear accelerators is the same. It has the same biological effect on the tumor. It also has the same ability to spare normal issue. This ability depends on the geometric strategies to avoid repeat beams crossing the same normal tissue. The two most popular forms of radiosurgery are based on either Cobalt-60 decay or linear accelerator beam. When Cobalt-60 is used, the radiosurgery instrument receives the commercial name of Gamma Knife. When the linear accelerator beam is used, the radiosurgery receives the popular name of LINAC radiosurgery. Again, both forms of radiosurgery have the same effect on the tumor.

Indications
Over the years, the use of radiosurgery for the treatment of pituitary tumors has been controversial. Extensive experience on the pituitary gland and tumor use of radiosurgery was developed with the Harvard cyclotron and the Berkeley syncyclotron. Destruction of the pituitary gland affords remarkable improvement of pain secondary to metastatic breast cancer. Thousands of patients underwent destruction of the pituitary gland in those two cyclotrons during the 50's and 60's. The data collected during those years are used today for radiosurgery treatment of pituitary tumors. Destruction of the pituitary for the treatment of pain is no longer performed because of better, more modern means of pain control.

Hormone secreting pituitary tumors such as prolactinomas, ACTH secreting tumors and GH secreting tumors respond well to radiosurgery, however, there is a long period after radio-surgery before the hormone level starts to fall to normal. Therefore, the tumor-related symptoms persist long after radiosurgery. Surgical resection, on the other hand, provides immediate control of the hormone hypersecretion. Because of this immediate control of the hormonal levels, microsurgery, usually transphenoidal, is the technique of choice for treatment of pituitary secreting tumors. Residual tumor, the portion of tumor infiltrating the cavernous sinus, or non-secreting pituitary tumor that is not compressing the optic pathways can be treated by radiosurgery. When there is compression of the optic apparatus, or the tumor is very close to the visual pathways, surgical resection is recommended. Recently, stereotactic radiotherapy has been developed to treat tumors in contact with optic apparatus. This technique affords better ability to spare normal brain than the conventional fractionated radiotherapy. Because of the exquisite visualization of the pituitary gland in relation to the tumor, radiosurgery also provides a less risk of affecting the production of other hormones than conventional radiation therapy.

Radiosurgery is a complement to microsurgery resection and it must be offered to the patient soon after surgery, usually immediately after demonstration of re-growth of the tumor. Radiosurgery has a high control rate of hormonal levels and less side effects to the normal brain than conventional fractionated radiation therapy.

In summary, radiosurgery is a non-invasive technique for treatment of residual pituitary adenomas or treatment of tumors in patients that are not fit for a microsurgery resection. Radiosurgery must be kept in mind during the follow up after surgical removal. When there is reoccurrence of the tumor, radiosurgery is an excellent option. Radiosurgery and stereotactic radiotherapy must replace conventional radiation therapy for the majority of the patients with pituitary adenomas. These two techniques differ substantially from conventional radiation therapy because they spare normal brain and the extent that other tissues in and around the skull are irradiated. This potentially allows for more effectiveness and less side effects.

Suggested Reading

1 Kjellberg RN, Kliman B: Radiosurgery therapy for pituitary adenoma. In the pituitary Adenoma, K.D. Post, I.M.D. Jacson, S Reichlin (eds). Plenum Publishing Co, New York, NY 1980.

2 Pollock BE, Kondziolka D, Lunsford LD, et al: Stereotactic radiosurgery for pituitary adenomas: imaging, visual and endocrine results. Acta Neurochir (Suppl.) 62:33-38, 1994.

3 Shalet, SM: Radiation and pituitary dysfunction. NEJM 328:130-131, 1993 Selch M, Solberg T, De Salles AAF, et al: Radiosurgery for benign tumors. In: Minimally Invasive Therapy of the Brain, AAF De Salles and R Lufkin, Thieme Medical Publisher, New York, NY 1996.

Gamma Knife Radiosurgery for Pituitary Adenomas

Mary Lee Vance, M.D., Edward R. Laws, Jr., M.D., Ladislau Steiner, M.D., Ph.D,
Melita Steiner, M.D., Bernhard Sutter, M.D., CJ Woodburn, Pamela Leake

Introduction

There are a number of aspects of Gamma knife radiosurgery that make it eminently suitable for the treatment of pituitary adenomas. Because most pituitary adenomas are benign lesions, it is thought that single fraction radiation is adequate therapy from a radiobiological perspective. Certainly having all the radiation given in one session is more convenient for the patient and is cost effective as well. Another advantage is that the focused radiosurgery should avoid damage to the hypothalamus, thus decreasing the risk of developing hypopituitarism from hypothalamic hormone deficiency. Focused radiosurgery also exposes a much smaller volume of brain to radiation, and smaller doses to brain are given, thereby decreasing the risk of seizures and deleterious effects on intellectual function. Finally, the very sharp and steep fall off from properly administered radiosurgery allows sparing of the optic nerves and optic chiasm, and, in many cases, sparing of intact normal pituitary gland.

Patterns of Care

Gamma knife radiosurgery can be employed as either primary or secondary therapy for pituitary tumors. By far, the majority of patients are treated secondarily after prior surgical resection, usually by the transsphenoidal approach. Gamma knife radiosurgery as primary therapy is suboptimal for hypersecretory pituitary adenomas because it does not produce an immediate decrease in excessive levels of growth hormone in acromegalics, of ACTH in Cushing's disease or of serum prolactin. Favorable effects may occur three to six months following radiosurgery, and are usually cumulative over time. Because these diseases are so harmful to the patient, most endocrinologists feel that treatment modalities that offer a prompt fall in hormonal levels to normal are superior.

Some intrasellar microadenomas (less than 10 mm in diameter) that are either non-functioning or associated with elevations in prolactin, may be successfully treated with primary Gamma knife radiosurgery, but long term results, are not yet available. The more common secondary application of Gamma knife radiosurgery is to treat tumors in which traditional microsurgery is unsuccessful in obtaining an endocrine "cure." For this reason, Gamma knife radiosurgery may be appropriate for some 40% of acromegalic patients, 15% to 20% of patients with Cushing's disease and 10% to 20% of patients with a prolactinoma. Gamma knife radiosurgery may also be appropriate for those patients who have initial remissions and then develop a recurrence (8% to 12 % of patients with acromegaly and Cushing's disease).

Other tumors suitable for secondary Gamma knife radiosurgery include clinically non-functioning adenomas that are incompletely removed, rapidly recurrent, or invasive in nature. There are some patients with intrasellar tumors that extend up to the level of the optic chiasm in whom transsphenoidal surgery successfully "debulks" the lesion such that subsequent Gamma knife radiosurgery may be administered to treat the residual tumor and to spare the optic apparatus.

Results

Table 1 represents our current experience in Gamma knife radiosurgery in 172 patients treated for pituitary tumors and related sellar and parasellar lesions. Results in patients with hypersecretory tumors have been generally satisfactory. Thirty patients with acromegaly have been treated and 21 have been followed for more than three months. Remissions have been documented from three to 30 months in four patients following the completion of Gamma knife radiosurgery, and we anticipate continued improvement in the remission rate as the time following treatment increases. Forty-one patients have been treated for Cushing's disease, and 25 of these have been followed for more than three months. Eleven of the 25 (44%) are in remission, with onset of remission occurring three to 14 months following Gamma knife radiosurgery. Although our 16 patients with prolactin secreting pituitary adenomas have all had a reduction in their serum prolactin levels, none has decreased to normal. Among five patients with Nelson's syndrome, one of four patients followed for more than three months has had remission of his illness. Among the large group with clinically non-functioning adenomas there has been excellent control, with many tumors decreasing in size. Two of these patients with recurring clinically non-functioning pituitary adenomas have had second treatments with Gamma knife radiosurgery and both remain under control. Tumor progression has occurred in a few patients, primarily those with clinically "silent" ACTH adenomas (positive ACTH on immunostaining, normal cortisol production).

These clinical results compare very favorably with those reported for conventional radiation therapy, and when adequate follow-up is available, we expect them to be superior.

Gamma Knife: Pituitary Disease
UVA Experience: 172 Patients

Diagnosis	# of Patients
Cushing's	41
Non Functioning	41
Acromegaly	30
Craniopharyngioma	26
Prolactinoma	16
Nelson's	5
Meningioma/Hemangiopericytoma	4
Metastic/Basal Cell/Sarcoma	4
Silent ACTH	2
Neurofibroma	1

Concerns and Complications

The major concern in the management of pituitary adenomas, regardless of treatment modalities, is the phenomenon of invasion of the sellar dura and the surrounding structures. Some tumors are quite large and extensively invasive, and obtaining adequate treatment plans for radiosurgery may be extremely difficult. Some of these tumors are relentlessly recurring and seem to defy any form of combination therapy. It is this type of tumor that is occasionally considered for a second treatment with Gamma knife radiosurgery.

Although the target tumor dosage has varied from 20 to 60 Gy and very careful limits on radiation dose to the optic nerves and chiasm have been maintained, there is still some uncertainty regarding the optimal dosage and optimal number of "shots". The new image-based computerized Gamma knife treatment plan software should improve our ability to deliver accurate and more effective radiosurgery, and continuous correlation of radiation dose with outcome should allow precise analysis of dose and conformational strategies.

With the possible exception of one minor partial visual field deficit, there have been no known complications in our patients. Follow-up in these patients has been careful and consistent, and we believe that all complications have been reported to us.

Conclusion

Gamma knife radiosurgery has become an indispensable part of our combined treatment program for the management of pituitary adenomas. In the future we believe that accurate imaging, accurate endocrinologic diagnosis, and careful planning will allow continuous improvement in results. The fact that many of our patients are very difficult cases with extensive and invasive tumors tends to underestimate the efficacy of this methodology in the management of lesions that are of optimal size and configuration. We anticipate that continued prospective follow-up of our patients will allow for rigorous analysis of the effects of Gamma knife radiosurgery and more definitive conclusions regarding this treatment for pituitary tumors.

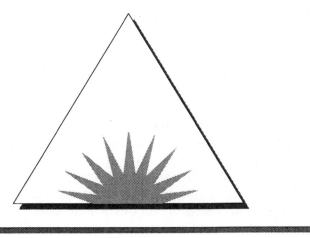

"Never let what you can't do interfere with what you can do."

Radiation Therapy of Acromegaly

Richard C. Eastman, M.D., Director, Division of Diabetes, Endocrinology and Metabolic Diseases. National Institutes of Health, NIDDK, Bethesda, Maryland

External beam irradiation with modern equipment is available at most major medical centers. It is an important treatment of acromegaly due to pituitary adenomas secreting growth hormone that cannot be cured surgically, and has predictable effects on the growth of the adenoma and on growth hormone levels.

Control of Growth of the Pituitary Adenoma

Further growth of the tumor is prevented in more than 99% of patients, with only a fraction of a percent of patients requiring subsequent surgery for tumor mass effects, such as loss of visual function due to pressure on the optic nerve by the tumor.

Effect on Growth Hormone Levels

Growth hormone levels fall predictably with time, and by 2 years are 50% lower than the level before treatment. By 5 years after irradiation the growth hormone levels have fallen to about 25% of the baseline level before treatment. A further fall in the growth hormone level is seen at 10 and 15 years after treatment. The percentage fall in growth hormone levels is not dependent on the size of the adenoma or on the pre-radiotherapy level of growth hormone. Patients respond equally well regardless of gender, history of previous surgery, and whether high prolactin levels are found. The fraction of patients achieving growth hormone levels less than 5 ng/mL approaches 90% after 15 years in our experience. Although the response to radiation is similar regardless of baseline growth hormone level, patients with initial growth hormone level greater than 100 ng/mL are significantly less likely to achieve growth hormone levels less than 5 ng/mL during long-term follow-up. Thus, surgery to remove part of an adenoma can significantly increase the long-term outcome if post-operative levels of growth hormone are below 100 ng/mL.

Effect on Pituitary Function

Hypopituitarism is the most common side effect of pituitary irradiation, and may be more likely in patients who have had surgery prior to irradiation. This complication does not appear to be more common in patients with acromegaly than in patients with other pituitary adenomas receiving similar treatment.

Side Effects

Side effects of irradiation are rare. Vision loss is extremely rare when the total dose is limited to 4680 rads given in 25 fractions over 35 days, with individual fractions not exceeding 180 rads. The reported cases have occurred almost entirely in patients who have received larger doses or higher fractional doses. The theory that patients with acromegaly are prone to radiation induced injury to the brain and optic nerves is not supported by a review of the reported cases. Other complications are also extremely rare.

Given the increased mortality of acromegaly, and particularly the risk of heat disease, our approach is to normalize IGF-I levels if possible. We recommend initial transsphenoidal adenomectomy, including partial removal of large adenomas with a low probability of surgical cure. Megavoltage irradiation is recommended to patients with persistent or recurrent growth hormone hypersecretion. Due to the delayed effects of irradiation on growth hormone secretion, we currently use bromocriptine and/or a somatostatin analogue to reduce growth hormone levels after radiotherapy. Medical therapy should be withdrawn at yearly intervals to determine whether continued medical therapy is required. Lifelong follow-up of pituitary function is indicated.

For a detailed discussion of radiation therapy for acromegaly, the reader should consult the following article:

Eastman RC, Gordan P, Glatstein E, Roth J. Radiation Therapy of Acromegaly. Melmed S (ED), Acromegaly, *Endocrinology and Metabolism Clinics of North America,* Volume 21:3, page 693, 1992.

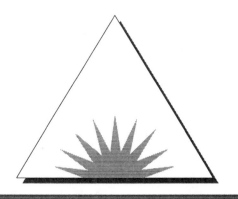

I am only one,
but still I am one.
I cannot do everything,
but still I can do something;
And because I cannot
do everything,
I will not refuse to do
the something that I can do.

The Nurse's Role ~ Surgical Management

The Endocrine Nurses Society

Tumors of the pituitary gland are often the cause of hyper or hypo secretion of one or more pituitary hormones. The goals of therapeutic intervention are: to restore or stop visual deterioration; to remove / inhibit the source of hormonal imbalance while preserving the normal pituitary tissue; to ultimately avoid substitution hormonal therapy; to prevent tumor recurrence. These goals can be achieved by medical treatment, surgery, radiation therapy or a combination.

The surgical approach to the removal of pituitary adenomas [hypophysectomy] depends upon the extent and shape of the tumor growth and may require two or more different surgical approaches.

Tumors within the pituitary gland [intrasellar], are more common and can be removed by microscopic surgery using the transsphenoidal approach. These microadenomas [<2mm] have specific locations within the pituitary gland depending upon their type and secretory capacity. Their location, color, consistency, and size, allows for the removal of the tumor tissue without disturbing normal glandular tissue, thus preserving normal pituitary function. Dumb-bell shaped or irregular shaped macroadenomas [>2mm] with suprasellar extension are more usually removed by the transcranial approach. Occasionally, both the transsphenoidal and transcranial approach are necessary. Preoperative radiographs [MRI,CT, plain films] will show the size of the tumor and help determine the type and extent of the surgical procedure required while stimulation and suppression tests evaluate the extent of pituitary hormonal dysfunctions.

Transsphenoidal surgery is performed under general anesthesia via an operating microscope with the patient in either a semi-sitting position, or supine with the head slightly tilted downwards. The incision is made at the inner aspect of the upper lip, and the sella turcica is entered via the sphenoid sinus. After the microadenoma is removed, the wound is sealed, to prevent ascending infection and leakage of cerebrospinal fluid [CSF], by either a fat graft taken from the anterior thigh, or by cartilage from the nasal septum. The gingival mucosa is sealed with loose catgut sutures. The nose may be packed for 24 - 48 hours. [It is more usual to pack the nose with nasopharyngeal tubes to allow for air flow, than without the tubes, although both methods are sited in the literature].

The effects of excessive hormones may affect the surgical technique: growth hormone secreting tumors cause enlargement of the nasal passages, mucosa and blood vessels, thus allowing easier passage through the nasal septum, but also causing extensive bleeding.

The frequency of complications is directly related to the size of the tumor, the surgical approach [complications are more common after transfrontal than after transsphenoidal surgery], and the experience of the neurosurgeon. The reported incidence of complications therefore also varies. CSF rhinorrhea, sinusitis, hemorrhage, central nervous system damage, diabetes insipidus, meningitis, appear to be the most common, with each occurring between 0.3 to 15% of all surgery. Lifelong hormonal replacement is necessary in 5 to 17% of all cases due to operative destruction of the pituitary gland. Mortality has been reported as less than 1%. Transcranial surgery is performed under a general anesthesia, with the incision made through the scalp, thus requiring the head to be shaved. The floor of the sphenoid sinus is opened and as the tumor is removed from the sella by the use of suction, malleable spoons and curettage, the suprasellar portion of the tumor falls into the sella, thus allowing it to be removed. Confirmation of complete removal is made by intraoperative radiography and hormonal sampling [growth hormone levels fall to normal within minutes]. However, in most macroadenomas, complete cure is hard to achieve as residual tumor is left behind especially around the cavernous sinus. The sella is closed using a piece of cartilage from the nasal septum, or fat from the thigh. The nostrils are packed with or without using nasopharyngeal tubes for easier breathing. Nasal packs are usually removed after 48 hours, the patients are ambulatory on the night of surgery and discharged on the fifth - tenth postoperative day. As transient diabets insipidus may be a complication of this surgery, a careful observation of the fluid balance, thirst and urine output, is essential.

Preoperative Nursing Care: Patient Education

The nurses role in preoperative care is to decrease the patient's anxiety by describing what to expect before, during, immediately after surgery, and for long term follow-up. While some issues are generic, concerns must be individualized according to the needs of the patient and the technique of the surgeon. Extensive examinations for both hormonal function and tumor size and location will be performed both pre and postoperatively. Preoperative hormonal testing assesses the secretory capacity of the tumor and damage by the tumor to other pituitary functions. Postoperative hormonal testing determines cure in the case of secreting tumors and residual function of the pituitary. [These tests are discussed elsewhere in this chapter]. The same tests are performed both pre and post operatively with particular attention to adrenal function assessment post operatively. Tumor size is assessed by x-rays and visual fields. Bacterial growth from the nose and mouth is assessed by swabbing for culture and sensitivity.

Some, but not all disease related signs and symptoms will be relieved by surgery and must be discussed in detail by the surgeon. Increased perspiration, skin oiliness and acne, headache, glucose intolerance, galactorrhea, sleep apnea, impotence or amenorrhea, from the effects of excessive growth hormone will be improved; enlargement of the facial sinuses may regress; visual field defects, hirsutism, arthralgias, colonic polyps, and enlargement of the heart, kidney and liver, and arterial hypertension may not change. Galactorrhea from excessive prolactin will improve, while resumption of menses and fertility may occur. Thyroid function disturbances from TSH production, will improve. Skin changes from excessive production of ACTH seen in Cushing's disease, will improve.

The patient can expect to be out of bed and ambulatory the day after the surgery or even the evening of surgery. Nasal packs will be in place for 48 hours which may necessitate oral breathing, and if so, the patient may experience dryness and thirst. Excessive thirst and urination is unusual and the nurse should be alerted since it could indicate post operative diabetes insipidus. Nasal discharge and post-nasal drip is to be reported to the nurse. The mouth may be sore if sutured, and mouth washes and dental floss can be used until brushing the teeth can be resumed after the incision has healed. Removal of fat from the thigh, or cartilage from the nose may give some discomfort. Transcranial surgery may cause headaches and itching from new hair growth and sutures. The sutures will be removed after 7 - 10 days and washing the head will be allowed while standing straight in a shower and not tilting the head. Details of any wound care will be given before discharge. Upper lip numbness and a decreased sense of smell causing a loss of taste are usual and can last for 3 months, therefore hot foods and liquids are to be avoided. Increased intracranial pressure is to be avoided for two months: bending is to be from the knees instead of from the waist; straining at stool is to be avoided by taking fiber or laxatives to prevent constipation; sexual activities can be resumed with caution; sneezing, coughing and nose blowing are to be avoided. Depending

The Nurse's Role: Surgical Management

upon the size and extent of the tumor's removal, hormonal replacement after the surgery may be temporary, permanent or may not be necessary.

While the thought of any type of brain surgery is very frightening, this surgery is localized as it does not encroach upon the brain functions per se, and therefore is not as dangerous, with thousands of these operations being performed yearly producing a low complication rate of less than 1 in 100. It is benign surgery, allowing ambulation the same day of surgery.

Postoperative Nursing Care

Monitoring for the lasting effects of anesthesia and for possible complications involving: neurologic status, changes in vision, disorientation, level of consciousness, decreased strength and the onset of diabetes insipidus, is maintained until the patient has been discharged. To assess for diabetes insipidus, a careful record of fluid balance must be maintained and the doctor alerted whenever the output exceeds the input, or the patient complains of excessive thirst or urination, or the urine specific gravity is low. Treatment of temporary, partial or total diabetes insipidus should be started immediately with intramuscular, subcutaneous or nasal vasopressin. CSF leakage is assessed by: monitoring the presence and amount of post nasal drip; testing nasal discharge for glucose, whose presence indicates that the fluid is CSF; monitoring the presence and severity of persistent, headaches. Most CSF leaks resolve with bed rest. Spinal taps may be necessary to relieve pressure, with surgical intervention rarely required. Frequent deep breathing to prevent pulmonary complications and coughing, is encouraged. Infection is monitored by assessing for meningitis: headache, elevated temperature, and neck rigidity. The effects of mouth breathing is made more comfortable by providing frequent oral rinses and petroleum jelly to the lips. Hormonal replacement, especially steroid coverage, may be necessary for several days, with steroids being tapered over 5 days.

Transsphenoidal surgery is the optimal approach for the surgical removal of pituitary tumors, resulting in improvement of quality of life and reduction in mortality and morbidity as a result of tumor growth. It is a relatively benign surgery with the patients being ambulatory the evening of the surgery. Permanent hormonal replacement may or may not be necessary, but the patients must be followed regularly after surgery to assess the success of the surgery, to monitor hormonal replacement and their response to treatment, and to detect tumor recurrence.

References

1   Fahlbusch R., Honegger J., Buchfelder M. :Surgical Management of Acromegaly. Endocrinology and Metabolism Clinics of North America 1992;21:669-89
2   Hardy J., Mohr G. Endocrine System. In Hardy J. [ed]: Hardy's Textbook of Surgery, 2nd Ed; pp 373 - 380 Philadelphia, J.B. Lippincott
3   Medical-Surgical Nursing, A Nursing Process Approach. pp 1529 - 1557 Philadelphia, W. B. Saunders Co. 1991
4   Healy P., Mourad L., American Nursing Review for Medical-Surgical Nursing Certification pp175-78; 265-79. Pennsylvania, Springhouse Corp.
5   Forrest A, Carter D, Macleod I, in Principles and Practice of Surgery. 2nd Ed; pp 338-44 Edinburgh, C. Livingstone 1991
6   Molitch M, :Clinical Manifestations of Acromegaly. Endocrinology and Metabolism Clinics of North America 1992;21:597-614
7   Melmed S: Acromegaly. N Engl J Med 322:966, 1990
8   Vance L: New Directions in the Treatment of Hyperprolactinemia. Endocrinologist 1997. 7:153-59

Section IV

Pediatric Issues

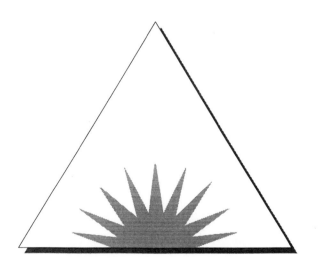

Second Edition

Pediatric Pituitary Tumors

Cheryl A. Muszynski, M.D., Division of Pediatric Neurosurgery,
Department of Neurosurgery, Beth Israel Medical Center, New York, New York

Introduction

The pituitary is a small, intracranial gland which secretes a number of different hormones that control growth and sexual development. Most pituitary tumors develop in the front, or anterior, portion of the pituitary gland (the adenohypophysis). The term, "pituitary adenoma," describes a tumor of the pituitary gland, the majority of which are benign and curable. Pituitary adenomas account for approximately 10% to 15% of all intracranial neoplasms in all age groups[16]. However, in the past, it has been well-documented that this type of adenoma occurs rarely in the pediatric age group[2,3,4]. In fact, only up to 10% of all identified pituitary tumors are found in children and adolescents[6,8,15,19,21,22,28,30]. More specifically, in 1982, Hoffman reviewed his experience with this entity at the Hospital for Sick Children. He reported an incidence of 1.2% of all supratentorial tumors treated over a 25-year period[11]. This figure is similar to the incidence of 2.6% subsequently described by Haddad and colleagues at the University of Iowa Hospitals and Clinics in 1991[9].

Unfortunately, the age ranges included in reported "pediatric" series have varied widely. For example, some series have included patients as old as 20 years, while others have limited the upper age limit to 17 or 18 years. Yet other reports include adults whose pituitary-related symptoms began during childhood. Consequently, it has been difficult to uniformly compare the different reported treatment outcomes. For the purpose of general discussion here, the "pediatric" age group will include all ages less than or equal to 18 years. The surgical management of pituitary tumors in this particular age group is the focus of this chapter.

The majority of pediatric pituitary tumors produce hormones ("functioning" adenomas), while the others do not ("non-functioning" adenomas). This is in contrast to adult pituitary tumors, the majority of which are non-functioning. In fact, the incidence of non-functioning adenomas is lower during the first three decades than it is later in life[5,17,29]. Despite this difference in "functional status" between pediatric and adult adenomas, there is no difference in the general characteristics between the two.

There are several types of functioning pituitary tumors, including those which produce prolactin (PRL), growth hormone (GH), corticotropin (ACTH), and those which are plurihormonal (producing more than one hormone type). Recently, Mindermann and Wilson reported that ACTH-releasing adenomas and prolactinomas varied in frequency before, during, and after puberty. More specifically, ACTH-releasing adenomas occur most commonly before puberty, whereas prolactinomas occur most frequently during and after this time period. However, this observation may in part reflect the fact that prolactinomas cannot cause endocrine symptoms in prepubertal children, since the endocrine substrates have not yet fully developed[26].

Initial treatment of symptomatic pituitary tumors may include medical and/or surgical therapy, depending upon the tumor type, size, and location, as well as the individual patient's age. One conventional way to consider these tumors is with respect to size. For example, a microadenomas defined as an adenoma less than or equal to 1 cm in diameter,[20,25,34] whereas a macroadenoma is one of any larger size. In general, radiation is not indicated as initial therapy for affected pediatric patients. However, in selected cases, stereotactic radiosurgery may subsequently be indicated for adjunctive therapy.

Clinical Presentation

In general, patients with pituitary tumors have one or more types of clinical presentations. The two most frequent types are signs/symptoms of (1) an endocrinopathy and (2) a mass lesion. The former presentation is characterized by the over- or underproduction of one or more pituitary hormones. The latter presentation is typified by headaches, visual loss, and/or pituitary insufficiency.

Patients with functioning pituitary tumors have signs and symptoms which vary, depending upon the type(s) of hormone(s) which are produced. Although the age at symptom-onset varies according to the adenoma subtype, several general priniciples have been identified. First, growth arrest commonly occurs with all pediatric pituitary adenomas, except GH-releasing ones[25]. Second, menstrual irregularities commonly occur with all pediatric pituitary adenomas except ACTH-releasing ones which cause Nelson's Syndrome[25].

Prolactinomas typically present with primary or secondary amenorrhea (lack of menstruation), oligomenorrhea (irregular menstruation), gynecomastia, galactorrhea (production of breast milk), visual loss, delayed puberty, hypogonadism/azoospermia, and/or short stature.

ACTH-releasing adenomas (causing Cushing's or Nelson's Syndromes) generally present with Cushingoid characteristics (centripetal obesity, moon faces, "buffalo hump", supraclavicular fat pads, hirsutism, acne, abdominal striae), short stature/growth arrest, mental status changes (irritability or psychosis), gynecomastia, hypertension, and/or glucose intolerance.

GH-releasing adenomas (causing acromegaly) typically present with rapid growth, enlargement of facial features (nose, lips, tongue, supraorbital ridges), enlargement of the hands and feet, hypogonadism, hypertension, menstrual irregularities and/or precocious puberty. Affected patients may also be afflicted by carpal tunnel syndrome, osteoarthritis, goiter, hyperhidrosis, colonic polyps, sleep apnea, and/or glucose intolerance.

Non-functioning adenomas represent the minority of pediatric pituitary tumors and often grow to be relatively large before detection. An individual with this type of tumor typically has signs and symptoms which are related to the mass effect exerted by these hormonally-silent adenomas.

An intermittent headache is another common complaint. Pituitary tumors may provoke or exacerbate headaches by different direct and indirect mechanisms. The former may consist of lateral erosion of the tumor into the cavernous sinus (which contains different divisions of the trigeminal nerve), or by involvement of the sellar dura. In these cases, headaches are typically located in the ipsilateral, frontal region. Another direct cause of headaches is pituitary apoplexy, which is characterized by the acute onset of a severe headache which coincides with hemorrhage of the tumor into itself. Indirect causes of headaches include pituitary insufficiency, dopamine-agonist-related side effects and acromegaly-associated cervical osteoarthritis[31].

Another type of tumor, located in the same intracranial region, but not of pituitary origin, is the craniopharyngioma. This is an epithelial tumor derived from the hypophyseal duct during the formation of Rathke's pouch. Craniopharyngiomas may afflict either children or adults. However, the majority occur in patients less than 18 years of age. Craniopharyngiomas are usually not discovered until they impinge upon adjacent structures. By that time, they are often very large and composed of solid and cystic materials. Associated symptoms include headaches, double vision, loss of peripheral vision, temperature regulation abnormalities, and/or pituitary insufficiency (undersecretion of pituitary hormones). The main goal of treatment is complete excision, whenever possible. Surgical removal may be accomplished by

Pediatric Pituitary Tumors

using either the transsphenoidal or the transcranial approach. During surgery, it is paramount that one preserve pituitary, visual and brain functions, Generally, radiotherapy is reserved for those patienplain ts who have residual craniopharyngioma postoperatively. Chemotherapy is infrequently used. However, when this treatment modality is indicated, bleomycin is typically instilled into the cystic portion of the tumor. This results in cyst capsule thickening, which is believed to make subsequent tumor removal relatively easier.

Another type of intracranial mass, located in the same vicinity, but not strictly of pituitary origin, is a Rathke's Cleft Cyst. This cyst is a residual cleft of Rathke's pouch which is a normal anatomic structure in the four-week old human embryo. Normally, by the seventh week of gestation, this pouch becomes obliterated at all but its uppermost (rostral) portion. The anterior wall of this residual portion, or cavity, develops into the anterior lobe of the pituitary gland. The back, or posterior, wall becomes the pars intermedia of the pituitary gland. In some individuals, a residual lumen, or Rathke's cleft cyst, remains between the anterior lobe and the pars intermedia of the pituitary gland. In general, these are small and asymptomatic fluid-containing cysts. However, infrequently, these cysts enlarge enough to extend into the suprasellar and/or sphenoid sinus regions. In these cases, the cysts may produce headaches, visual problems and/or pituitary insufficiency. In general, the goals of treatment include careful cyst wall excision and cyst drainage.

Diagnostic Evaluation
Initial diagnostic evaluation of pituitary tumors includes neurological and neuro-ophthalmologic exams, serum levels of pituitary hormones and radiographic imaging. Although sellar radiographs, tomograms, pneumoencephalograms and contrast-enhanced computed tomographic (CT) scans were utilized in the past, magnetic resonance imaging (MRI) of the brain (with special attention to the sellar region) is currently the diagnostic procedure of choice. This imaging modality assesses for integrity and size of the sellar floor, signal changes within the pituitary gland, as well as for supra- and parasellar extension of the intrasellar, pituitary mass.

Treatment Options
Pituitary tumors may be treated by medications, surgery, radiation therapy, or by a combination of these strategies. The optimal treatment regimen chosen for an individual depends upon his or her age as well as upon the tumor's type, size and location. Although treatment plans vary from one patient to the next, the goals generally remain the same. These include the correction of any endocrinopathy and relief of symptoms and signs resulting from the tumor's mass effect. It is essential to coordinate the recommendations of knowledgeable endocrinologists and neurosurgeons to provide high-quality care to these patients.

Surgery
Surgery is indicated for the following symptomatic patients:
(1) Those with hormonally-active (functioning) pituitary tumors who have failed an appropriate trial of medical therapy.
(2) Those with hormonally-inactive (non-functioning) pituitary tumors.

Microsurgical transsphenoidal resection is the preferred approach for pituitary tumors (micro- and macroadenomas) which are confined to the sella turcica or have a regular suprasellar extension. Another indication for this approach is pituitary apoplexy which is considered a neurosurgical emergency. In all of the above cases, the goal of surgery is complete removal of adenomatous tissue while sparing normal pituitary gland and respecting adjacent neurovascular structures. In general, after endotracheal anesthesia is administered, a lumbar subarachnoid drain is placed and connected to a closed sterile drainage system. This allows for the intraoperative infusion of sterile saline, which may aid in the removal of the suprasellar portion of tumor. Typically, the lumbar drain is removed before the patient is awakened. However, in some cases, the drain will remain in place for a few days postoperatively.

Although the transsphenoidal procedure is technically the same as that which is performed in adults[10], several anatomical issues are unique to the pediatric age group. First, the sphenoid sinus is frequently "conchal" in type, i.e., it is filled with cancellous bone[27]. Therefore, a high-speed diamond drill is required to adequately expose the sella[23]. Second, pediatric patients typically have generously-sized intracavernous sinuses located in the anterobasal sellar dura which must be respected during dural opening. In selected cases, when complete intrasellar exploration fails to identify obvious tumor, a subtotal hypophysectomy may be indicated.

Although a much less frequent finding, pediatric pituitary tumors may extend intracranially to involve contiguous structures. In these cases, a transcranial approach would be recommended. This procedure involves temporary removal of a portion of the skull to gain adequate access to the tumor.

At Beth Israel Medical Center's Institute for Neurology and Neurosurgery (I.N.N.), we use new imaging technologies that provide unprecedented views into the human brain. One of these is the computerized image-guided system, which has a hand-held navigating instrument, enabling the surgeon to use computer-generated information during surgery. Another is the stereotactically-guided surgical microscope which offers unsurpassed intraoperative localization accuracy. In the very near future, intraoperative MRI will be available to provide "real-time" feedback, to ensure precise surgical resection, and thereby, to optimize our treatment results. These new instruments have dramatically expanded the current options available to patients with pituitary tumors.

Surgical Complications
In the majority of cases, surgery is accomplished with minimal morbidity and no mortality. Typically, normal pituitary tissue, including the pituitary stalk, is well preserved. However, as with any surgical procedure, it is important to be aware of the very small, but real, potential for complications. These include hemorrhage, infection, pituitary insufficiency, diabetes insipidus (excess urination), CSF rhinorrhea, hydrocephalus and/or cerebral vasospasm. The average reported incidence of such complications is 3.6%[36]. By and large, surgery is a safe and effective means of resecting pituitary tumors.

Outcome
Following transsphenoidal surgery, "success rates" (i.e., control of disease without requirement for adjuvant treatment) have varied, depending upon the adenoma subtype.

For ACTH-releasing adenomas, success rates range from 61% - 100 %[1, 5, 7, 13, 20, 29, 37]. In fact, patients in this group who went into initial remission were often later found to be cured[24, 29, 35].

For prolactinomas, success rates range from 28% - 74%[5, 20, 29]. In general, postoperative outcome of patients in this group correlates with tumor size. Microadenoma patients have a high cure rate following resection alone. However, macroadenoma patients often require adjuvant medical and/or radiotherapy to subsequently achieve good responses[12,18,29,33].

For GH-releasing and for endocrine-inactive adenomas, success rates range from 12% - 85%[5,20] for the former and from 40% - 50 % for the latter[5,29]. Tumor recurrence rates range from 10% - 50%[5,14,25,29,34] and vary according to the adenoma subtype.

Conclusions
♦ The presence of *primary amenorrhea* and/or *short stature* should prompt an evaluation for a pituitary adenoma.

Pediatric Pituitary Tumors

- Menstrual irregularities in girls are associated with different types of pituitary adenomas, not just with prolactinomas.
- ACTH-secreting adenomas are the most common subtype found in childhood.
- Early diagnosis of pituitary tumors is essential to reduce the incidence of local extension and to optimize treatment results.
- The ultimate treatment plan is one which carefully meets the needs and addresses the goals of a given, individual patient.
- For appropriate candidates, transsphenoidal resection of pituitary tumors is safe and effective. Successful adenomectomy may obviate the need for chronic medical therapy and allow for the development of normal fertility.
- The unique features of pediatric pituitary tumors warrant further study with genetic and molecular biological studies.

References

1 Chandler WF, Schteingart DE, Lloyd RV, McKeever PE, Ibarra-Perez G. Surgical treatment of Cushing's disease. J Neurosurg. 66:204-212, 1987.
2 Costin G. Endocrine disorders associated with tumors of the pituitary and hypothalamus. Pediatr Clin North Am. 26:15-31, 1979.
3 Dastur DK, Lalitha US. Pathological analysis of intracranial space-occupying lesions in 1000 cases including children. Pituitary adenomas, developmental tumors, parasitic and developmental cysts. J Neurol Sciences. 15:397-427,1972.
4 David M, Bernard-Weil E, Pradat P. Adenomes hypophisaires de l'enfant. Revue Neurol. 106:334-336, 1962.
5 Dyer EH, Civit T, Visot A, Delalande O, Derome P. Transsphenoidal surgery for pituitary adenomas in children. Neurosurgery. 34:207-212, 1994.
6 Fraioli B, Gerrante L, Celli P. Pituitary adenomas with onset during puberty. T Neurosurgery. 59:590-595, 1983.
7 Friedman RB, Oldfield EH, Nieman LK, Chrousos GP, Doppman L, Cutler GB, Loyiaux DL. Repeat transsphenoidal surgery for Cushing's disease. J Neurosurgery. 71:520-527,1989.
8 Gaini SM, Giovannelli M, Forni C, Villani R,Scuccimarra A, Carteri A, Iraci G. Pituitary adenomas in infancy and childhood. In: Villani R, Giovannelli M, Gaini SM, eds. Modern Problems in Paediatrics. Basel: Karger. 220-225, 1977.
9 Haddad SF, Van Gilder JC, Menezes AH. Pediatric pituitary tumors. Neurosurgery. 29:509-514, 1991.
10 Hardy, J. Transsphenoidal microsurgical removal of pituitary microadenoma. In: Krayenbuhl H, Maspes PE, Sweet WH, eds. Progress in Neurological Surgery. Basel: Karger. 200-216, 1975.
11 Hoffmann HJ. Pituitary adenomas. In: American Association of Neurological Surgeons, eds. Pediatric Neurosurgery: Surgery of the Developing Nervous System. New York: Grune and Stratton. 493-499, 1982.
12 Hubbard JL, Scheithauer BW, Abboud CF, Laws ER. Prolactin- secreting adenomas: the preoperative response to bromocriptine treatment and surgical outcome. J Neurosurgery. 67:816-821, 1987.
13 Johnson J, Chrousos GP, Nieman LK, Doppman JL, Cutler GB, Oldfield EH. Transsphenoidal microsurgery for Cushing's disease in children(abstr). Presented at the 61st Annual Meeting of the American Association of Neurological Surgeons, Boston, April 24-29, 1993.
14 Kane LA, Leinung MC, Scheithauer BW, Bergstralh EJ, Laws ER Tr., Groover RV, Kovacs K, Horvath E, Zimmerman D. Pituitary adenomas in childhood and adolescence. J Clin Endocrinol Metab. 79:1135-1140, 1994.
15 Koos WT, Miller MH. Intracranial tumors of infants and children. Stuttgart: G. Thieme Verlag. 213-220, 1971.
16 Kovacs K, Horvath E, Asa SL. Classification and pathology of pituitary tumors. In: Wilkins RH, Rengachary SS, eds. Neurosurgery. New York: McGraw-Hill. 834-842, 1985.
17 Kovacs K, Horvath E. Tumors of the Pituitary Gland. In: Hartmann WH, Sobin LH, eds. Atlas of

Tumor Pathology. Washington, D.C.: Armed Forces Institute of Pathology. 206,1986.

18 Laws ER Jr., Fode NC, Randall RV, Abboud CF, Coulam CB. Pregnancy following transsphe-noidal resection of prolactin-secreting pituitary tumors. J Neurosurg. 58:685-688, 1983.

19 Laws ER Jr., Scheithauer BW, Groover RV. Pituitary adenomas in childhood and adolescence. Frog Exp Tumor Res. 30:359-361, 1987.

20 Laws ER Ir. Pituitary Tumors-Therapeutic Considerations: Surgical. In: Barrow DL, Selman WR, eds, Neuroendocrinology, Concepts in Neurosurgery. Baltimore: Williams & Wilkins. 5:395-400, 1992.

21 Lucas C, Guibout M, Taquet P, Grisoli F, Giraud F. Aspects diagnostiques et evolutifs de l'adenome a prolactine chez l'enfant. Arch Pr Pediatr. 37:79-86, 1980.

22 Ludecke DK, Herrman HD, Schulte FJ. Special problems with neurosurgical treatment of hormone-secreting pituitary adenomas in children. Frog Exp Tumor Res. 30:362-370, 1987.

23 Maira G, Anile C. Pituitary adenomas in childhood and adolescence. Can J. Neurol Sciences. 17:83-87, 1990.

24 Mickle TP. Cushing's Disease in childhood. In: Marlin AE, ed. Concepts in Pediatric Neurosurgery. Basel: Karger. 9:65-76, 1989.

25 Mindermann T, Wilson CB. Pediatric pituitary adenomas. Neurosurgery. 36:259-269, 1995.

26 Mizutani T, Teramoto A, Aruga T, Takakura K, Sanno N. Prepubescent pituitary null cell macroadenoma with silent macroscopic apoplexy: case report. Neurosurgery. 33(5):907- 910, 1993.

27 Moss-Salentijn L. Anatomy and embryology. In: Blitzer A, Lawson W, Friedman WH, eds. Surgery of the Paranasal Sinuses. Philadelphia: W.B. Saunders. 1-22, 1985.

28 Odom GL, Davis CH, Woodhall 8. Brain tumors in children: Clinical analysis of 164 cases. Pediatrics. 18:856-870, 1956.

29 Fartington MD, Davis DH, Laws ER Tr, Scheithauer BW. Pituitary adenomas in childhood and adolescence. Results of ranssphenoidal surgery. TNeurosurgery. 80(2):209-216, 1994.

30 Richmond IL, Wilson CB. Pituitary adenomas in childhood and adolescence. J Neurosurgery. 49:163-168, 1978.

31 Riskind PN. Headaches and pituitary tumors. Massachusetts General Hospital Neuroendocrine Center Bulletin. 1(2):4, 1996.

32 Sane K. Problems in the treatment of children with brain tumors. Frog Exp Tumor Res. 30:1-9, 1987.

33 Scamoni C, Balzarini C, Crivelli G, Dorizzi A. Treatment and long-term follow-up results of prolactin-secreting pituitary adenomas. J Neurosurg Sci. 35:9-16, 1991.

34 Stephanian E, Lunsford LD, Coffey RJ, Bissonette DI, Flickinger JC. Gamma knife surgery for sellar and suprasellar tumors. Neurosurgery Clinics of North America. 3(1):207-218, 1992.

35 Styne DM, Grumbach MM, Kaplan SL, Wilson CB, Conte FA. Treatment of Cushing's disease in childhood and adolescence by transsphenoidal microadenomectomy. N Engl J Med. 310:889- 893, 1984.

36 Tindall GT, Woodard EJ, Barrow DL. Transsphenoidal excision of macroadenomas of the pituitary gland. In: Rengachary SS, Wilkins RH, eds. Neurosurgical Operative Atlas. Baltimore: Williams & Wilkins. 1: 287-298, 1991.

37 Wilson CB, Dempsey LC. Transsphenoidal microsurgical removal of 250 pituitary adenomas. J Neurosurgery. 48:13-22, 1978.

Pituitary Tumors in Childhood

Constantine A. Stratakis, M.D., Dsc, Staff Scientist, NICHD, NIH,
Assistant Professor, Pediatric Endocrinology,
Clinical Genetics & Metabolism, Georgetown University

Introduction

In every 20 tumors seen in children, only one is endocrine. However, among the tumors of the endocrine glands, those of the pituitary are the most frequent: pituitary adenomas and other tumors represent one fifth of all endocrine neoplasms seen in childhood.[1]

Almost all pituitary tumors in childhood are benign. The tumors arising from the gland are characterized as "adenomas" whereas those arising from the surrounding tissues bear different names depending on the type of their cells, Among the latter the most frequent are craniopharyngiomas and teratomas. The adenomas are also characterized as "macroadenomas" if they have a size that exceeds 1 cm, and "microadenomas", if their size is smaller than 1 cm. This is an important distinction among the various pituitary tumors since their prognosis largely depends on their size.

The following pituitary gland tumors can occur in childhood, each one named after the pituitary hormone that they produce: prolactinomas, corticotropinoma, somatotropinoma, gonadotropinoma, thyrotropinoma. Two relatively frequent tumors do not produce any hormones but, rather, cause dysfunction of the pituitary gland due to their expansion: these are chromophobe adenoma, craniopharyngioma. Definitive diagnosis of these tumors is based on staining of pathological specimens obtained during surgery, with the exception of patients with prolactinomas, in whom the diagnosis is largely biochemical.

It is not known what is causing these tumors to appear at such a young age, but certainly genetics plays a role. For example, certain pituitary tumors constitute part of inherited genetic syndromes that are collectively called the syndromes of multiple endocrine neoplasia (MEN), There are at least two types of these syndromes (MEN type and MEN type-II); it is MEN-I that has been associated with pituitary adenomas in childhood. Another MEN type is Carney complex. This disease (named after Dr. Carney who first described it) is also inherited; it is associated with a variety of other nonendocrine tumors (skin, breast and heart myxomas, and spotty skin pigmentation). Neurofibromatosis and other genetic conditions have also been associated with tumors of the pituitary gland. Certain pituitary tumors (craniopharyngiomas and various cystic or solid lesions known as "teratomas" form early in the development of the embryo, indicating that additional genetic mechanisms (not necessarily inherited) are present and may lead to their formation.

Clinical Presentation

All pituitary tumors may cause symptoms arising from pressure on the adjacent structures. Headaches, visual disturbances, and manifestations from one or more pituitary hormone deficiencies can be the presenting symptoms. If the tumor is producing a hormone by itself, then there is the combination of one pituitary hormone excess (for example, hypercortisolism due to a pituitary corticotropin-producing adenoma will lead to Cushing's syndrome) and multiple pituitary hormone deficiencies (in the same example of the patient with Cushing's syndrome, hypercortisolism will be accompanied by decreased growth and thyroid function due to the absence or incomplete secretion of the pituitary-derived growth hormone and thyrotropin, respectively).

Pituitary Patient Resource Guide

There is one exception to this rule: relatively high prolactin levels can be found in a patient that does not have a prolactin-producing pituitary tumor. This is because any pituitary tumor has the potential of interrupting hypothalamic control of prolactin secretion by the pituitary. Under normal circumstances, the hypothalamus is responsible for suppression of prolactin secretion,

Menstrual dysfunction and galactorrhea can be seen in female adolescent patients with hyperprolactinemia. Intracranial hypertension and hydrocephalus may be found in patients with pituitary tumors. The usual finding an ophthalmologic examination is very characteristic defects of the visual fields because most suprasellar pituitary tumors impinge on the crossing fibers of the optic nerves. Other changes in vision depend an the location of the tumor.

Deficiency of one or more pituitary or hypothalamic hormones may result from pressure from the expanding pituitary tumor. Depending on the hormone affected, different symptoms may arise. The most frequently affected hormone is somatotropin or growth hormone (GH). Deficiency of this hormone leads to poor growth, hypoglycemia, or both in younger children. The deficiency is diagnosed by measuring the plasma GH concentration after stimulation with medicines such as arginine, insulin, dopamine, or glucagon.

Deficiency of corticotropin (ACTH) leads to secondary adrenal insufficiency characterized by weakness, orthostatic hypotension hyponatremia, and hypoglycemia in younger children. It is a life-threatening condition that must be diagnosed early. Diagnosis is made by measuring plasma cortisol 1 hour after adrenal stimulation with an intravenous bolus of ACTH. Pituitary ACTH deficiency produces adrenal atrophy and a diminished cortisol response.

Gonadotropin [luteinizing hormone (LH) and follicle-stimulating hormone (FSH)] and thyrotropin (TSH) deficiencies may also occur in patients with pituitary tumors. Gonadotropin deficiency manifests as pubertal arrest or regression in children already in puberty or as delayed or absent puberty ill younger children. Plasma LH and FSH are low for the age in these children, and bone age, indicating the level of skeletal maturation, is delayed. Thyrotropin deficiency manifests as poor growth, diminished performance at school, constipation, cold intolerance, dry skin, and other symptoms of hypothyroidism. Measurements of serum total thyroxine (T_4), free T_4, and TSH are required for the diagnosis.

Extension of a pituitary tumor into the hypothalamic paraventricular nucleus may result in vasopressin (AVP) deficiency. This leads to inability to concentrate urine and dehydration. The disease is called diabetes insipidus and is characterized by polyuria, polydipsia, and extensive electrolyte abnormalities. It should be contrasted with the better known diabetes mellitus, which is the common form of diabetes known and is caused by insulin deficiency. Diabetes mellitus is not a complication of children with pituitary tumors. The diagnosis of diabetes insipidus may be confirmed by a water deprivation test.

Certain hypothalamic tumors (e.g. hamartomas) can present with precocious puberty and/or hyperprolactinemia due to compression of the pituitary stalk and disruption of the normal inhibition of puberty and/or prolactin, secretion exerted by the hypothalamus. Hamartomas are frequent in genetic syndromes associated with craniofacial anomalies and abnormalities of the extremities; patients with these genetic defects and/or positive family history should be screened for these tumors by magnetic resonance imaging (MRI).

Diagnostic Evaluation of Patients with Pituitary Tumors
In all patients, magnetic resonance imaging (MRI) of the head and/or the hypothalamic pituitary unit is necessary. Biochemical teats that are needed vary per tumor type: For patients with corticotropinomas, a dexamethasone suppression test (DST), serum corticotropin (ACTH), urinary free cortisol (UFC) levels and ovine (o) corticotropin-releasing hormone

stimulation (oCRH) test. For patients with prolactinomas, a serum prolactin (PRL) level. For those with thyrotropinomas, a thyrotropin releasing hormone (TRH) test; for those with somatotropinomas, serum growth hormone (GH) and insulin-like growth actor -I (IGF-I) levels and an oral glucose suppression test (oGST). For patients with gonadotropinomas, a-submit, luteinizing hormone (LH), LH ß-submit, and follicle-stimulating hormone (FSH) levels before and after stimulation with thyrotropin-releasing hormone (TRH). For patients with suspected non-secreting tumors, signs of pituitary stalk dysfunction and pituitary insufficiency are investigated.

Treatment of Pediatric Patients with Pituitary Tumors

Standard guidelines exist for the various types of tumors.[4] Surgery is recommended for masses that enlarge rapidly and threaten vision, regardless of the type of the tumor. Smaller tumors can be removed by transsphenoidal surgery. Larger tumors with suprasellar extensions can be removed by craniotomy or combined craniotomy and transsphenoidal surgery. Frequently, complete tumor excision is not feasible, and mere debulking is attempted.

Bromocriptine and pergolide, drugs with potent dopamine agonist activity, are the treatment of choice for prolactinomas (4), Bromocriptine doses ranging from 5 to 20 mg per day, with a gradual increase in dosage to avoid initial side effects such as nausea and orthostatic hypotension, are frequently sufficient to correct the hyperprolactinemia and cause regression of the tumor. Pergolide is a hundred fold more potent than bromocriptine, but experience with its clinical use is still limited. Years of treatment with dopamine agonists may be required for permanent cure. Bromocriptine, usually at higher doses (up to 25 mg/day), is occasionally helpful in the treatment of somatotropinomas and chromophobe adenomas.

Transsphenoidal surgery is a low-risk procedure (4, 5). Rare complications include total hypophysectomy and panhypopituitarism, cavernous sinus hemorrhage, transient or permanent diabetes insipidus or inappropriate antidiuretic hormone secretion syndrome, cerebrospinal fluid leaks, meningitis and blindness. Patients with pituitary function deficiencies are treated with appropriate replacement therapy (4-6).

The pituitary adenomas and the craniopharyngiomas are usually radioresistant. However, radiotherapy in doses as high as 5000 cGy divided into 200-cGy fractions is given for the treatment of corticotropinomas and somatotropinomas if surgery has been unsuccessful. Accordingly, radiotherapy of craniopharyngiomas after subtotal excision may decrease the incidence of recurrences.

Corticotropinomas respond relatively well to radiation, with about 70% to 80% of children cured after 1 to 2 years therapy. An alternative to radiation therapy is bilateral adrenalectomy. However, patients are then committed to life-long glucocorticoid and mineralocorticoid replacement. In approximately 15% of patients so treated, Nelson's syndrome (i.e. pituitary ACTH-secreting macroadenoma) develops within the 10 years after the adrenalectomy. Then, if the visual system is threatened, transsphenoidal surgery or radiation therapy is indicated.

Medications that inhibit adrenal secretion such as mitotane, or other steroidogenesis enzyme inhibitors such as aminoglutethimide, metyrapone, tristane, and ketoconazole may be employed to control the hypercortisolism in patients with Cushing's syndrome and inoperable or recurring pituitary tumors. Patients tolerate most of these drugs poorly, although ketoconazole is relatively well tolerated and frequently used. This drug has some hepatotoxicity, and liver function should be monitored in patients receiving it. Skin rash is a common complication of aminoglutethimide treatment.

When pituitary tumors are associated with pituitary hormone deficiencies, replacement treatments should be instituted. The deficiencies may develop after surgery. The replacement treatments include recombinant growth hormone (rGH) for GH deficiency, hydrocortisone for adrenal insufficiency, and thyroxine for hypothroidism. Testosterone enanthate and one of the estradol/progestin combinations (oral contraceptive pills) may be employed for the treatment of male and female hypogonadism, respectively, vasopressin is the treatment of choice for diabetes insipidus.

Prognosis

The prognosis for patients with pituitary tumors is generally good. These tumors are benign, although some have a tendency to invade adjacent structures. In the most recent report of pediatric patients with non-ACTH-secreting pituitary adenomas, those with microadenomas had a 70% operative cure rate and a 65% long term cure rate. The recurrence rate for microadenomas was 25%. Macroadenoma patients had a 33% operative cure rate, a 55% long term cure rate, and a recurrence rate of 33%. In the same series, macroadenoma patients required more aggressive adjuvant therapy and had higher rates of postsurgical pituitary dysfunction. Macroadenomas or craniopharyngiomas with suprasellar extensions are frequently difficult to remove completely and require adjuvant radiotherapy. Treatment of these tumors by surgery and/or irradiation may add to the endocrine morbidity. Monitoring of visual function is crucial. Most patients with ACTH-secreting tumors do well because of their relatively smaller tumors; thus, in our and other centers, the operative success in these tumors exceeds 90%, ACTH-secreting macroadrenomas, however, are more difficult to cure, just like the other tumors of the pituitary gland that exceed 1 cm in size.

Surgery or irradiation is rarely needed far hypothalamic hamartomas. The early identification of these tumors is necessary for timely treatment of the associated central precocious puberty with a GnRH-analog.

References

1   C.A. Strarakis, G.P. Chrousos. Endocrine Tumors. In: "Principles and Practice of Pediatric Oncology" Ed. by P.A. Pizzo & D. G. Poplack, 3rd Editian, J.B. Lippincott Co., Philadelphia, PA, 1996, pp947-976.

2   Hung W: Clinical Pediatric Endocrinology. St. Louis, Mosby Year Book, 1992.

3   Stratakis CA, Carney JA, Lin J-P, et al. Carney Complex, a familial multiple neoplasia and lentiginosis syndrome: analysis of 11 kindreds and linkage to the short arm of chromosome 2. J. Clin. Invest. 97 : 599, 1996.

4   Klibanski A, Zervas NT: Diagnosis and management of hormone-secreting pituitary adenomas. N Engl J Med 324 : 822, 1991.

5   Magiakou MA, Mastorakos G, Oldfield EH et al. Cushing syndrome in children and adolescents; presentation, diagnosis and therapy N. Engl. J. Med. 331 : 629, 1994.

6   Kane LA, Leinung MC, Scheithauser BW, et al. Pituitary adenomas in childhood and adolescence. J. Clin. Endocrinol. Metab. 79 : 1135, 1994.

~ A Superior Attitude ~

" The longer I live, the more I realize the impact of attitude on life. Attitude, to me, is more important than facts. It is more important than the past, than education, than money, than circumstances, than failures, than successes, than what other people think, say or do. It is more important than appearance, giftedness, or skill. It will make or break a company...a school...a team...a home. The remarkable thing is we have a choice everyday regarding the attitude we will embrace for that day. We cannot change our past...we cannot change the fact that people will act in a certain way...we cannot change the inevitable. The only thing we can do is plan on the one thing we have, and that is our superior attitude. I am convinced that life is 10% what happens to me and 90% how I react to it. A superior attitude will produce superior results."

Section V

Psychosocial Aspects of Pituitary Disease

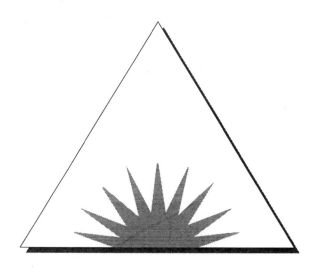

Second Edition

The Emotional Aspects of Pituitary Disease

Michael A Weitzner M.D., H. Lee Moffitt Cancer Center

It comes as no surprise that the most neglected effect of pituitary disease is the emotional distress that results from the massive disruption that occurs in one's life and the impact the illness has on one's loved ones and significant others. The impact of the emotional effects of pituitary disease was not lost on Harvey Cushing, perhaps one of the most influential surgeons of the 20th century, particularly with respect to the pituitary gland. Although not a trained psychiatrist, he greatly appreciated the impact that hormonal alterations from pituitary disease had on well-being and emotional functioning. In fact, he had stressed the need to study the emotional side effects of endocrine disorders as well as the impact that hormonal alterations had on preexisting coping patterns. Unfortunately, not much research has been conducted in this area. It is only in the last decade, the "Decade of the Brain," that the relationship between brain structures, neurohormones, neuropeptides, and emotions has become clearer.

Much research has been done in the last 10 years and our understanding of how the brain works has increased exponentially over the last several years. Through the increased use of functional brain imaging (i.e., PET [positron emission tomography]), we have learned just how truly interrelated all cortical and subcortical areas (i.e., midbrain and brainstem) are. We also recognize how important the frontal lobes are to our overall mental and brain functioning. The frontal lobes are our "governing bodies" for behavior and they may be affected not only by direct insults such as trauma or space-occupying lesions, but also by problems that arise in other, more distant parts of the brain, such as the hypothalamus and pituitary gland. It is safe to say, then, that behavior is comprised of two components: those related to environmental influences (i.e., family, work, etc.) and biological influences (i.e., frontal lobe function and effects from the limbic system, the seat of our primitive, base emotions). Environmental influences on behavior determine and mold the way people express and control their emotions. These influences are not consistent in everyone since people come from different family and social backgrounds. As a result, our ability to tolerate stress and frustration are different. Therefore, the ways in which people handle the "emotional side effects" of hormonal alterations resulting from pituitary disease will also be different, dependent on how people have handled stress and their emotions in the past.

From the biological perspective, the hypothalamus and pituitary gland play an important role in certain aspects of emotional functioning. We know that the two are responsible for maintaining the internal milieu. They are responsible for coordinating electrolyte balance, blood glucose levels, body temperature, metabolic rate, autonomic tone, aspects of sexual functioning, our day-night cycles (e.g., circadian rhythms), and regulation of our immune system. The hypothalamic-pituitary axis also has close connections with the certain limbic structures (the more primitive areas of our brain) which have important roles in the regulation of four types of behavior: (1) memory and learning; (2) regulation of drive; (3) emotional coloring of experience; and (4) higher control of hormonal and autonomic tone. As mentioned above, the impact that the hypothalamic-pituitary axis has on these functions is determined not only by the degree of acute or chronic psychological stress that is present but also how a person has learned to deal with that stress.

The hypothalamic-pituitary axis also has an impact on frontal lobe functioning and, therefore, behavior and affect. We have a greater appreciation, through recent research, of the frontal lobes and their importance in regulating behavior. Consequently, it has become clearer to what degree they are responsible for motivation and drive. Apathy is a term that has come to be used to reflect this absence of motivation and drive. However, apathy has also been used to describe a flat affect or emotional unresponsiveness, suggesting depression. Defining apathy in this way creates much ambiguity since a person's emotional state and the motivation that person has to do things are not the same. Much research has been done to further define apathy. As a result of research with neuropeptides and neurotransmitters, apathy has emerged as a recognized syndrome. Since the hypothalamus and pituitary have an indirect role on motivation, this syndrome of apathy has a direct bearing on pituitary disease and may explain many of the symptoms people with pituitary disease experience during the course of their treatment and recovery.

Apathy has three components: (1) observable behavior, such as decreased goal-directed behavior; (2) emotional content, such as a decreased emotional reaction to situations and distress; and (3) thought content, as evidenced by decreased goal-directed thoughts, goals for the future, interests, and curiosity. It is not simply the lack of emotion that defines apathy; it is the presence of diminished emotional responsiveness to goal-related events. It is, therefore, the "not caring" that defines apathy. This problem is particularly difficult to assess and manage. The primary reason for this difficulty relates to the fact that the patient suffering from apathy rarely refers him- or herself for an evaluation of apathy. This may be because the person experiencing it does not recognize it for what it is. At other times, particularly when in its milder form, the patient does comment about the apathy, but then it is not taken seriously by the family or the health care professional. Many times it is discounted by families, patients, and health care professionals as depression or "she(he) is just feeling sorry for her(him)self." However, apathy may add further stress to a family that is already heavily stressed by the illness. It can also place a tremendous burden on the spouse or significant other who must take on additional responsibilities of the household, personal and family relationship that would have been done by the person with apathy.

How, then, is the hypothalamic-pituitary axis involved in these emotional and behavioral changes? Many of these neuropsychiatric disturbances seen in pituitary disease are directly related to the size of the tumor and the effect the tumor has on surrounding brain structures as the tumor extends beyond the sella turcica. Hormonal alterations occurring as a result of the tumor also play an important role in the etiology of these neuropsychiatric symptoms. Forward extension of the tumor may involve the frontal lobes directly by causing compression of normal brain tissue. This scenario would cause involvement of areas responsible for higher level executive and cognitive functions, resulting in the following problems: (1) impaired problem-solving behavior; (2) problems with focused attention and concentration; (3) difficulty completing tasks due to an inability to do tasks in an ordered fashion; and (4) decreased control of emotions. People tend to be more irritable and depressed-appearing. Forward extension may also occur laterally to the temporal lobes. Problems, here, tend to be more personality-focused, with increased irritability, intensification of previously dominant personality traits, coping mechanisms, and adaptive styles.

As mentioned above, emotional and behavioral problems are also the result of hormonal alterations. There is much research which has documented the psychiatric effects of hyperprolactinemia, hypercortisolism, and increased levels of growth hormone. A common syndrome to all of these altered hormonal states is depression. To varying degrees, irritability and personality change are also observed. The most common personality change observed is an exaggeration of a previously well-adapted character trait. For example, the person who was somewhat obsessive (i.e., orderly, regimented, etc.) at work and relaxed at home would now be so regimented to everyone else's exasperation. Or, take the person who was high-strung before the pituitary tumor and is now hyper-irritable and snappy all the time. More research is being done to determine exactly what the increased levels of hormone are doing on a neurotransmitter level in the brain.

Thus, the common denominator in these emotional and behavioral problems seen in people with pituitary disease appears to be the disturbance of neurotransmission or neuromodulation at the level of the hypothalamic microenvironment. The hypothalamus is strategically placed between neural systems associated with the amnesia syndromes (i.e., hippocampus, amygdala, mammillary bodies, mesiodorsal thalamus, and basal forebrain). It is the center of neuroendocrine, autonomic, and homeostatic regulation and has a major role in the expression of emotional behavior. It also has a connection to the limbic lobes. Finally, many hypothalamic peptides are thought to serve as neuromodulators as well as having a role in anterior pituitary function. Normal patterns of secretion are likely to be easily disrupted by pituitary tumors and/or their treatment. Treatment for these emotional and behavioral problems is available but is rather intricate, oftentimes involving the use of different medications which affect different neuro transmitters. Medications are also only part of the treatment. Individual and family counseling is often necessary to help the person and the family system adapt to this major disruption. Families are often emotionally exhausted by the emotional roller-coaster rides the person with pituitary disease experiences. Without professional help, previously well-adapted and functioning families are destroyed not by the tumor itself, but the emotional havoc wrought in its wake. This is preventable; it only takes a mind willing to see "the forest through the trees."

References

1   Fava GA, Sonino N, Morphy MA (1993) Psychosomatic view of endocrine disorders. Psychotherapy and Psychosomatics 59, 20-33.

2   Cummings JL (1993) Frontal-subcortical circuits and human behavior. Archives of Neurology 50, 873-880. 3. Marin RS (1996) Apathy: Concept, syndrome, neural mechanisms, and treatment. Seminars in Clinical Neuropsychiatry 1, 304-314.

Psychosocial Aspects of Endocrine Disease

Nicoletta Sonino, M.D., Division of Endocrinology
Institute of Semeiotica Medica, University of Padova, Italy

This article was originally published by Karger in *Psychotherapy and Psychosomatics*, 1997. Reprinted with permission.

Introduction

Harvey Cushing was a pioneer in the psychosomatic approach to endocrine disease. He outlined major issues of interest in endocrinology: (a) the study of the role of psychic traumas' in the pathogenesis of some endocrine conditions (we are not blind to the fact that there may lurk in the background some primary derangement of the nervous system itself), (b) the effect on the psyche and nervous system of chronic states of glandular overactivity or underactivity, currently subsumed under the rubric of organic affective disorders, as well as he fight against the psychic incapacitation's of the malady by patients, (C) the ailment of residual symptoms after adequate treatment (it is even more common for a physician or surgeon to eradicate or otherwise treat the obvious focus of disease, with more or less success, and to leave the mushroom of psychic deviations to vex and confuse the patient for long afterwards, if not actually to imbalance him[1]. These aspects have been highlighted by recent research evidence and have been partially considered previously[2,3]. They are summed up together with the scanty data of new research evidence for an undated psychosocial comprehension of endocrine disease. Indeed, despite an upsurge of interest in areas of psychoneuroendocrinology dealing with the limbic-hypothalamic control of hormonal function, the relationship of endocrine disease to psychological distress has been largely neglected in clinical practice.

Life Events

Short-term acute, experimental stresses have become the focus of a large volume of endocrine research[4]. However the validity of laboratory stresses as models for those of real life has been questioned, and the extension and applicability of laboratory results to long-term situations is purely inferential. Many kinds of psychological stress, both acute and chronic, have been shown to involve the hypothalamic-pituitary-adrenal axis. Psychological factors may either raise or lower the level of pituitary-adrenal activity Some important variables include the quality of emotional reaction, the style and effectiveness of psychological defenses, and whether the threat is of an acute or chronic nature[5]. Chronic stress incorporates several elements, including life events. By 'life events' are meant discrete changes in the subjects social or personal environment that should be external and verifiable rather than internal or psychological. They may play a substantial role in uncovering a person's vulnerability to a particular physical or psychiatric disorder[6]. This has been demonstrated for some endocrine conditions by structured methods of data collection and control groups confirming clinical observations scattered throughout the literature.

Several intriguing issues have emerged in studying Cushing's Syndrome. Stressful life events in the year before the first signs of disease onset were investigated in 66 consecutive patients with Cushing's Syndrome of various etiologies and in a control group of 66 healthy subjects matched for sociodemographic variables, using Paykel's Interview for Recent Life Events[7]. The patients with Cushing's Syndrome reported significantly more losses, undesirable and uncontrolled events than controls. The results did not depend on the well-known relationship between life events and depression, since there were no differences between patients with and without major depression. A subdivision between patients with pituitary-dependent (Cushing's Syndrome) and pituitary-independent (primary adrenal hyperfunction or ectopic ACTH production) forms, compared with their matched controls, indicated a causal role for stressful life events exclusively in Cushing's Syndrome[7], supporting the hypothesis of a limbic-hypothalamic involvement in the pathogenesis of this condition[8]. The results in Cushing's Syndrome are remarkably similar to those obtained comparing depressed patients with the general population, and in particular to those of a study performed with the same methods, in the same geographic area[9]. This adds to other analogies between Cushing's Syndrome and non-endocrine major depression, and calls for further investigation on the pathogenetic mechanisms of both conditions.

Life events have been investigated in 70 patients with Graves' Disease by the same rigorous method employed for Cushing's Syndrome[10], and recently in a sample of 100 patients[11], and found to be significantly more frequent than in controls. The same conclusions were drawn by mailing a questionnaire about life changes to 219 patients with Graves' Disease and 372 control subjects[12], and by a self-reporting questionnaire recalling life events, daily stress and coping in 95 patients compared to their matched controls[13]. Stressful life events may affect the regulatory mechanism of immune function in a number of ways[4,14]. Within the complex pathogenesis of autoimmune thyroid hyperfunction, these studies, as well as several clinical uncontrolled observations, emphasize the role of emotional stress.

Unfortunately, the contribution of recent life events to the onset of endocrine disorders such as hyperprolactinemia and polycystic ovary syndrome has not been investigated in a controlled way by reliable probes. The coexistence of life stress and affective disturbances has been shown to particularly affect the pulsatile release of plasma LH in hypothalamic amenorrhea[15] and to trigger the onset of rapid weight gain in women[16], suggesting the need for a structured psychodiagnostic approach in the assessment of neuroendocrine responses to environmental stimuli.

Quality of Life

Depressive symptoms have been associated with almost all endocrine diseases, and in a few of them (Cushing's Syndrome, Addison's Disease, hyperthyroidism, hypothyroidism, hyperprolactinemia) they may often reach the intensity of a major depressive disorder and the quality of organic mood syndrome. It is noteworthy that major depression affects Cushing's Syndrome more than any other endocrine and non-endocrine medical condition[17,18] with no significant difference between pituitary dependent and pituitary independent forms[17]. Other mental manifestations, ranging from anxiety to cognitive impairment and psychotic disturbances may occur, even though to a lesser degree than depression[19,20]. Psychological symptoms may have a profound influence on quality of life (i.e., function in daily life, productivity, emotional stability and well-being) and on how the endocrine disease process is experienced.

While the psychological implications of GH deficiency in childhood (disturbances in identity formation, social withdrawal, impaired self-esteem, distorted body image) have been emphasized in several investigations, only recently has attention been focused on the compromised quality of life of adults with GH deficiency[21-23]. They were found to have difficulties in leading a normal professional and private life[24]. Both physical and psychological improvement upon recombinant GH treatment was observed in double-blind, placebo-controlled, cross-over studies concerned with GH-deficient adults[25]. The high prevalence of depression, hostility, anxiety and irritability in the symptom complex of hyperprolactinemia and their variable response to either psychotherapy or pharmacological intervention (bromocriptine vs. antidepressants) deserves more consideration in the perspective of patients' long term well-being.

Psychological symptoms are often among the prodromes of endocrine disorders, as shown for depression in Cushing's Syndrome and Graves Disease[17]. It is not clear whether they represent the first signs of hormonal derangements, due to the sensitivity of the brain to such changes, or whether they constitute a predisposing factor for hypothalamic-pituitary activation. Depression in Cushing's syndrome may be an example of the former, anxiety and phobic disorders in hyperthyroidism or early neurotic traits in hyperprolactinemia may be examples of the latter. In this view, an endocrine etiology should be taken into account in patients not responding to standard psychiatric treatments.

Hirsutism is widely recognized to exert great emotional impact upon patients, even when amounts of excess hair are small and medically insignificant. Although it does not entail major affective disturbances, unlike Cushing's Syndrome, hyperthyroidism, and hyperprolactinemia, quality of life appears to be compromised. In a recent investigation, women with hirsutism belonging to the spectrum of disorders from idiopathic hirsutism to polycystic ovary syndrome reported significantly more social fears than a normal control group[27]. In addition to pharmacological and/or cosmetic measures, a role for psychological approaches more specific than simple reassurance was therefore suggested. On the other hand, patients who complain of hirsutism with no objective evidence provide an example of abnormal illness behavior in endocrinology, which may cause substantial invalidism. In adult female patients with congenital adrenal hyperplasia, quality of life was investigated as to the critical issue of partnership and sexuality[28]. Patients reported impaired body image and lack of female identification compared to healthy controls. There were no significant differences among the various clinical forms of this condition. Further longitudinal research may help identify specific problems and improve the quality of psychological care for such patients.

Response to Treatment

A treatment primarily directed to the physical condition may be more effective than psychotropic drugs in organic affective syndromes associated with endocrine disease. Examples are provided by the favorable effects of steroid synthesis inhibitors (i.e., metyrapone and ketoconazole) upon depression in Cushing's Syndrome or antithyroid agents on anxiety in hyperthyroidism. Clinical endocrinologists may thus tend to underestimate psychiatric symptoms as readily suppressible by adequate medical or surgical treatment. However, disappearance of psychiatric symptoms upon proper endocrine treatment is not always the case[19,20]. In our experience and in previous investigations using definite diagnostic criteria for depression. About 70% of patients fully recovered from their depression after successful treatment of Cushing's Syndrome, whereas there were no substantial changes in the others or even worsening in some[17]. In those who actually deteriorated, the value of appropriate psychiatric intervention was underscored. It is of interest to note that one of them responded to an antidepressant drug she had been exposed to unsuccessfully while being hypercortisolemic. Similarly, while phobias and hyperthyroidism frequently coexist, and detection and treatment of hyperthyroidism were found to also solve patients' long-standing agoraphobia[29], successful management of thyroid hyperfunction may not always be sufficient to overcome an anxiety disorder. Since anxiety itself may increase a person's vulnerability to hyperthyroidism, it is important to evaluate the coexistence of phobias and hyperthyroidism on an individual basis[30].

Establishing etiological priorities in affective disorders associated with endocrine disease is a complex task that requires considerable clinical skills, and becomes necessary when the patient responds only partially to ongoing treatment. On the other hand, long-standing endocrine disorders may imply a degree of irreversibility of the pathological process and induce highly individualized affective responses based on each patients' psychological assets and liabilities. Unrealistic hopes of cure may foster discouragement and apathy. A psychosomatic approach could be therefore important in the convalescence and rehabilitation phase.

Conclusion

As outlined by the above examples, the interrelationship between hormonal abnormalities and psychological factors is complex and should be viewed in a multifactorial frame of reference. A first simple implication would be for the clinician to be reminded of the necessity for the same routine analysis of his patient's mental status that is commonly given to the alimentary, circulatory, excretory, neuromuscular and other functions[1]. Yet, a new interest in a global approach to the endocrine patient should be stimulated by research advances in the understanding of behavioral-neural-endocrine-immune system interactions[14]. In the perspective of integrated psychoneuroimmunology, some diseases may be better interpreted as the final common pathway of different pathophysiological mechanisms. In this sense, a paradigmatic case is provided by the 'mysterious' chronic fatigue syndrome, in which the quality of life is highly compromised. and both minor immunological and endocrine abnormalities have been described[31]. A contribution to the psychosocial understanding of endocrine disease may also be offered by the research domain of chronoendocrinology and its use of chrononeuroendocrine markers, such as melatonin[32].

Patients have become increasingly aware of the issues raised in this brief review. Their difficulties in coping with endocrine illness have led to the foundation of several patients' associations in recent years.

Acknowledgement

The present study was supported by grant 545/01/94 from Regione Veneto (Venice, Italy).

References

1   Cushing H: Psychic disturbances associated with disorders of the ductless glands. Am J Insanity 1913;69:965-990.
2   Sonino N, Fava GA, Fallo F, Boscaro M: Psychological distress and quality of life in endocrine disease, Psychother Psychosom 1990;43;140-144.
3   Fava GA, Sonino N, Morphy MA: Psychosomatic view of endocrine disorders. Psychother Psychosom 1993;59:20-33.
4   Stratakis CA, Chrousos GP: Neuroendocrinology and pathophysiology of the stress system. Ann NY Acad Sci 1995;771:1-18.
5   Vingerhoerts AJJM, Assies J: Psychoneuroendocrinology of stress and emotions. Psychother Psychosom 1991;55:69-75.
6   Theorell T: Critical life changes. A review of research. Psychother Psychosom 1992;57:108-117.
7   Sonino N, Fava GA, Boscaro M: A role for life events in the pathogenesis of Cushing's disease. Clin Endocrinol 1993;38:261-264.
8   Kriger DT: Pathophysiology of Cushing's disease. Endocr Rev 1983;4:22-43.
9   Fava GA, Munari F, Pavan L, Kellner R: Life events and depression. J Affect Disord 1981;3:159-165.
10 Sonino N, Girelli ME, Boscaro M, Fallo F, Busnardo B, Fava GA: Life events in the pathogenesis of Graves' disease. A controlled study. Acta Endocrinol (Copenh) 1993;128:293-296.
11 Radosavljevic VR, Jankovic SM, Marinkovic JM: Stressful life events in the pathogenesis of Graves'disease. Eur J Endocrinol 1996;134:699-701.
12 Winsa B, Adami HO, Bergstrom R, Gamstedt A, Dahlberg PA, Adamson U, Jansson R, Karlsson A: Stressful life events and Graves' disease. Lancet 1991;338:1475-1479.
13 Kung AWC:Life events, daily stresses and coping in patients with Graves' disease. Clin Endocrinol 1995;42:303-308.
14 Ader R, Cohen N, Felten D: Psychoneuroimmunology: Interactions between the nervous system and the immune system. Lancet 1995;345:99-103.
15 Facchinetti F, Fava M, Fioroni L, Genazzani AD, Genazzani A: Stressful life events and affective disorders inhibit pulsatile LH secretion in hypothalamic amenorrhea. Psychoneuroindocrinology 1993;18:397-404.

16 Ferreira MF, Sobrinho LG, Pires JS, Silva MES, Santos MA, Sousa MFF: Endocrine and psychological evaluation of women with recent weight gain. Psychoneuroendocrinology 1995;20:53-63.

17 Sonino N, Fava GA, Belluardo P, Girelli ME, Boscaro M: Course of depression in Cushing's syndrome: Response to treatment and comparison with Graves' disease. Horm Res 1993;39:202-206.

18 Dorn LD, Burgess ES, Dubbet B, Simpson SE, Fridman T, Kling M: Psychopathology in patients with endogenous Cushing's syndrome: 'Atypical' or melancholic features. Clin Endocrinol 1995;43:433-442.

19 Stern RA, Robinson B, Thorner AR, Arruda JE, Prohaska ML, Prange AJ: A survey study of neuropsychiatric complaints in patients with Graves' disease. J Neuropsychiatry 1996;8:181-185.

20 Leentjens AFG, Kappers EJ: Persistent cognitive defects after corrected hypothyroidism. Psychopathology 1995;28:235-237.

21 Rosen T, Wiren L, Wilhelmsen L, Wiklund I, Bengtsson BA: Decreased psychological well being in adult patients with growth hormone deficiency. Clin Endocrinol 1994;40:111-116.

22 Wallymahmed ME, Baker GA, Humphris MD, MacFarlane IA: The development, reliability and validity of a disease specific quality of life model for adults with growth hormone deficiency. Clin Endocrinol 1996;44:403-411.

23 Bengtsson BA: Growth hormone deficiency in adults: A new indication for recombinant human growth hormone. J Intern Med 1996;239:283-286.

24 Takano K, Tanaka T, Saito T, and the Connittee for the Study group of Adult GH deficency: Psychosocial adjustment in a large cohort of adults with growth hormone deficiency treated with growth hormone in childhood: Summary of a questionnaire survey. Acta Paediatr Scand 1994;399 (supl):16-19.

25 Bengtsson BA, Eden S, Lonn L, Kvist H, Stokland A, Lindstedt G, et al: Treatment of adults with growth hormone (GH) deficiency with recombinant human GH. J Clin Endocrinol Metab 1993;76:309-317.

26 Sobrinho LG, Almeida-Costa JM: Hyperprolactinaemia as a result of immaturity or regression: the concept of maternal subroutine. Psychother Psychosom 1992;57:128-132.

27 Sonino N, Faba GA, Mani E, Belluardo P: Quality of life of hirsute women. Postgrad Med J 1993;69:186-189.

28 Kuhnle U, Bullinger M, Schwarz HP, Knorr D: Partnership and sexuality in adult female patients with congenital adrenal hyperplasia. First results of a cross-sectional quality-of-life evaluation. J Steroid Biochem Molec Biol 1993;45:123-126.

29 Emanuele MA, Brooks MH, Gordon DL, Braithwaite SS: Agoraphobia and hyperthyroidism. Am J Med 1989;86:484-486.

30 Matsubayashi S, Tamai H, Matsumoto Y, Tamagawa K, Mukuta T, Morita T, Kubo C: Graves' disease after the onset of panic disorder. Psychother Psychosom 1996;65:277-280.

31 Demitrack MA, Dale JK, Straus SE, Laue L, Listwak SJ, Druesi MJP, et al: Evidence for impaired activation of the hypothalamic pituitary-adrenal axis in patients with chronic fatigue syndrome. J Clin Endocrinol Metab 1993;73:1224-1234.

32 Webb SM, Puig-Domingo M: Role of melatonin in health and disease. Clin Endocrinol 1995;42:221-234.

Psychosocial Aspects of Endocrine Disease

149

Diurnal Endocrinology and Sleep Disorders

Douglas C. Aziz, M.D., Ph.D., Specialty Laboratories
Santa Monica, California

Diurnal and Circadian Rhythms

The term diurnal rhythm designates the reproducible day-to-day changes in endocrine hormone secretion and serum concentrations. This diurnal variation is a function of both endogenous (internal pacemakers) and exogenous stimuli. Exogenous stimuli than can affect the diurnal variation in hormone secretion include sleep-wake cycles, light-dark cycles and postprandial (meal) effects. By definition, the circadian rhythm is the endogenous endocrine pacemaker that varies on a daily periodic basis in the absence of sleep, regular light-dark cycles and regular feeding. These cycles can be disrupted for a variety of reasons and affect mental and physical attitude and sleep patterns. The disorders of sleep associated with pituitary tumors are well described. Most transmeridian travelers have experienced "jet lag" because the light-dark and sleep-wake cycles are not synchronized with the endogenous circadian rhythms. Studies involving sleep deprivation, abrupt changes in light-dark cycles, photic effects, shift-workers and rapid time zone changes (jet lag) have elucidated the relative contribution of endogenous circadian rhythm versus other factors affecting the diurnal rhythms.[1,2]

The endogenous circadian period is not exactly 24 hours. In "free run" experiments in which subjects remain awake, eat an identical snack hourly, and remain in an environment of constant temperature, light and social cues, subjects naturally develop a rhythmic circadian period of approximately 25 hours. In natural daily environments, the endogenous clock is reset daily by light-dark cues to entrain the diurnal rhythm to 24 hours. Evidence for resetting the endogenous clock is demonstrated in experiments where light pulses are presented in early subjective night and are interpreted as late dusk, delaying the succeeding rhythm; light pulses presented late in subjective night are interpreted as early dawn and cause the next phase to advance.[2]

Diurnal Variation in Pituitary Hormone Concentration

Plasma growth hormone (GH), prolactin, thyroid-stimulating hormone (TSH), luteinizing hormone (LH), adrenocorticotropin hormone (ACTH) and melatonin are all elevated during nighttime sleep. Plasma GH exhibits a low stable concentration interrupted by bursts of secretion. The plasma concentration is extremely pulsatile, demonstrating abrupt and profound increases immediately followed by sharp decreases. A major surge occurs in the first 2 hours after sleep onset and is associated with deep slow-wave sleep, followed by less intense pulses during sleep and wakefulness.[2] Secretion is blunted when subjects are sleep deprived, but can be induced when subjects nap during the day.

Plasma prolactin concentration follows a sinusoidal pattern with a major and prolonged increase after the first few hours of sleep which does not subside until 1-2 hours after awakening. Sleep deprivation blunts the response, but the evening following a sleep-deprived night is associated with concentrations higher than in controls.[3] An endogenous circadian rhythm is a minor component of the diurnal variation. Like GH, a nap during the day will induce prolactin secretion.

The elevation in plasma ACTH concentration occurs much later in the night than GH or prolactin and peaks in the early morning. There is a constant, almost linear decrease in plasma ACTH concentration during the day and evening, reaching an ebb several hours after the onset of sleep. Rhythmicity of ACTH and other hormones of the corticotropic axis persists during sleep deprivation, light-dark experiments and changes in meals, including fasting and continuous glucose infusion, indicating that the corticotropic axis has a strong natural circadian component.[1] Serum cortisol concentrations, which parallel plasma ACTH concentrations, have a diurnal amplitude variation. Modulation of concentration is mediated through changes in pulse amplitude rather than pulse frequency.[1] Sleep-deprivation has a small effect in reducing the amplitude by 10%–20%. Because of the strong endogenous circadian pacemaker, the cortisol rhythm can take 5-10 days to fully recover from abrupt shifts (6-8 hours) in light-dark and sleep-wake cycles. A more rapid shift can be achieved with critically timed bright light exposure.

TSH normally exhibits low concentrations during the day, increases abruptly at 8:00 pm by approximately 75%, remains elevated throughout the night and abruptly decreases on awakening. Low-amplitude pulsatile fluctuation in the TSH concentration occurs throughout the 24-hour period. Sleep-deprivation causes either no change, a slight increase or a slight decrease in nighttime TSH concentrations. On the evening following the sleep-deprived night, TSH concentrations are depressed, even below daytime concentrations.[3]

Prepubertal children exhibit episodic low amplitude and low frequency gonadotropin-releasing hormone (GnRH) and luteinizing hormone-releasing hormone (LHRH) pulses, which persist throughout the day and night. Episodic secretion of GnRH results in pulsatile secretion of the pituitary gonadotropins, LH and FSH. The low amplitude and low frequency pulses increase in amplitude and frequency with the onset of puberty. The diurnal rhythm becomes more pronounced as the child approaches puberty, with LH amplitude increasing during sleep in the peripubertal stage. Later in puberty the pulses increase throughout the day and are quite variable with slowing of pulse frequency and increase in amplitude during the night.[4] The pubertal diurnal variation persists in sleep-deprived subjects, albeit with reduced magnitude.

In the adult male, testosterone exhibits a diurnal variation with an amplitude of about 50% of the mean. The nocturnal rise of testosterone appears to be independent of sleep. In elderly men (>age 70 years), the diurnal variation in LH is lost but continues for testosterone.

In women, the early follicular phase of the menstrual cycle is characterized by large and infrequent LH pulses which slow nocturnally. Pulse amplitude reductions and pulse frequency increases during the midfollicular phase are less affected by sleep. During the late follicular phase, pulse amplitude again increases, and no diurnal modulation is observed. In the luteal phase, the diurnal variation returns with nocturnal slowing of the pulses. Higher LH concentrations that occur in premenopausal women as they approach menopause are due to increases in pulse amplitude.[5]

Melatonin and the Pineal Gland

Light perceived by the eyes stimulates a multisynaptic pathway in which signals are transmitted through the supra chiasmatic nucleus (SCN), spinal cord, and superior cervical ganglion to the pineal gland where melatonin is secreted into the circulation during darkness. Blind individuals who are unable to synchronize the light-dark cycle or individuals who suffer from delayed onset sleep insomnia benefit from exogenous melatonin. Melatonin is used in the resynchronization of diurnal rhythms in transmeridian travelers.[6]

The interaction between melatonin and the hypothalmic-pituitary axes is complex. Increased circulating melatonin causes inhibition of GnRH, and treatment of men with testosterone causes a fall in the melatonin concentration. Most patients with pituitary tumors, independent of the secretory (ACTH, prolactin, GH) or non-secretory nature of the adenoma, do not have altered melatonin secretory rhythms. However, some patients, particularly those with large tumors, can have an abolished melatonin rhythm or abnormally high diurnal variations in melatonin. These tumors may have invaded into the neural connections between the hypothalmus and the spinal cord, disrupting the normal retinal-pineal synaptic pathway.[6]

Sleep Disorders

Sleep disorders include the "delayed sleep phase syndrome" which accounts for about 10% of all patients who report difficulty sleeping, where patients have difficulty initiating sleep, but have normal sleep duration and architecture. Less common is the "advanced sleep phase syndrome" where patients are hypersomnolent in the evening, fall asleep early and wake up early and refreshed[2]. The "hypernychthemeral syndrome" causes insomnia due to a free-running sleep-wake cycle. The proximate cause of the hypernychthemeral syndrome can be due to a defective entrainment mechanism. The circadian pace maker, perhaps related to melatonin secretion is not set to the normal daily light-dark cycle. Blindness or interruption of the retinal-pineal neural pathways alters the diurnal variation in melatonin secretion and can cause patients to experience unentrained sleep patterns.

References

1   Van Cauter E. Diurnal and ultradian rhythms in human endocrine function: a minireview. Horm Res 1 990;34:45-53.
2   Schwartz WJ. A clinician's primer on the circadian clock: its localization, function, and resetting. Adv Intern Med 1993;38:81-1 07.
3   von Treuer K, Norman TR, Armstrong SM. Overnight human plasma melatonin, cortisol, prolactin, TSH, under conditions of normal sleep deprivation, and sleep recovery. J Pineal Res 1996;20:7-14.
4   Tenover JS, Matsumoto AM, Clifton DK, Bremner WJ. Age-related alterations in the circadian rhythms of pulsatile luteinizing hormone and testosterone secretion in healthy men. J Gerontol 988;43:MI 63-9.
5   Reame NE, Kelch RP, Beitins IZ, Yu M, Zawacki CM, Padmanabhan V. Age effects of follicle-stimulating hormone and pulsatile luteinizing hormone secretion across the menstrual cycle of premenopausal women. J Clin Endocrinol Metab 1996;81:1512-8.
6   Webb SM, Pulg-Domingo M. Role of melatonin in health and disease. Olin Endocrinol 1995;42:221-234.

Emotional Aspects of Hyperprolactinemia

L.G. Sobrinho, M.D., Department of Endocrinology, Portuguese Cancer Institute, Lisboa, Portugal

Like all other hormones, prolactin is a circulating substance that acts as a messenger within a complex network of information, connecting every cell within a living organism such that some form of coherent and purposeful functioning is achieved.

Hormonal levels, or variations thereof, may induce neural changes that may, ultimately, translate into changes in behavior, emotions and feelings. On the other hand, environmental changes, once perceived by the sensory organs and interpreted by the nervous system, evoke adaptive responses that may include measurable changes in circulating hormonal levels.

The relationships between hyperprolactinemia and emotions can be looked at from three points of view:

♦ Effects of hyperprolactinemia on the central nervous system.
♦ Effects of the environment on prolactin secretion.
♦ Emotional changes associated with the mass effect of a pituitary tumor and with the knowledge by the patient that he/she has a tumor in the "brain."

I. Effect of Hyperprolactinemia on the Central Nervous System

Prolactin and the Brain

Prolactin *does* act upon the central nervous system and produces behavioral changes.

Since prolactin does not cross the blood-brain barrier (vessels in the brain are sheathed in such a way that only selected circulating substances enter the nervous tissue), peripheral prolactin is likely to enter the cerebro-spinal fluid (CSF) via the choroid plexuses (specific structures localized in the cerebral ventricles that secrete the CSF and transport some substances to the brain) where the specific binding for prolactin is twenty fold that in the hypothalamus and/or by retrograde transport through the portal vessels.

Prolactin concentrations in the cerebrospinal fluid are about 20% of that in the blood and fluctuate in parallel with it. Prolactin binding sites within the central nervous system have been identified in the hypothalamus, choroid plexuses and, to a lesser extent, in the substantia nigra, a structure of the midbrain containing an important number of dopamine producing neurons. There is no evidence of specific prolactin binding in other regions of the brain.

There is also a prolactin synthetic pool in the brain, separate from that of the anterior pituitary. The main region where prolactin is produced is the hypothalamus, although its concentration there is four orders of magnitude below that found in the pituitary. The role of this neural prolactinergic system is unknown. It is nevertheless interesting that prolactin, a recognized hormone, is also a neurotransmitter, or modulator of neurotransmission. To make the situation even more complex prolactin is also synthetized by cells of the immune system that are, simultaneously, targets for its actions.

Prolactin modulates the activity and receptor density of dopamine and exerts a modulatory effect on central dopamine transmission. The administration of prolactin or a state of hyperprolactinemia stimulate the turnover of dopamine in some brain structures and inhibit it in others. In humans, hyperprolactinemia increases hypothalamic dopaminergic tone.

Prolactin also appears to increase the central opiate tone. Rats with transplantation- induced hyperprolactinemia present with analgesia, reduced response to electric shock and reduced core temperature, effects that can be reversed by naloxone, an opioid antagonist. These observations are consistent with the findings, in a similar model of hyperprolactinemic rats, of an increased expression of the proopiomelanocortin (a precursor of b-endorphin, an opioid) gene in the arcuate nucleus and of increased concentration of b-endorphin in hypophyseal portal blood.

Opioids markedly reduce hypothalamic dopamine and stimulate prolactin secretion, suggesting the possibility of a positive feed back system in which prolactin increases the secretion of opioids that, in turn, increase he secretion of prolactin (for specific references and further information pertinent to this and to the following part see ref[1].

Metabolic and Behavioral Actions of Prolactin

Most biological functions of prolactin are, across species, associated with metabolic and behavioral adaptation to parenthood and inhibition of sexual behavior. A few examples of metabolic effects of prolactin that are adaptive for the success of the parental function are:

1 - Increase in food intake by female rats, an effect also observed in birds, with consequent increase in the deposition of fat and weight gain which, as mentioned above, fulfils an adaptive role in building reserves for feeding the offspring.

2 - Increase in the mobilization of fat in the puerperal period and of its uptake by the breast.

3 - Priming of the breast and stimulation of the production of milk in mammals and of the crop sac secretion in birds.

4 - Increase in the mesenteric circulation in birds (thereby increasing the temperature of the skin) and promotion of the brood spots (featherless spots of the abdominal skin), such that the heat transfer to the eggs is maximized during hatching.

Deposition of fat and weight gain are essential in the adaptation for motherhood also in women. It occurs in pregnancy, but also in pseudopregnancy and as a common early finding in the natural history of prolactinomas, both in women[2] and in men[3]. These latter associations clearly emphasize that, however important the placental hormones may be (and are) in the deposition of fat during pregnancy, this essential adaptive function is also secured by other mechanisms, prolactin secretion being one of them.

Maternal behavior

Prolactin is unnecessary for the expression of maternal behavior since such behavior is seen in hypophysectomized, virgin, female rats when exposed to pups. However, the latency period of this effect is considerably shortened by the administration of prolactin. Non hypophysectomized estrogen-progesterone primed adult female rats given bromocriptine respond slowly to foster young whereas a similar group to which prolactin is added respond much faster. The latency to display full maternal behavior, i.e., retrieving and grouping all test pups and crouching, is about 6 days in the former group and 2 days in the latter. Also, the administration of bromocriptine to young prepubertal male rats (who respond much faster when exposed to pups than postpubertal ones and have slightly elevated prolactin levels during this period of heightened sensitivity) significantly prolongs the latency to behave maternally. Again, administration of prolactin reverses the inhibitory effect of bromocriptine and restores the lower latency of the maternal response. In hamsters, one single postpartum administration of bromocriptine induces eating of the pups by the dams. In rabbits, prolactin stimulates the production of a pheramone by the nipple which facilitates the nipple search behavior by the pups.

Just as prolactin is an effector substance in the induction of maternal behavior, also its secretion is stimulated whenever such behavior might be appropriate. Upon exposure to pups the secretion of prolactin by intact rats is strongly stimulated. Therefore, the relationships between prolactin release and maternal behavior can be looked at as a recursive process of mutually-reinforcing influences.

Mating

Hyperprolactinemia markedly reduces the levels of sexual behavior in mammals and in birds. This observation is consistent with the increased opioid and dopaminergic tones induced by hyperprolactinemia. Both directly suppress the secretion of gonadotrophin releasing hormone (GnRH). Naltrexone provokes only a slight and transient effect in normalizing GnRH secretion, in hyperprolactinemic women, suggesting that opioid mechanisms, albeit important, are redundant in the hypogonadism of hyperprolactinemia. Prolactin also directly inhibits the secretion of gonadotrophin-releasing-hormone in some systems but not in others.

Other behavioral effects

Other observed effects of prolactin such as facilitation of learning capacity (which is reduced either by dopamine or opioid antagonists), induction of novelty-induced grooming behavior, reduction of pain sensitivity and of the incidence of gastric ulcers induced by physical stress may reflect the above-mentioned effects of prolactin on the dopaminergic and opioid systems.

Psychological Correlates of Hyperprolactinemia in Humans

There is a wide agreement that patients with hyperprolactinemia present with an unusual prevalence of depressive disorders (for review see ref. 4). When women with hyperprolactinemia due to a pituitary adenoma were compared to nursing mothers it was found that depressed mood, loss of interest in usual pleasures, decreased libido and irritability predominated in the adenoma group as compared to the others. These symptoms ameliorated in some patients following surgical removal of the adenoma[5]. Similar findings were reported in another study[6] in which women with pathological hyperprolactinemia scored higher than puerperal controls for depression and anxiety. However, both groups had elevated "hostility" scores. As pointed out by the authors, some hostility (towards strangers) is part of the adaptive psychological program of motherhood along with the increased infant-directed acceptant behavior.

In a study containing 103 women with pathological hyperprolactinemia and 82 controls, sexual dysfunction was observed in 58% of the patients and 27% of the controls. Bromocriptine had a positive effect on the condition in 54% of the patients. Hypoestrogenism did not appear to play a major role in the sexual dysfunction of hyperprolactinemia. Estrogen levels were equally low in women with and without sexual dysfunction and estrogen containing medications had been taken by 35 of the patients without any effect. Slight intermittent dyspareunia was described in only 3 patients, a complaint that is semiologically distinct from low libido and anorgasmia[7]. Headaches are also unusually common in hyperprolactinemia, even in the absence of demonstrable pituitary tumor[4,8].

In men with pathological hyperprolactinemia the impairment of the sexual function is even more remarkable than in women. As testosterone secretion is often impaired in these patients it is difficult to dissociate a direct behavioral effect of prolactin from the consequences of their hypogonadal state. The physiology of sexual dysfunction appears to be complex and the results of the treatment are unpredictable. Bromocriptine corrects the condition in about half of the patients but, when it does, the results can be observed before any marked increase in testosterone concentrations[9]. The hypogonadism of hyperprolactinemia results both from the negative effect of prolactin on the secretion of LH (see above) and to the mass effect of a pituitary tumor that disrupts the portal circulation. This latter factor explains why the correction of the hyperprolactinemia in patients with macroprolactinomas does not usually normalize testosterone secretion[10].

II. Effects of the Environment on Prolactin Secretion.

Hyperprolactinemia may be driven by interactional demands. Parenting by males (in which the influence of a previous pregnancy does not confound the observations) has been described to be associated with increased prolactin levels both in avian and primate species[4,11]

Nonpuerperal women have been described to develop hyperprolactinemia or production of milk in specific conditions of maternal role playing:

1. In primitive cultures, when a woman dies shortly after giving birth, and in the absence of a wet nurse, the child is taken care of by a non puerperal woman, often the grandmother. These women have been described to produce milk in response to the suckling by the infant. While the actual production of milk has not been quantified, it is possible that, in the context of grief and of the absolute need to feed the child, some women may be recruited to develop a neurohormonal response such that the production of milk is facilitated[4].

2. A group of 240 women who adopted newborns and wanted to nurse them was studied and reported [12]. All produced some milk in response to suckling. In 63 % of them the supplement given was inferior to 454 g/day, suggesting that the secreted milk may have had some nutritive value. Sixteen percent could nurse the children without any supplement after the first month. Five entered a state of amenorrhea after they started nursing Although prolactin values were not measured, this study demonstrates that an adaptive biological response involving production of substantial amounts of milk may be elicited in the absence of a previous pregnancy.

3. There are, in the psychoanalytical literature, several detailed descriptions of women who, in the context of actual or threatened separations, developed breast engorgement and lactation. One of the published reports bears the suggestive title of "Lactation as a denial of separation"[13]. In another case a woman, a menopausal grandmother in psychotherapy, developed galactorrhea in association with the wish to breast feed her infant grandchild and re-establish, in fantasy, close symbiotic ties with her own mother[14].

4. A paradigmatic example of prolactin changes conditioned be environmental and psychological factors is pseudopregnancy. Pseudopregnancy in humans is a psychotic disorder characterized by the delusional belief of being pregnant. These patients persist in their belief even when confronted with unequivocal evidence that they are wrong. This condition is now uncommon in industrialized cultures but was once rather frequent and is said to have epidemiological significance in some places of Africa. It is usually triggered by an environmental event acting upon an unsophisticated personality. Its psychodynamics has been described as representing a state of profound helplessness in which the person regresses to an early mother-to-child relationship in which the distinction between the roles of the mother and child is blurred. A profound depression follows the resolution of the psychotic state and the acceptance that the fantasy of pregnancy does not hold true.

Whatever the credit the reader wants to give to psychoanalytical formulations, the undisputed fact is that the delusional state is associated with bodily changes that mimic true pregnancy - marked weight gain, abdominal protuberance, breast engorgement, galactorrhea and amenorrhea. Pseudopregnancy is a unique example of a condition in which external events, acting upon predisposed persons in a specific cultural setting, evoke a cluster of neuroendocrine effects that closely mimic the normal adaption to pregnancy. The abnormality lies in the fact that the "pregnancy" the organism is adapting to exists only as a mental construct of the patient. This construct must be connected to some transductional mechanisms that evoke an otherwise normal neuroendocrine response in the absence of its usual triggering system - the cascade initiated by the placental hormones.

The neuroendocrinology of pseudopregnancy has been studied by several authors (for review, see 4). The most consistent finding is a slight to moderate increase in prolactin values. Even when the values are within the reference range they are close to the its upper limit[15].

5. In a systematic study of siblings of patients with prolactinomas interviews and endocrine studies (at least five morning samples on 5 different days) were performed on 37 sisters and 17 brothers of women with prolactinomas. All males had normal prolactin levels at all times. The sisters were compared with 72 controls matched for age and socio-economic class. It was found that 23 of the 37 sisters and 27 of the 72 controls (a total of 50 women) had been brought up under conditions of paternal deprivation (as defined by absence of the father or exposure to an alcoholic, violent one, before the age of 9). These women had significantly higher mean prolactin levels than the others (14.7 ng/ml v. 9.4 ng/ml; $p < .001$). A closer analysis of the data revealed that most women in both groups had similar, normal, prolactin levels. The differences in the means were due to a significantly higher number of outliers in the deprived group. In this group, 12/50 had average serum prolactin values above 20 ng/ml (one of themplain with pharmacological and imagiological evidence of prolactinoma) as opposed to 3/59 of the others. When corrected for paternal deprivation, no differences in the prolactin levels were observed between women from the sisters and the control groups suggesting that the differences observed were related to environmental rather than genetic factors[16].

6. Women with an history of recent weight gain (more than 5 Kg in the last year) in the absence of change in dietary, exercise or smoking habits and in the absence of a well defined endocrine disease (e.g., Cushing's syndrome) were found to have mean serum prolactin levels (measured hourly for 24 hours) that, although within the normal range, were significantly higher (14.6 v. 8.4 ng/ml; $p = .012$) than that of controls. Galactorrhea was significantly more common in the group that gained weight. This group scored higher for depression in the MMPI and SCL90 test than controls[17,18]. Moreover, important life-events almost always preceded the weight gain while they were much less common in the controls.

These observations suggest that rapid, unexplained, gain of weight in women bears several similarities to pseudopregnancy - the weight gain itself, galactorrhea, marginally elevated prolactin levels, depressive mood and triggering by an external event - and, probably, likewise consists of a state of activation of a neuroendocrine "maternal" subroutine.

Psychogenic Factors in the Genesis of Prolactinomas

Prolactinomas are the most common adenomas (an adenoma is, by definition, a benign tumor) of the pituitary. Their genesis is unknown. Although no genomic abnormality has, so far, been consistently identified, it is accepted that one or more abnormalities in the DNA of its cells is/are responsible for their overgrowth and hyperactivity. Clinically silent pituitary adenomas are fairly common in the general population (1.5% to 26.7% in autopsy series of persons who died from all causes), 42% of which are prolactinomas[19]. However, clinically significant prolactinomas affect no more than 2/1000 of the female population[20].

There are epidemiological characteristics of prolactinomas suggesting that psychological events *precede* the clinical onset of the disease[2].

The clinical onset of the disease commonly follows an important interactional event. This temporal relationship between life events and the appearance of the symptoms was also described for ACTH producing adenomas responsible for Cushing's Disease[21].

Emotional Aspects of Hyperprolactinemia

At least as intriguing as the close temporal association between life events and onset of the symptoms is the fact that most women with prolactinoma or idiopathic hyperprolactinemia (i.e., hyperprolactinemia without imagiological evidence of a pituitary tumor) were reared, in their childhood, either without their father or with an alcoholic, violent one. These observations, initially published in 1980[2], were subsequently confirmed by all authors that addressed the question (for revisions up to 1991 see 4, subsequent series[22,23]). Whatever the causal links involved, it is clear that hyperprolactinemia in a woman can hardly explain the death, estrangement or alcoholism of her father some 10-20 years before. Rather, conditions in early life, possibly related to a prolongation of the early symbiotic relationship between mother and child, in the absence of a father that provides support for both and an alternative model and love object for the child, predispose some girls to react with hyperprolactinemia to specific events later in life. For the interested reader, a more detailed description of this model was published elsewhere[24].

The mechanisms that mediate the sequence - early organization of the personality neuroendocrine reactivity to life events characterized by hyperproduction of prolactin pituitary adenoma, are unknown. The very sequence itself is somewhat unconventional in current endocrinological thinking. However, the sequence - adaptation to stimulus hyperplasia functioning adenoma, has been well characterized in several glands, including the pituitary, as in the case of mice transgenic for GHRH (Growth Hormone Releasing Hormone) that eventually develop GH producing pituitary adenomas following continuous exposure to endogenous GHRH[25]. A similar evolution, in a patient with spontaneous, endogenous, hyperproduction of GHRH was reported[26]. Other examples, in humans, are the development of diffuse goiter, first, and of thyroid adenomas later, as a response to low iodine intake in endemic goiter areas. Also, the hyperparathyroidism due to parathyroid hyperplasia in patients with chronic renal failure occasionally proceeds towards autonomous adenoma (the so-called "tertiary hyperparathyroidism").

Even in the pituitary, a pathological description of the evolution, in inadequately compensated patients with Addison's disease, from diffuse hyperplasia to full blown ACTH-producing pituitary adenomas, through an intermediary state of "tumorlets" has been reported[27].

III. Emotional Changes Associated with the Mass Effect of a Pituitary Tumor and with the Knowledge by the Patient that He/She has a Tumor in the "Brain."

Large pituitary tumors may affect neural structures in the vicinity and produce loss of vision. Less commonly a voluminous mass may provoke, among other symptoms, altered states of consciousness, sleepiness and changes in appetite regulation. These symptoms depend exclusively on the volume and localization of the tumor and, therefore, are common to all pituitary expansive lesions. Specific for prolactinomas, however, is the fact that considerable regression in the symptoms may be obtained by medical therapy with dopaminergic agonists, due to the marked and often rapid effect of these drugs in reducing tumor size.

It is obvious that the disclosure, to a patient, that she/he has a "tumor" within the head may have a major emotional impact. The overall effect depends on the personalities of the patient and physician, the relation of trust between them and on the way the information is conveyed. It certainly also depends on cultural settings. There is no guaranteed recipe for a good patient-to-doctor relationship, but a couple of hints may be helpful. The first is the following, admittedly personal, attitude:

The patient is entitled to an accurate explanation about her/his situation and prognosis. However, the doctor must be aware that, just like beauty is in the eyes of the beholder, information is in the ears of the listener. A word like "tumor", while technically appropriate when applied to an adenoma, does not rule out malignancy, a dire, if incorrect, association some patients quickly make. Explanations involving many technical details and quotations may be required by some patients but not be easily followed by others who may feel (correctly or not) that long explanations may serve the purposes of diluting out meaningful information and/or of trying to transfer to the patient the share of responsibility that a professional should not alienate. In sum - bare essential information must be provided with a wording appropriate to the patient's culture and degree of anxiety; all questions must be answered honestly; details should be given only when specifically required.

The second hint is to keep in mind and, in a matter-of-fact way, convey to the patient the basic information that is applicable to most patients with prolactinomas (the "default" scenario): - Prolactinomas are almost always benign tumors. Medical treatment with dopamine agonists such as bromocriptine, cabergoline or others reduces the size of the adenoma in most patients, often to an unmeasurable size. All studies demonstrate that, even without treatment, small prolactinomas are stable and hardly ever increase either in size or in endocrine activity over the years.

In the few patients in whom there are reasons to believe that the "default" scenario will not apply, an individualized, frank and sensible approach becomes necessary.

Conclusions

Prolactin acts upon the central nervous system affecting behavior, emotions and feelings. Hyperprolactinemia may induce depressive states and reduced sexual desire and response, effects that are, in part, reversible when the prolactin levels are normalized by treatment. On the other hand, hyperprolactinemic states, including prolactinomas affect preferentially persons with a background characterized by paternal deprivation in childhood. Therefore, some psychological difficulties felt by these patients may precede the disease and have roots that are independent of their current endocrine state. This possibility must be considered when, as often occurs, an endocrinologically successful treatment meets with rather poor amelioration in the overall well-being of the patients. Unfortunately, there is no specific form of therapy for these common emotional problems. However, a physician familiar with the complexity described above may, often, find his/her way to some specific needs of the patients without being blinded by a reductionist approach to an endocrine disorder that may be only part of a more complex disease.

References

1   Sobrinho (1997) Basic science aspects of prolactin modulation of brain and behavior. *In* Halbreich U (Ed) Hormonal modulation of brain and behavior, American Psychiatric Press, Inc., New York (in press).

2   Nunes MCP, Sobrinho LG, Calhaz-Jorge C, M.A. Santos, J.C. Mauricio, M.F.F. Sousa (1980) Psychosomatic factors in patients with hyperprolactinemia and/or galactorrhea. Obstetrics & Gynecology 55, 591-5.

3   Hulting AL, Muhr C, Lundberg PO, Werner S (1985) Prolactinomas in men: Clinical characteristics and the effect of bromocriptine treatment. Acta Med Scandinav 217, 101-9.

4   Sobrinho, LG (1991) Neuropsychiatry of prolactin. Baillière's Clinical Endocrinology and Metabolism. 5; 119-42.

5   Rothchild E (1985) Psychologic aspects of galactorrhea. Journal of Psychosomatic Obstetrics and Gynecology 4; 185-96.

6   Mastrogiacomo I, Fava M, Fava GA, Kellner R, Cetera C, Grismondi G (1983) Post-partum hostility and prolactin. International Journal of Psychiatric Medicine 12; 128-94.

7   Sobrinho LG, Sá-Melo P, Nunes MCP, Barroso LE, Calhaz-Jorge C, Oliveira LC, Santos MA (1987) Sexual dysfunction in hyperprolactinaemic women. Effect of bromocriptine. Journal of

Psychosomatic Obstetrics and Gynaecology 6; 43-8.

8   Kemman E, Jones JR (1983) Hyperprolactinemia and headaches. American Journal of Obstetrics and Gynecology. 145; 668-71.

9   Buvat J, Lemaire A, Buvat-Herbaut M, Fourlinnie JC, Racadot A, Fossati P (1985) Hyperprolactinemia and sexual function in males. Hormone Research 22, 196-203.

10 Berezin M, Shimon I, Hadani M (1995) Prolactinoma in 53 men; clinical characteristics and modes of treatment (male prolactinoma) Journal of Endocrinological Investigation 18;436-41.

11 Garcia V, Jouventin P, Mauget R (1996) Parental care and the prolactin secretion pattern in the King penguin: an endogenously timed mechanism? Hormones and Behavior 30; 259-65.

12 Auerbach KG and Avery JL (1981) Induced lactation. American Journal of Diseases in Children. 135; 340 - 3.

13 Aruffo R (1971) Lactation as a denial of separation. Psychoanalytical Quarterly 40;100-22. episodic gonadotropin and prolactin secretion in human pseudocyesis. Acta Endocrinologica 124; 501-9.

14 Zeitner RM, Frank MV, Freeman D (1980) Pharmacogenic and psychogenic aspects of galactorrhea: a case report. American Journal of Psychiatry 137; 111-2.

15 Bray MA, Muneyyirci-Delale O, Fofinas GD, Reyes FI (1991) Circadian, ultradian, and prolactin secretion in human pseudocyesis. Acta Endocrinologica 124; 501-9.

16 Sobrinho LG, Nunes MCP, Calhaz-Jorge C, Afonso AM, Pereira MC, Santos MA (1984) Hyperprolactinemia in women with paternal deprivation during childhood. Obsterics & Gynecology 64; 465-8.

17 Ferreira MF, Sobrinho LG, Pires JS, Silva MES, Santos MA, Sousa MFF (1995) Endocrine and psychological evaluation of women with recent weight gain. Psychoneuroendocrinology 20; 53-63.

18 Ferreira MF , Sobrinho LG , Santos MA , Sousa MFF , Moberg KU (1997) Rapid weight gain, at least in some women, is an expresion of a neuroendocrine state characterized by reduced hypothalamic dopaminergic tone. Psychoneuroendocrinology (in press).

19 Molitch M, Russel EJ (1990) The pituitary "incidentaloma". Annals of Internal Medicine 112; 925-31.

20 Miyai K, Ichihara K, Kondo K, Mori S (1986) Asymptomatic hyperprolactinemia and prolactinoma in the general population - mass screening by paired assays of serum samples. Clinical Endocrinology (Oxf) 25; 549-54.

21 Sonino N, Fava GA, Boscaro M (1993) A role for life - events in the pathogenesis of Cushing's disease. Clinical Endocrinology (Oxf) 38: 261 - 4.

22 Assies J, Vingerhoets AJJM, Poppelaars K (1992) Psychosocial aspects of hyperprolactinemia. Psychoneuroendocrinology 17; 673-9.

23 Intebi AD, Beraldo L, Zukerfeld R, Katz D, Diez RA (1996) Traumatic events in childhood and psychological aspects in hyperprolactinemia. Program & Abstracts of the 10th International Congress of Endocrinology, S. Francisco, USA, P2 - 474, pg 523.

24 Sobrinho LG, Almeida-Costa JM (1992) Hyperprolactinaemia as a result of immaturity or regression: the concept of maternal subroutine. Psychoterapy & Psychosomatics 57, 128 -32.

25 Asa S, Kovacs K, Stefaneanu L, Horvath E, Billestrup N, Gonzalez-Manchon C, Vale W (1992) Pituitary adenomas in mice transgenic for growth hormone releasing-hormone. Endocrinology 131: 2083 - 9.

26 Zimmerman D, Young WF, Ebersold MJ, Scheithauer BW, Kovaks K, Horvath E, Whitaker MD, Eberhardt NL, Downs TR, Frohman LA (1993) Congenital gigantism due to growth hormone-releasing hormone excess and pituitary hyperplasia with adenomatous transformation. Journal of Clinical Endocrinolology and Metabolism 76; 216 - 22.

27 Scheithauer BW, Kovacs K, Randall RV (1983) The pituitary gland in untreated Addison's disease. Archives of Pathology and Laboratory Medicine 107; 484-7.

Hormones and Sexuality

Sandy Hotchkiss, MSW, BCD

Editor/Publishers Note: *Some of the information on which this article is based may not yet be fully debated and agreed to within the scientific community. However, multiple lines of suggestive studies indicate that the information provided may well be the best knowledge available at the time of publication.*

"Men are from Mars; women are from Venus," the modern catchphrase goes, a shorthand way of conceptualizing the differences between the sexes. Men are by nature aggressive and preoccupied with sex, we tell each other, "poisoned" at times by the singular hormone that defines their masculinity. Women, on the other hand, are natural-born nurturers, unfortunately subject to predictable "raging hormonal influences" that are the stereotypical hallmark of their gender. Intuitively, not to mention by experience, we all know it is much more complicated than that. And indeed it is.

Beyond the "Big Three" sex hormones—testosterone, estrogen, and progesterone are a cast of other endocrine characters—peptides and neurotransmitters, as well as hormones—that all exert powerful influences on our sexuality in sickness and in health, for better or for worse, till death do us part. Some, such as pheromones, dopamine and serotonin, have begun to creep into the periphery of our awareness as medical science advances and collides with popular culture, while others, such as oxytocin, vasopressin, prolactin (known to many pituitary-tumor patients) and the alphabet-soup hormones DHEA, PEA and LHRH are primarily the turf of medical researchers, animal labs and arcane professional journals.

Knowledge is power, however, and the more we know about the way our bodies work, the better advocates we can be for our own health and well-being. Information not only helps us make sense of our experience, it also makes us better able to communicate with our doctors so that we are more likely to get what we need—and want.

Understanding of the intricate relationship between hormones and sexuality has exploded in recent decades, but there remain many questions yet to be answered. What is known may astound you, however, and challenge beliefs you have considered axiomatic. Did you know, for example, that sexuality is such an integral part of human nature that it is evident even before birth? That erections in male fetuses have been observed on ultrasound, that females lubricate vaginally in the womb, and some may even have minimenstrual periods shortly after birth, the result of sudden estrogen withdrawal when separated from their mothers during delivery? From the uterus to the grave, we are sexual beings, governed by complex biochemicals that act, react and interact to determine much of what we hold to be most meaningful in life.

To begin our exploration of the relationship between hormones and sexuality, let us review what we know about those hormones most commonly associated with sex. Testosterone, the "male" hormone, is actually responsible for the aggressive sex drive in both men and women. Manufactured in the testicles, ovaries and adrenal glands, its concentrations are 20 to 40 times higher in men than in women, but it can transform into estrogen, the "female" hormone, in both sexes.

Contrary to popular opinion, testosterone has less to do with potency and frequency than it does with the specific drive for genital sex and orgasm. It increases sexual thoughts and fantasies, but it also makes us want to be alone—or at least totally in control of sexual situations. As such, it favors masturbation over intercourse, and the necessary elements that compel us to partner sex come from other hormonal substances. Surprisingly, testosterone does not have a strong effect on erection (except indirectly, by fueling desire) and even decreases tactile sensitivity, especially in the penis. If a man with normal testosterone levels experiences low sex drive or erection problems, giving him testosterone supplements not only won't help him but may make his problem worse. So it is wise to have levels of free (metabolically active) testosterone checked before embarking on hormone treatment.

Just as testosterone serves as an aphrodisiac for both sexes, it also has antidepressant capabilities. This may seem strange given testosterone's well-deserved reputation as a trigger for aggression, competitiveness and violence, but it's all a matter of degree—and interaction with other hormones. Anger and irritability occur in men when testosterone spikes, and their levels oscillate every 15 to 20 minutes, as well as following daily, seasonal and annual rhythms. Sometimes testosterone increases during sex, sometimes not. In women, testosterone promotes assertiveness and self-confidence, but combined with the female androgyn progesterone, as occurs in the premenstrual phase of the monthly cycle, it contributes to irritability and aggressive behavior. In excess amounts over time, testosterone can change a woman's body, relocating fat and muscle, creating a broader chest, narrower hips, smaller breasts, an enlarged clitoris, a mustache and beard.

Should your testosterone level be on the low side, there are several ways to increase it naturally. Think about or have sex more often, eat more meat, exercise more vigorously and, if you can, win. Yes, winning competitions actually raises testosterone levels, while losing causes them to dip. Another reason to work on that tennis game.

Now we turn to the female hormones, estrogen and progesterone. Estrogen is the quintessential stuff that makes women look, smell and feel so different from men. Produced primarily by the ovaries but also by the brain and fat cells (where it may be stored), estrogen stabilizes mood, lubricates and maintains the sexual and reproductive apparatus and governs what is known as the receptive sex drive, the desire to go along with what the male initiates. Women also have three other sexual "gears" that are ruled by various hormones or hormone combinations: active, or aggressive, which is testosterone-driven ; preceptive, or seductive, which is fueled by a combination of estrogen and three other helpers (oxytocin, progesterone and LHRH); and aversive, the not-tonight-I-have-a -headache mode that results from a nasty concoction of progesterone, prolactin, vasopressin and serotonin, four antagonists that on their own could spoil an otherwise promising evening but in combination will completely pull the plug on a woman's desire for sex.

These last four hormones are all natural "sex offenders," interfering in various ways with sexual desire. Progesterone, which is produced by the ovaries and the adrenal glands, is the hormone that increases during the last two weeks of the menstrual cycle until it drops abruptly, causing bleeding to begin. It kills off libido in both sexes by reducing testosterone levels and is especially deadly in synthetic forms. Progesterone in men is so malevolent that it has been used to chemically castrate child molesters and other sexual predators. Studies have shown that within the first month of treatment with MPA, a particularly powerful form of synthetic progesterone, testosterone levels can drop over 90 percent, but that even when they don't, sexual arousal is decreased. Megace, another synthetic progesterone used to treat prostate cancer, has been shown to cause marked loss of sex drive in up to 70 percent of male patients who receive this treatment.

In females, however, progesterone is a more "paradoxical" hormone, particularly when it occurs naturally. It may complement sexual desire and interest by increasing receptivity and proceptivity (in combination with estrogen) and by offering a mildly sedative effect at low levels. It also contributes to making women more nurturing, particularly toward their own children. At higher levels and in combination with testosterone, it can make women irritable and aggressive and is a mild depressant. It is the major ingredient in the Norplant implant and other, oral contraceptives.

Progesterone creates some of its worst sexual havoc via its impact on other players in the hormonal drama, so in order to tell the story, we must first become acquainted with the rest of the cast.

While testosterone and estrogen are the male and female leads, the real star of the show is Dehydroepiandrosterone, or DHEA, the most powerful chemical in our internal world. This is the chief hormone produced by the fetus, in amounts 200 to 400 times greater than progesterone and testosterone, and more than 800 times higher than fetal levels of estrogen. DHEA blood levels peak around age 25 and decline steadily thereafter, but in adult men, DHEA blood levels are 100 to 500 times greater than testosterone.

A steroid hormone manufactured mainly in the adrenals but also by the ovaries, testicles and brain, DHEA is regulated by the pituitary hormone ACTH (Adrenocorticotrophic hormone). DHEA cycles throughout the day in a volatile pattern of unpredictable peaks and valleys that respond not only to environmental triggers but also to our emotions.

DHEA is a natural aphrodisiac that boosts sex drive, particularly in women. At increased levels, libido rises, just as sexual activity causes DHEA to increase in the brain. Oral contraceptives, among other medications, lower DHEA, and it drops drastically under stress, which may explain the mechanism by which acute or chronic stress reduces sex drive and why men lose erections when they worry about performance. Conversely, transcendental meditation and other stress-reduction techniques, as well as regular, vigorous exercise over an extended period of time, will raise DHEA blood concentrations.

DHEA as a hormonal supplement shows some promise for treatment of low sexual desire in women. However, insufficient research has been completed to qualify DHEA for FDA approval, and although it is available in health food stores, the government has published warnings to the public about using this substance without medical supervision. Recent findings indicate that DHEA supplements may lead to liver damage, even when taken briefly, and there may also be cancer risks. Because it boosts testosterone levels in women, there is additional concern about masculinizing effects, so it is not wise to start experimenting on one's own. The antidepressant medication Bupropion, marketed as Wellbutrin, is widely available and may do the same job without compromising femininity. By increasing DHEA levels, it enhances libido, more so in women than in men.

Moving down the playbill, another character who can spice up the action is Phenylethylamine, or PEA, a naturally occurring amphetamine-like substance that produces the feeling of a mind-altered state. PEA is the spirited ingenue of the cast who "percolates" during arousal, excitement and orgasm, lending a sweetly nervous quality to sex. Rather adolescent in character, PEA can cause depression when low and anxiety, disturbed sleep and even psychosis when high. In optimal range, it is an antidepressant in both sexes and a stimulant to sexuality. Abnormally high PEA levels seem to occur more often in women than in men, typically rising at or near ovulation. Although synthetic forms of amphetamine derivatives similar to PEA are sold over the counter or by prescription as appetite suppressants, and PEA is present naturally in chocolate and diet soft drinks, this is definitely a substance to be treated with respect. It is suspected to be the cause of "love addiction," and the use of PEA-like stimulant drugs for the treatment of sexual dysfunction has been known to cause "crazy behavior." Should you be tempted to experiment a bit on your own with an unrestrained chocolate binge, be forewarned: although PEA is present in chocolate, it is metabolized so quickly that it doesn't have time to have much effect on our libido.

No tale worth telling is without its conflict between good and evil, and the story is made even more compelling when the good guys have a bit of a dark side and the bad guys a few redeeming qualities. And so it is with our hormonal drama. The good guys include oxytocin and vasopressin, two peptides secreted by the posterior pituitary, and a neurotransmitter called dopamine. The sex offending bad guys are another neurotransmitter called serotonin and the pituitary hormone prolactin.

Oxytocin and vasopressin could be considered the yin and yang of sexually active pituitary peptides. Both are "bonding agents" which propel us to deep and satisfying intimate connection, "chemical commitment," as it were. Oxytocin, the affectionate wife and mother, has almost no power in the absence of estrogen but is operative in both sexes, increasing sexual receptivity and causing uterine contractions during child birth and orgasm in females, and increasing penile sensitivity and speeding ejaculation in males. Oxytocin makes us want to touch; it reduces stress, but it also makes us forgetful and diminishes the capacity to think and reason.

Vasopressin, on the other hand, is the faithful and rational husband, working closely with testosterone to modulate male sexual behavior by muting the intensity of certain feelings and narrowing the emotional range. In contrast to oxytocin, it appears to improve memory, cognitive powers and concentration and enhances lovemaking in men by facilitating attention to sexual cues and increasing focus on the here-and-now. Primarily a man's chemical, it depends on testosterone for its sexual effects. In female sexuality, it inhibits receptive (but not preceptive) sex but may be essential for triggering orgasm in both sexes.

These two are all tame, domesticated bliss when compared to the raw pursuit of pleasure—not just sex but any pleasure—represented by the neurotransmitter dopamine. This chemical is Dionysus at the orgy, Ferris Bueller on his day off, Cyndi Lauper and the girls just having fun. In a nutshell, dopamine makes you happy, increasing sex drive and facilitating orgasm while actually reducing cravings for alcohol and other abused substances. Without electrochemical reinforcement of dopamine in the brain, we become subdued and listless, unable even to anticipate pleasure and unresponsive to customary sexual cues and triggers. Testosterone increases dopamine (as does cocaine, the anti-Parkinsonian drug L-dopa, and the antidepressant Wellbutrin), but too much of a good thing can also be bad. Excessive dopamine can cause schizophrenia—and premature ejaculation, a sexual disorder which has recently been found responsive to manipulation of another neurotransmitter, serotonin.

In our hormonal drama, serotonin plays the part of dopamine's arch-nemesis, for whatever dopamine can create in the way of urgent sexuality, serotonin can undo by blunting impulsive pleasurable arousal and inhibiting orgasm in both sexes. At higher levels, serotonin says, "Let's just be friends", but at low levels and particularly for men in combination with alcohol, it can be as much a monster as Dr. Jekyl's Mr. Hyde: sexually aggressive, indiscriminate, violent and mean.

The ability to inhibit the reuptake of serotonin in the brain has created a whole new generation of antidepressant medications that can make you feel peaceful and good but can also destroy your sex life. Prozac and its progeny (Zoloft, Paxil, Luvox, Effexor) may initially improve desire and responsiveness by soothing anxiety, but once a higher serotonin set point has been established, sexual excitement and responsiveness subside.

Women generally have more serotonin than men to begin with, and together with their lower testosterone levels, there is a natural depression of both sexuality and aggression relative to men. Unlike men, who can become dangerous when serotonin levels drop too low, lower serotonin levels in women are associated with being more readily arousable and easily orgasmic and with taking more initiative. Serotonin has been found to have a preferential relationship with estrogen, facilitating both progesterone and our final sex offender hormone, prolactin.

Prolactin is the prude who teaches health class, piously pronouncing that these precious body parts are for procreation, not pleasure. Prolactin, secreted by the pituitary, creates breast milk and is also involved in the production of sperm and the maintenance of genital tissue. It tends to mute sensation and alertness in general and can cause mild depression and fatigue. While it does not diminish the enjoyment of sex, at high levels, such as are found in nursing mothers and people with prolactin-producing pituitary tumors, it is deadly to desire, sabotages orgasm and can cause impotence in men. When dopamine and prolactin meet in battle, dopamine usually wins, restoring lost libido. Estrogen, oxytocin and progesterone, however, boost prolactin, which in chronically high levels lowers testosterone. On its own, however, testosterone, like dopamine, lowers prolactin, while stress, vigorous exercise and high protein meals all cause it to rise.

There is one final chemical that plays an important role in our sexual functioning by regulating the relationship between estrogen and testosterone. Synthesized in the hypothalamus, LHRH (leutinizing hormone-releasing hormone) triggers the production of testosterone and oversees the production and release of LH (leutinizing hormone) and FSH (follicle-stimulating hormone), two key players in conception and menstruation. Keenly sensitive to environmental triggers as well as visual, emotional and sexual cues, LHRH fluctuates dramatically. If, for example, a man's testosterone levels are too low or he is exposed to visual sexual stimuli such as an attractive woman or erotic material, LHRH levels will increase to activate production of testosterone. If testosterone levels are too high, LHRH can convert excess testosterone to estrogen, restoring balance. Stress and danger decrease LHRH, reducing the body's ability to self-regulate the primary sex hormones.

LHRH has been found to mildly increase sexual desire and has been used to treat low libido, impotence, low testosterone and anovulation (the failure to ovulate). Secreted in cycles of approximately 90 minutes duration, LHRH illustrates an important principle in hormone treatment. Because the natural behavior of many hormones such as LHRH is to surge and dip in "pulsatile" fashion, total hormone levels are often less important than changes in levels. Consequently, constant replacement doses do not always achieve the desired effect because they fail to duplicate the natural hormonal rhythms that are sensitive to environmental input and intermittent peak intensities to stimulate sexual response. In the future, pills and injections may be replaced by pumps and time-release pellets that more closely mimic nature.

Having met the cast of characters, we are now ready to watch how the plot unfolds. As the curtain rises, LHRH, the director, introduces us to the manly Testosterone and his two cronies, Dopamine the Depraved and Vasopressin the Wise. They make an odd trio, but they have been fast friends since their early teens. Dopamine is Testosterone's favorite drinking buddy, and when these two get together, the good times really roll. They bring Vasopressin along just to make sure things don't get too out of hand. There's something about Vasopressin that makes Testosterone feel more in control, and if there's one thing Testosterone likes, it's being in control. Another thing he really likes is sex, and right now, that's the first thing on his mind.

Lately, he tells his friends, he's been having some problems at home. His wife, Estrogen, is a mystery to him, and just when he thinks he has her figured out, she seems to turn into a different person. Sometimes, she's easy to get along with and just wants whatever he wants. He likes that. Sometimes, she has a mind of her own and chases him around the bedroom. He kind of likes that, too. But other times, she won't have anything to do with his romantic overtures and can be a real pain to live with. He doesn't like that at all. Now he's starting to wonder if it's the company she keeps.

For openers, there's that crazy sister of hers, Progesterone. She comes for a visit every month and stays for about two weeks, which is way too long as far as he's concerned. While she's in the house, there's no peace. The woman doesn't seem to get along with anybody, although he has to admit she's good with the kids. Dopamine and Vasopressin keep their distance when she's around, and Testosterone himself just tries to lay low, waiting for his sister-in-law to leave and his wife to become her easygoing self again. But recently he's noticed that Progesterone's not the only one who turns his wife against him. She's been hanging around with his old girlfriend Serotonin, and the two women have been spending alot of time with that pompous priest Prolactin. Now Estrogen seems to have no interest in sex at all. Testosterone is miffed; he and Serotonin always had a good thing going, until Dopamine persuaded him that she was spoiling their fun. Still, they had parted on good terms—so what's she doing now interfering with his marriage? It's enough to make his blood boil, and when he's in this mood, everybody had better look out because things can get pretty nasty.

Vasopressin is worried. He was best man at Testosterone and Estrogen's wedding, and he does not like to see their marriage heading for trouble. Estrogen has always treated him well, and he has his own reasons for disliking Serotonin, who is fond of putting him down. What to do? he wonders. He knows Testosterone is counting on him for some answers.

Vasopressin turns to Dopamine, approaching him cautiously. He may be the only one who can pull Testosterone out of this black mood, but Vasopressin has to be careful. Dopamine can be a real pal, but sometimes, the guy just seems out to get him. Right now, Dopamine is daydreaming about his girlfriend, Oxytocin. Now there's a pair, thinks Vasopressin. Who would have ever thought that a party animal like Dopamine would fall for a sweet little thing like Oxytocin? She'd rather cuddle than make out, but they seem to be good for each other, as long as Vasopressin's around to make sure his buddy doesn't get too whipped.

Dopamine gets high just thinking about his girlfriend and how good she is to them all. Ever since Estrogen introduced her around, she's been everybody's friend. Maybe she could speak up on Testosterone's behalf, he suggests fondly.

Fat chance, says Testosterone, still in his foul mood. He knows that Oxytocin has been going to church with Estrogen and Serotonin, and when Prolactin has the devotion of the ladies, he is a force to be reckoned with. From his pulpit, he rails against the pleasures of the flesh and condemns women who behave seductively. Sex is to be enjoyed only in the missionary position, he preaches, and women don't need orgasms to conceive children, which is the only reason for them to have sex at all. Testosterone heard one of his sermons once, and it was enough to make him impotent for awhile. As Prolactin's power rises, Testosterone feels himself shrivelling again.

He has to face it, his buddies are short on solutions. In desperation, he turns to the one person who may have an answer, his mother, DHEA. She is not only wise in the ways of love, but because of his reverence for mothers in general, she also has Prolactin's respect as well. There is something almost magical about DHEA's ability to inspire women sexually, and as long as Progesterone is out of town, DHEA can exert her influence without interruption. She's happy to advise her son.

First, she reminds him that while Prolactin has defeated him in the past, the priest is no match for Testosterone when he is able to rally Dopamine and Vasopressin to an action plan promoting pleasure over piety. Secondly, if Serotonin's influence can be overcome, then Estrogen will be herself again and the problem will be solved. Take advantage of Progesterone's absence, she counsels him, and why not introduce Estrogen to that perky little PEA? Spending time with her is bound to make the mellow Ms. Serotonin seem dull by comparison.

So Testosterone follows his mother's advice and everything goes as DHEA has predicted (of course). Estrogen stops attending church with Serotonin and instead goes lingerie shopping with PEA. Even little Oxytocin tags along, always eager to be with her beloved Estrogen. With Serotonin out of the picture, Vasopressin starts to feel more sure of himself; he encourages Testosterone to be more assertive, and Testosterone gets over the meanies. Estrogen and Testosterone party with Dopamine and Oxytocin, and before the night is over, everything is back to normal in the Testosterone household. Vasopressin smiles and closes the bedroom door on the loving couple. There's nothing like wedded bliss, he muses.

And that would be the happy ending to the story if it weren't for the wild-eyed Progesterone, who pays another visit a few weeks later to wreak havoc on their sexual harmony. With a little help from Serotonin, she restores Prolactin to power, brings Testosterone and Vasopressin to their knees and humbles even the mightly Aphrodite herself, DHEA. And as if that weren't enough, she has one last fiendish trick up her sleeve: the power to convince the director, LHRH, that the entire plot has been too dominated by the male point of view. So he recasts Testosterone in the Estrogen role, looking for some balance. Progesterone laughs maniacally and exits stage left, leaving behind a bloody mess. But she'll be back, and the story repeats until the final curtain.

Disease and disaster, as many of us know too well, can drastically rewrite this script, disrupting the dynamic balance of key characters, overpowering the sexual antagonists or eliminating some of the players altogether. When this happens, we often find ourselves trapped in a mystery waiting to be solved. We hold the clues, but others must help us find the solutions to our sexual dilemmas.

The endocrinology of sexuality is an infant science, searching for knowledge in molecules so infinitessimal that one whole person's worth can fit on the head of a pin. In that tiny universe, Mars and Venus are but the launching points, and we are the pioneers.

The author wishes to thank Theresa L. Crenshaw, M.D., whose 1996 book The Alchemy of Love and Lust (New York, G.P. Putnam's Sons, hardcover, $24.95) synthesized the current research on hormones and sexuality and provided most of the information for this article.

Men, Sex, and Pituitary Tumors

Dan Freed - Patient

Editor/Publishers Note: *Some of the information on which this article is based may not yet be fully debated and agreed to within the scientific community. However, multiple lines of suggestive studies indicate that the information provided may well be the best knowledge available at the time of publication.*

Pituitary tumors often cause sexual problems. This can be one of the most troubling aspects of the disease. Pituitary patients and their sexual partners need information and guidance to deal with these problems. Yet discussion of sexual issues is often lacking in literature written for patients, and many doctors are neither well-informed nor comfortable talking about sexual dysfunction.

This article presents what I hope are useful facts, thoughts, and suggestions about the sexual effects of pituitary tumors on men, based on my personal experience as a pituitary patient and on my amateur dabbling in the medical literature.

Sex and the Pituitary

How could a tumor on the pituitary, a small gland inside the skull, affect sexuality? Most people only know the pituitary (if they have ever heard of it at all) for its role in promoting growth during adolescence. As most pituitary patients know, however, the pituitary secretes eight different hormones which control diverse bodily functions including growth, metabolism, lactation, and reproduction.

Two of the pituitary hormones are crucial for normal sexual and reproductive function. These are *luteinizing hormone* (LH) and *follicle-stimulating hormone* (FSH). These hormones are secreted into the bloodstream, where they travel to the *gonads* (sex glands—testes in men, ovaries in women) and stimulate the production of sex hormones and reproductive cells. Without LH and FSH, the gonads do nothing.

In men, LH stimulates the production of *testosterone*, the primary male sex hormone, and FSH stimulates the production of sperm cells. Testosterone is largely responsible for male sexual behavior and secondary sex characteristics (such as beard growth). A deficiency of testosterone is called *hypogonadism*, and it can cause a variety of sexual problems.

Most types of pituitary tumors can cause hypogonadism, although the exact reason is not known with certainty. According to one estimate, it occurs in about 30% of men with growth-hormone-secreting tumors (acromegaly), about 70% of men with non-secreting tumors, and about 90% of men with prolactin-secreting tumors (prolactinomas).[1] Furthermore, an excess of prolactin (*hyperprolactinemia*) can itself cause sexual problems, for reasons that are not currently well understood.[2-5] Men with prolactinomas, therefore, suffer a double blow to sexuality: too little testosterone and too much prolactin. ACTH-secreting tumors (Cushing's Syndrome) may also cause sexual problems.[6]

So what are the effects of these hormonal imbalances on a man's sex life?

Sex and Food: An Analogy

Talking about sex can be difficult. There are many taboos, misconceptions, and false expectations. Talking about sexual problems can be even more difficult. To make things easier, I'm going to draw an analogy between sex and food.

This is not a new analogy. Sex and food are often compared. Both involve basic biological drives—the drive to reproduce and the drive to stay alive. Poets and advertisers make frequent use of the analogy; consider the love letter whose author "hungers" for his lover, or the consumer in a TV ad who "lusts after" a piece of cheesecake.

I'm going to use this analogy to help talk about sexual problems. There are far fewer taboos, misconceptions, and false expectations about food than there are about sex, and so sometimes it's easier to illustrate a point about sex by first making the analogous point about food.

Desire vs. Ability

There is an obvious difference between the *desire* to do something and the *ability* to do it. This difference applies to any biological drive. Diseases can affect desire, ability, or both.

Consider food. The desire to eat is known as hunger, or appetite. The ability to eat requires the ability to chew, salivate, swallow, and digest. Diseases can rob you of your appetite, so that you don't want to eat, or they can render you incapable of swallowing food or keeping it down, so that you can't eat.

The desire for sex has a variety of names: desire, lust, arousal, "horniness." etc. Psychologists and physicians often use the word *libido*. The ability to have sexual intercourse requires, in men, the ability to get an erection, achieve orgasm, and ejaculate (though there are many sexual activities that require none of these). The word *potency* is often used for these sexual abilities. There is good evidence that pituitary tumors can rob men of *both* desire *and* ability. Some of this evidence is discussed later.

Desire without Ability, and Vice Versa

It is very important to understand that desire and ability are not the same thing. It's possible to have desire without ability, or ability without desire. When it comes to sex, desire and ability are often confused for each other, so it's helpful to talk about food first.

It's possible to be hungry but unable to eat. Some diseases can make it difficult to keep food down, for example; your appetite is good and you eat with gusto, but you can't absorb it. Other diseases can render you incapable of swallowing or salivating, again without diminishing appetite. This can be a very frustrating situation.

Similarly, it's possible to feel sexual desire but not get an erection. This is easily misunderstood. Many people, both men and women, interpret the lack of an erection (or the failure to ejaculate) as indicating a lack of sufficient desire, but this is incorrect. Alcohol, for example, can interfere with erections. This has been known for a long time; Shakespeare fans may recall the scene from *Macbeth* in which the Porter describes the sexual effects of drinking: "it provokes the desire, but it takes away the performance."

It's also possible to eat without being hungry. This is a common experience; social obligations or scheduling constraints often require us to eat when we're not hungry, and most of us can usually manage it. Making love without feeling desire is possible as well; men can sometimes force themselves through sexual encounters for which they have little enthusiasm and still "perform" adequately. The motivation may, again, be a perceived obligation or a scheduling constraint.

Desire Can Affect Ability, and Vice Versa

Though desire and ability are not the same thing, they are not entirely independent either. A lack of desire may interfere with ability, and a lack of ability may inhibit desire. It's fairly obvious how lack of desire can undermine ability. If you try to eat when you're not hungry, you might not be able to keep it down; you may even find it difficult to swallow in extreme cases. Similarly, it may be difficult or impossible to perform sexually if desire is lacking.

What's less obvious is that it can work in reverse: a lack of ability can lead to reduced desire. How does this work? If engaging in some activity repeatedly results in an unpleasant experience, eventually you won't feel like engaging in that activity anymore. This principle is sometimes used by psychologists to break people of bad habits (like smoking), an approach known as *aversion therapy*.

This explains how problems with sexual potency can lead to problems with libido. Repeated failures in sexual experiences, with the associated embarrassment and frustration, can cause a loss of interest in sex. This is a danger faced by anyone with a sexual problem. It can create a vicious circle of declining desire and ability that is difficult to escape.

Desire vs. Appeal

Now that the distinction between desire and ability is clear, there's another important distinction to make: between *desire* and *appeal*. It's possible to find something (or someone) very appealing without desiring that thing (or person). It's easier to understand this distinction by considering food first.

Imagine you're at a restaurant and you've just finished a large meal. You're pleasantly full and have no interest in dessert. Then the waiter rolls the dessert cart to your table. The desserts look delicious and smell even better. You listen to the waiter's description of each dessert and imagine how good they must taste. You wish you had saved some room. But eventually you ask for the check, because you're simply not hungry. You make a mental note to come back to this restaurant someday to try the desserts.

Clearly, food can appeal to your senses even when you're not hungry. Sometimes the appeal can be strong enough that you force a dessert into a full stomach, though you probably won't really enjoy it if you do.

Likewise, a sexual partner can appeal to your senses, even when you have no desire for sex. This is easily misunderstood. A man's partner is likely to assume that if he has no desire, then he must not find her appealing. In other words, she assumes that the problem is with her ability to provoke desire in him, rather than in his capacity to feel desire. And, even worse, he might make the same incorrect assumption. Obviously, this misunderstanding can be disastrous to a relationship.

Reflexive Responses

When dealing with basic biological drives, there can be automatic responses to certain stimuli. These responses, like the reflex to flinch when an object is thrown at your face, are involuntary and don't involve any conscious thought. They can occur even without desire. Good-smelling food may cause you to salivate, even if you're not hungry. Similarly, erotic stimuli can cause erections without evoking desire.

There is actually some direct experimental evidence of this kind of reflexive sexual response in men with low testosterone (hypogonadism) due to a pituitary tumor or some other disease. Several researchers[7-9] have shown erotic films or photos to hypogonadal men and measured their erectile response. The result is quite surprising, as summed up by one author:[8]

> Our studies of hypogonadal men have shown that in the laboratory, erections to erotic films occur to a normal extent, even though the men...are experiencing a marked loss of sexual interest.[4]

This reflexive response is easily misinterpreted. It could lead a man, or his partner, to incorrectly conclude that "there's nothing wrong with him." If he responds sexually to racy movies, but not to her, it seems to prove that his sexuality is intact but he's not interested in her. In truth, his response to the movie is "hard-wired" and proves very little.

Sex and Food: Limits of the Analogy
While the analogy between sex and food is useful, it has its limits. For one thing, you must eat to live, but nobody ever died from lack of sex. There are several other ways in which sex is different from—and move complicated than—food.

♦ Sexual desire can be more fragile than appetite for food. Stress, fear, embarrassment, and relationship problems can all kill sexual desire rather quickly.
♦ Sexual ability is more dependent on desire than eating ability is dependent on hunger. It's easier to eat a meal without an appetite than it is to get an erection without desire. To put it another way: it's easier to "force it down" than to "force it up."
♦ There are many social pressures and myths regarding sex. For example, it's often believed that "normal" men *always* want sex, and are just waiting for an opportunity. This is silly; nobody *always* wants *anything*. A person who was *always* hungry would be considered to have a problem; why should unceasing sexual appetite be considered normal?

The myths surrounding sex make sexual problems especially difficult. These myths are discussed—and dismissed—in a book I would highly recommend: *The New Male Sexuality*, by Bernie Zilbergeld.[10] I'll have more to say about this book later.

Assessing Sexual Problems
Pituitary tumors can affect both sexual desire and sexual ability. Sexual feelings and behaviors are complicated and difficult to judge objectively. They are also strongly affected by the dynamics of a relationship, or the lack of a relationship. How can a man with a pituitary tumor tell what sexual effects the tumor is having on him?

It is very important to understand that the sexual effects of hypogonadism and hyperprolactinemia vary enormously from one patient to another. Even more important, the effects can vary enormously from one time or situation to another for the same patient. Some doctors, failing to understand this, ask their patients if they are "impotent." as though it were an all-or-nothing choice. It's much more likely that the patient has a mixed and confusing history of erection or ejaculation problems in certain situations but not others.

Some examples will be helpful. These are taken from case histories of men with prolactinomas studied at the Masters and Johnson Institute.[11]

> Subject D...began to ejaculate inconsistently with a partner 10 years prior to his presentation for therapy. He never had difficulties ejaculating while masturbating....[H]e met his present partner 2 years ago. He had no difficulty ejaculating with her until she recently moved into his apartment.

> Subject C...discovered that [his wife] was having an affair. During the attempted reconciliation, he began to lose his erections upon insertion. He then became impotent and his wife left him....He met his present girlfriend and had intercourse with her daily for 90 days without difficulty. Following this period he lost his erections on about half the coital attempts. When the erection was maintained, he typically had difficulty ejaculating. [p. 868]

The fact that a man with a pituitary tumor can perform adequately in some sexual situations does not mean that he is unaffected by the tumor. Both of these men's sexual problems were inconsistent and strongly affected by complications within their relationships. It is also worth noting that Subject D's problems had been going on for 10 years before he sought help. This is sadly typical.

Assessing Sexual Desire

Sexual desire (libido) is purely subjective, and therefore very difficult to assess. Research studies on libido in men with hypogonadism have mostly relied on the patients' own evaluations of their feelings. Some objective measures can be defined, such as frequency of intercourse. However, this is affected by relationship dynamics, for men in ongoing relationships, or by opportunity, for men not in ongoing relationships. For men who are not in any sexual relationship, a good measure of libido is frequency of masturbation.

Perhaps the only way to be certain of the effects of a pituitary tumor on libido is to compare the patient's feelings and behavior before treatment to those after treatment. Several researchers have done this, and found that libido improved considerably after treatment.[7, 11, 12, 13] This should be encouraging to all men with pituitary tumors.

Assessing Sexual Ability

As has already been discussed, sexual ability is strongly influenced by libido. However, it is possible to evaluate sexual ability separately. One technique used by researchers is to measure erections during sleep, a phenomenon known as *nocturnal penile tumescence* or NPT (no kidding). NPT occurs without consciousness, so libido is not a contributing factor.

Healthy males of all ages, while sleeping, get erections about 3-5 times during the night. These erections occur during dreams, regardless of whether or not the dream has sexual content.[10] Hypogonadal men have fewer and less pronounced sleep erections than normal men; if the hypogonadism is cured, normal sleep erections return.[7, 9, 12, 13] The reduction in sleep erections only occurs if the hypogonadism is relatively severe, and hyperprolactinemia alone does not produce the effect.[9]

NPT is measured by having the patient spend a night sleeping with a mechanical strain gauge attached to his penis (no kidding). While the device is painless, the procedure isn't exactly for everyone. A man can get similar information by noticing how often he awakes in the morning with an erection. Despite the common belief that morning erections are caused by a full bladder, they are actually the result of simply happening to wake up in the midst of a sleep erection.

Morning erections are a good objective indicator of sexual health. One study found that hypogonadal men awoke with erections only 2% of mornings. After the hypogonadism was cured, this jumped to 31%.[12] Another good indicator is the frequency of "spontaneous erections" during the day, which occur without any obvious stimulus. A study of hypogonadal men found that spontaneous erections hardly ever occurred before treatment; after treatment, they occurred about once a day.[7]

Summary: Sexual Effects of Pituitary Tumors

The effects of pituitary tumors on a man's sex life can be summarized as follows:

- He may experience reduced desire for sex.
- He may engage in sex or masturbation less frequently.
- He may have trouble getting or maintaining an erection.
- He may have trouble reaching orgasm and/or ejaculating.
- He may have fewer erections during sleep and upon waking in the morning.
- He may have fewer spontaneous erections during the day.
- He may notice that, despite these changes, some erotic stimuli still produce an erection.

Pituitary Patient Resource Guide

All of these symptoms may or may not occur. If they occur, they may occur consistently or inconsistently, often or seldom, predictably or unpredictably, in all situations or only certain situations. They may develop gradually or suddenly. They may appear, disappear, and reappear again.[11] It can be confusing and frustrating, and much patience is required.

So what can be done about these problems? There are two answers: get medical treatment and learn coping skills.

Medical Treatment

Pituitary tumors require careful, ongoing medical treatment. One of the primary goals of treatment is to restore normal levels of all hormones. For resolving sexual problems in men, it is most important to eliminate hypogonadism and, if present, hyperprolactinemia.

When hyperprolactinemia is present, it is generally treated first. This is because lowering the prolactin level to normal often causes the testosterone level to rise to normal without further treatment. This occurs in the majority of patients,[14] but is by no means certain.[1, 2]

Hyperprolactinemia is usually treated with medication. There are currently two drugs available in the USA for this purpose: bromocriptine (brand name Parlodel) and cabergoline (brand name Dostinex). Both drugs have an excellent track record; they eliminate hyperprolactinemia in the large majority of patients.

Hypogonadism may be treated directly by testosterone replacement therapy. Testosterone may be delivered by injections or skin patches. Until recently, skin patches had to be applied to the scrotum, but patches are now available that can be applied to more convenient and comfortable locations.

As many pituitary patients are well aware, restoring hormone levels to normal is often a lengthy process, requiring multiple modes of treatment, dosage adjustment, and a certain amount of trial and error. Meanwhile, the sexual problems continue to affect the patient's life. It is crucial, therefore, to know how to cope with sexual problems as effectively as possible.

Coping With Sexual Problems

When coping with sexual problems, there are three basic goals:

1. *Minimize the emotional toll on the patient.* Depression, stress, guilt, humiliation, and other painful emotional reactions to sexual dysfunction are common. These can make the problems worse.

2. *Minimize the emotional toll on the patient's partner and on the relationship.* The patient's sexual problems may make his partner feel unloved, unattractive, hurt, and angry. The relationship may be damaged or even destroyed as a result.

3. *Maximize the sexual enjoyment that is still possible.* The sexual effects of a pituitary tumor are not absolute; some desire and ability are usually retained. It's better to concentrate on enjoying what you can do than on grieving over what you can't.

Psychotherapy, and sex therapy in particular, can help with all of these goals. The benefit of therapy has been demonstrated in several studies of men with prolactinomas.[4,5,11] One study of 8 patients[11] reported that "every patient found some benefit from sex therapy in that it facilitated increased frequency of and improved performance in sexual interactions" (p. 869).

Here are some suggestions for men who are coping with the sexual effects of a pituitary tumor. These are based on advice from therapists and my own experience. I offer these suggestions with humility, since I am a long way from having mastered coping skills.

♦ Remember that all is not lost. There are many things you can do to improve your situation.

♦ Don't punish yourself. You have a disease. It's no reflection on your character or your worth as a man.

♦ Don't push yourself. It won't bring you or your partner any pleasure.

♦ Tell your partner what you're thinking and feeling: what you do and don't want sexually, what you do and don't feel you're capable of doing, what you're worried about, etc. This isn't easy. It's hard to ask yourself these questions, harder still to answer them, and even harder to communicate the answers to your partner. But it's very important.

♦ Tell your partner how you feel about her. Make sure she knows that you still love her and still find her appealing. Be specific. Make her understand that the problem is your disease, not her lovability or attractiveness.

♦ Experiment. Some sexual activities may work better than others. Some might work better for you, others might work better for your partner. Be flexible.

♦ Consider seeing a therapist. Counseling may be more effective if your partner comes with you.

I would also suggest that you—and your partner—read Bernie Zilbergeld's book, mentioned earlier.[10] If you've read his original book (*Male Sexuality*, 1978), be sure to get the new (1992) book. He has added lots of important material, including two new chapters on problems of sexual desire. The book is full of information and very specific suggestions on resolving problems. It is clearly written, nontechnical, compassionate, and often very funny.

I hope that these suggestions are helpful, and I hope that this article has been informative.

Appendix: Doctors and Sex

Doctors can be amazingly bad at dealing with sexual issues. In fact, it can be downright comical. To illustrate, here are some examples from my own experience.

One neurosurgeon initiated his discussion of sexual problems with the following question: "So, is your... um... sex thing working?" I asked for clarification. After some beating around the bush, he finally asked, "Can you... you know... ejaculate?" I said I could. He then quickly changed the topic, as though that had settled the entire matter.

As I became more aware of the sexual effects of my tumor, I decided it might help to consult a psychotherapist or sex therapist. I asked an endocrinologist for a referral, naively assuming that since endocrinological diseases have a huge impact on emotions and psychological state, endocrinologists must work closely with mental health professionals on a regular basis. Wrong! After a week, I had heard nothing from the endocrinologist, so I obtained a referral elsewhere and visited a psychiatrist who specializes in sexual problems.

A few days later, the endocrinologist called me to discuss a change in my medication. Then he said, "Oh, by the way, you wanted some sort of referral for sex therapy? Why do you want that?" I explained that I thought it would be helpful (it seemed obvious to me), and that, in fact, I had already seen a therapist. He then asked, suspiciously, "What did he do to you?" I assured him that we had simply talked!

References

1 Ambrosi B, Giovine C, Nissim M, Gaggini M, Bochicchio D, Travaglini P, Faglia G. Treatment of hypogonadism in men with prolactinomas. In *Therapy in Andrology: Pharmacological, Surgical, and Psychological Aspects*, edited by GF Menchini Fabris, W Pasini, and L Martini, Excerpta Medica (Amsterdam), 1982, pp. 92-99.

2 Nagulesparen M, Ang V, Jenkins JS. Bromocriptine treatment of males with pituitary tumours, hyperprolactinaemia, and hypogonadism. *Clinical Endocrinology*, Vol. 9, 1978, pp. 73-79.

3 Carter JN, Tyson JE, Tolis G, Van Vliet S, Faiman C, Friesen HG. Prolactin-secreting tumors and hypogonadism in 22 men. *New England Journal of Medicine*, Vol. 299, 1978, pp. 847-852.

4   Bancroft J, O'Carroll R, McNeilly A, Shaw RW. The effects of bromocriptine on the sexual behaviour of hyperprolactinaemic man: a controlled case study. *Clinical Endocrinology*, Vol. 21, 1984, pp. 131-137.

5   Buvat J, Lemaire A, Buvat-Herbaut M, Fourlinnie JC, Racadot A, Fossati P. Hyperprolactinemia and sexual function in men. *Hormone Research*, Vol. 22, 1985, pp. 196-203.

6   Corrigan EK. Cushing's syndrome. In *The Pituitary Patient Resource Guide, First Annual North American Edition*, Pituitary Tumor Network Association (Encino, CA), 1995, pp. 149-156.

7   Kwan M, Greenleaf WJ, Mann J, Crapo L, Davidson JM. The nature of androgen action on male sexuality: a combined laboratory-self-report study on hypogonadal men. *Journal of Clinical Endocrinology and Metabolism*, Vol. 57, 1983, pp. 557-562.

8   Bancroft J. Hormones and Sexual Behavior. *Journal of Sex and Marital Therapy*, Vol. 10, 1984, pp. 3-21.

9   Carani C, Granata AR, Fustini MF, Marrama P. Prolactin and testosterone: their role in male sexual function. *International Journal of Andrology*, Vol. 19, 1996, pp. 48-54.

10 Zilbergeld B. *The New Male Sexuality*. Bantam Books (New York), 1992.

11 Schwartz MF, Bauman JE, Masters WH. Hyperprolactinemia and sexual disorders in men. *Biological Psychiatry*, Vol. 17, 1982, pp. 861-876.

12 O'Carroll R, Shapiro C, Bancroft J. Androgens, behaviour and nocturnal erection in hypogonadal men: the effects of varying the replacement dose. *Clinical Endocrinology*, Vol. 23, 1985, pp. 527-538.

13 Burris AS, Banks SM, Carter CS, Davidson JM, Sherins RJ. A long-term, prospective study of the physiologic and behavioral effects of hormone replacement in untreated hypogonadal men. *Journal of Andrology*, Vol. 13, 1992, pp. 297-304.

14 Molitch ME. Prolactin. In *The Pituitary*, edited by S Melmed, Blackwell Science (Cambridge, MA), 1995, pp. 136-186.

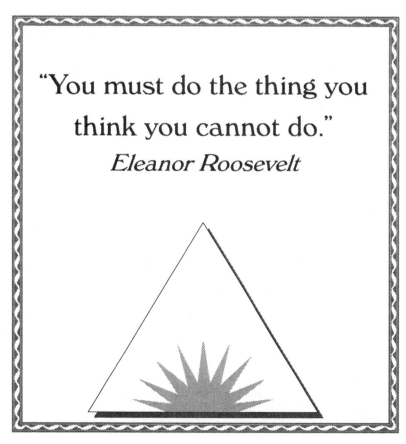

"You must do the thing you think you cannot do."
Eleanor Roosevelt

Pituitary Tumors and the Reproductive System

Christina Wang, M.D., Director, Clinical Study Center, Harbor-UCLA Medical Center,

Functioning and non-functioning pituitary tumors affect the reproductive system. The pituitary tumor may compromise the function of the remaining pituitary gland resulting in decrease in other hormones normally secreted by the pituitary. After pituitary surgery or irradiation, normal pituitary cells may be damaged which will lead to the deficiency of other pituitary hormones. The symptoms of hormone deficiency may become apparent only after many months or years.

In the human, the testes and the ovary are mainly controlled by two pituitary hormones: luteinizing hormone (LH) and follicle-stimulating hormone (FSH). In men, LH controls the secretion of the male hormone testosterone from the testes. FSH regulates the production of sperm by the testes. In women, FSH helps the follicle (which contains the egg) to develop and to produce female hormones including estradiol. LH in the female controls the rupture of the follicle releasing the mature egg (ovulation). It also promotes the function of the corpus luteum to produce another female hormone, progesterone. Progesterone from the corpus luteum supports early pregnancy.

Possible Reproductive Problems in Men with Pituitary Tumors:

If the pituitary hormone LH is low, testosterone production by the testes is decreased. Low testosterone levels are associated with decreased sexual function, in particular, loss of sexual desire. Other long-term effects of low testosterone include decrease in beard growth, loss of body hair, decrease in muscle mass and strength, osteoporosis and decrease in red cell mass. Deficiency in testosterone can be remedied by replacement in the form of intramuscular injections of the hormone dissolved in oil once every 2 to 3 weeks. Transdermal delivery systems are also available which can be applied to the scrotum or other parts of the body. Newer preparations of the male hormone under development include: sublingual natural testosterone tablets, longer acting intramuscular injections, and creams/gels. Before testosterone replacement, a thorough physical examination including a rectal examination to exclude prostate disease must be done. Blood tests are recommended to exclude liver dysfunction, lipid abnormalities and prostate disease. Regular follow-up to assure adequate replacement is required after stabilization of the dose at 6 monthly or yearly intervals. Testosterone replacement will not make a man fertile. Deficiency of the secretion of FSH may be an additional cause of low sperm production. If fertility is desired, an endocrinologist should be consulted and hormone replacement should be altered to human chorionic gonadotropin as a substitute for LH and human menopausal gonadotropin for FSH as necessary. Recombinant human FSH and LH may be available soon.

Possible Reproductive Problems in Women with Pituitary Tumors:

Prolactin can be secreted by a pituitary tumor either alone or sometimes together with growth hormone (see section on Prolactinomas). This increase in prolactin may cause menstrual irregularities and milk production by the breast (galactorrhea). Bromocriptine, or the recently approved carbergoline, is highly effective in decreasing prolactin levels to the normal range and can restore normal reproductive function in both women and men.

Untreated acromegaly or Cushing's Disease can also be associated with the occurrence of excessive and coarse body hair in women (hirsutism). Hirsutism in Cushing's Disease is due to excessive production of male hormones by the adrenal glands. Hirsutism in acromegaly can be due to excessive production of male hormones (androgens) from the ovary or the adrenals.

In acromegaly the associated increase in production of insulin-like growth factor 1 (IGF-I) in these organs may be one of the causes of excess androgens. The hirsutism associated with Cushing's Disease or acromegaly will usually decrease in severity with lowering of cortisol or growth hormone levels that occur after treatment of the pituitary tumor.

Most frequently, in association with secreting or non-secreting tumors, the levels of the other pituitary hormones such as luteinizing hormone and follicle stimulating hormone are decreased. This will lead to abnormal development of the ovarian follicles, decreased ovarian hormone secretion (estrogens and progestins) and disturbed ovulation. If the female hormone secretion is low, symptoms such as vaginal dryness, skin changes, smaller and softer breasts, and other long-term risk factors such as loss of bone mass (osteoporosis) and increased risks of coronary heart disease may develop. Estrogen replacement therapy should be used with progestins to counteract the effect of estrogens alone on the endometrium. Combinations of estrogens and progestins can be used in cyclical manner or continually. The schemes of hormone replacement therapy are the same as those used for post-menopausal women. If the woman desires fertility, then she should consult an endocrinologist or reproductive endocrinologist. The endocrinologist should be consulted since the pituitary tumor may enlarge during pregnancy and treatment of the tumor should be completed before pregnancy occurs. If there is no ovulation, induction of ovulation can be initiated with follicle stimulating hormone (human menopausal gonadotropins or human follicle stimulating hormone) to induce the development of the follicles containing the egg and luteinizing hormone (human chorionic gonadotropin) to induce ovulation. If pregnancy occurs, progestins are used to support the endometrium until the embryo is implanted into the endometrium. These hormones should be administered in a sequential manner and must be monitored by ultrasound examination of the ovary, and blood hormone levels, usually under the supervision of a reproductive endocrinologist. The success of ovulation induction is usually high in patients with pituitary tumors.

Pregnancy in the Panhypopituitary Patient

George T. Koulianos, M.D., Director, Reproductive Endocrinology and Infertility, Mobile Infirmary Medical Center, Clinical Assistant Professor, University of South Alabama

Introduction

Panhypopituitary women are infertile due to an absence of the pituitary hormones Follicle Stimulating Hormone (FSH) and Luteinizing Hormone (LH). These hormones are necessary for normal ovarian function, estrogen production and ovulation. The typical panhypopituitary patient is infertile and does not experience regular menstruation unless she receives estrogen and progestin therapy. Ovulation requires appropriate replacement of FSH and LH.

Infertility Evaluation

Prior to the medical initiation of ovulation, other factors, which may be contributing to a couples inability to conceive, must be excluded. The basic evaluation includes a semen analysis and hysterosalpingogram (HSG). The semen analysis is the single most important test in the evaluation of the male and provides an accurate assessment of the number of sperm, the percentage of sperm that are motile, the size and shape of individual sperm and the volume of the ejaculate. If an abnormal semen analysis is noted, further evaluation would be needed prior to beginning ovulation induction.

An HSG provides the physician with information about the uterine cavity and condition of the fallopian tubes. With the patient placed as for a pelvic examination, a small tube is placed into the cervical canal. X-ray dye is then injected slowly, and the flow of dye into the uterine cavity, out through the tubes and into the pelvis can be seen on a TV screen. A permanent record of the study is made by taking several x-rays. It is important to confirm that the fallopian tubes are normal prior to ovulation induction and any suggestion of scar tissue (pelvic adhesions) would require laparoscopic evaluation. Laparoscopy is an out-patient surgical procedure that allows direct visualization of the ovaries, fallopian tubes and uterus.

To conceive, panhypopituitary patients require ovulation induction with human menopausal gonadotropins (hMG). HMG (Perganol, Humagon, or Repronex) is a potent fertility drug containing equal amounts of the pituitary hormones, FSH and LH and allows the physician to exogenously replace the FSH and LH that these women lack. hMG is given as a daily injection and during treatment patients require careful monitoring. Unfortunately, hMG therapy can be expensive with a typical cycle costing $600.00 to $1200.00 for medication alone. For the panhypopituitary patient this expense can be even higher. Fortunately, many although not all insurance carriers cover a portion if not the entire cost of treatment. Pregnancy rates in women with low or absent FSH and LH requiring hMG to induce ovulation are similar to those of normally ovulating women but more that one course of treatment may be needed to attain pregnancy. Helping a couple deal with the frustration of repeated partial success (ovulation) but ultimate failure (negative pregnancy test) requires a physician with time, sensitivity and compassion.

Most patients require 7 to 15 days of stimulation to obtain a mature follicle(s), this period may be extended if the ovary is slow to respond. This is especially true in the panhypopituitary patient. Throughout treatment the follicle size is monitored with vaginal ultrasound and blood estrogen. A follicle is a fluid filled structure which houses the ripening egg. Once the follicle is mature and the estrogen is appropriate ovulation is induced with human chorionic gonadotropin *(hCG)* and the couple either has intercourse or an insemination is scheduled.

Potential side effects of this treatment include breast tenderness, hot flashes, swelling or rash at the injection site, abdominal bloating, mood swings, and mild twinges of abdominal pain. The most serious side effect is hyperstimulation syndrome where the ovaries enlarge and can become extremely tender. Severe cases can frequently be avoided with careful monitoring and withholding hCG. Despite intensive monitoring, multiple pregnancies can occur with a 25% incidence of twins and an approximately 5% incidence of higher order gestation.

Growth Hormone

On occasion, panhypopituitary women can respond poorly to hMG therapy. In the past, the only option for these responders was increasing the dosage of hMG and duration of treatment. These patients can use dozens of ampules of hMG and still respond poorly with either a small number of follicles and/or low blood estrogen value. Recently it has been suggested that Growth Hormone (GH) can modulate ovarian function by decreasing the amount of hMG needed to induce ovulation and increasing peak estrogen levels. This may be especially important for the panhypopituitary patient who is GH deficient. Since GH only exerts a permissive role by allowing FSH and LH to work on the ovary, only small amounts are needed.

Pregnancy

Once pregnant the placental tissue will produce sufficient amounts of the pregnancy hormone hCG to stimulate ovarian progesterone production and maintain the pregnancy. Most pregnancies require careful physician monitoring of the patient's panhypopituitism. A team approach is often utilized and includes the endocrinologist and obstetrician. The onset of labor may be compromised since there is an absence of the pituitary hormone oxytocin. Oxytocin stimulates the uterus to contract and its absence may make normal vaginal delivery impossible necessitating a cesarean section.

Conclusion

Panhypopituitary patients are rare and challenging. Pregnancy is usually possible with ovulation induction with hMG and poor responders with GH. Once pregnant careful attention is needed and delivery may require ceasarean section. Thanks to new innovation in infertility therapy, we are now better equipped to meet these challenges.

Suggested Readings

1 Katz, E., Ricciarelli, F., Adashi, B. The potential relevance of growth hormone to female reproductive physiology and pathophysiology. Fertility and Sterility 1993, 59:8-34.
2 Blumenfeld, Z., Lunenfeld, B. The potentiating effect of growth hormone on follicle stimulation with human menopausal gonadotropin in a panhypopituitary patient. Fertility and Sterility 1989, 52:328-331.
3 Koulianos GT, Degelos, SD, Castracane VD: Effect of exogenous growth hormone in a panhypopituitary patient undergoing ovulation induction with hMG. Presented at the 53rd Annual Meeting of the Society for Reproductive Medicine, Cincinnati OH, October, 1997.
4 Lanzone, A., Fortini, A., Fulghesu, A.M., et al. Growth hormone enhances estradiol production follicle-stimulating hormone-induced in the early stage of follicular maturation. Fertility and Sterility 1996, 66:948-953.

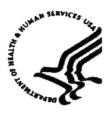

DEPARTMENT OF HEALTH & HUMAN SERVICES

NATIONAL INSTITUTES OF HEALTH

The National Institutes of Health (NIH) is conducting clinical studies that include evaluation and treatment of:

- Cushing's syndrome
- Acromegaly
- TSH-producing pituitary tumors
- Prolactinoma
- Hypopituitarism
- Non-functioning pituitary tumors
- Diabetes insipidus/hyponatremia
- Gonadotropin-producing pituitary tumors
- Pediatric Pituitary Tumors

The NIH is a state-of-the-art facility for:

- Diagnosis of pituitary tumors
- Pituitary imaging
- Pituitary surgery

All patients are admitted as participants in research protocols. Admission and care at the NIH Clinical Center are free of charge. In certain cases, travel expenses to and from the NIH Clinical Center may be reimbursed. Have your physician write a letter of referral to one of the following institutes if you would like more information:

- Cushing's disease, gonadotropin-producing tumors, diabetes insipidus, prolactinoma, pediatric tumors: NICHD referrals, National Institutes of Health, Bldg. 10, Rm. 10S261, 10 Center Drive, MSC 1834, Bethesda, MD 20892-1834, Fax: (301) 402-1073

- TSH-producing pituitary tumors, acromegaly, and pituitary tumors related to multiple endocrine neoplasia type I: NIDDK referrals, National Institutes of Health, Bldg. 10, Rm. 8S235, 10 Center Drive, MSC 1770, Bethesda, MD 20892-1770, Fax: (301) 480-4517

Section VI

Patient Input

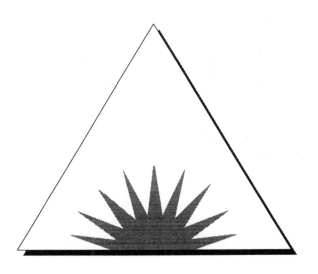

Second Edition

Taking Control of Her Life
Tara Pritchard - Patient

Although I have told my story many times now, it still does not seem real. I had always been very healthy. Until recently most of my medical concerns were minor. In December of 1994 I had a full hysterectomy. I experienced many female difficulties and finally decided after having my two children, it would be better for all the family to end the roller coaster ride of mood swings and physical discomfort. Surgery went well but soon it seemed I was having new troubles. I gained weight that I could not control, constantly fatigued, I could not concentrate. For the next two years I was in and out of my doctor's office for tests, with no resolve. Things grew even worse. This is list of my symptoms:

- Heart pounding.
- Hair lost shine & thinning.
- Dry skin.
- Constipation.
- Not sleeping well.
- Loss of concentration.
- VERY, very tired.
- Depression.
- Tremors (feel as though I am shaky but have pretty steady hand).
- Urination during the night.
- Breasts feel full and enlarged but no discharge.
- Throat feels tight and swollen.
- Dizzy spells.
- Eyes hurt- pressure feeling from behind the eyes. Vision has deteriorated in the last 2 years.
- Weight gain!! 14 pounds in 6 months. No change in diet.
- Large muscles hurt and sore. (feels like lactic acid, will hurt one day and gone the next).
- Severe migraines - Some last for 3 days.
- No interest in intimacy.

I gained more weight, lost more concentration, lost strength, began to experience heart palpitations. I was cold all the time, my hair lost all shine and was thinning. I could not stand all day or walk up stairs; my muscles shook and felt like rubber. At this point I was scared and frustrated! I had spent nine years body building and competing! My doctor said all was fine. It was not fine! I did not get into competitive shape and condition by accident. At this point many of my friends and acquaintances had noticed and commented on the deterioration.

I was on a business trip and while I was waiting for my plane I had another heart palpitation. It lasted for at least three minutes. I thought maybe I was having a heart attack. I promised God if I got home OK I would kick in that wonderful "type A" personality He gave me. I went back to my doctor. She ran more tests. To shorten the story many of my test results were very low, such as thyroid. She sent me to a heart doctor and they had me wear a monitor for 24 hours. My average heart rate while active was only 64 bpm. During sleep I experienced episodes when my heart rate dropped to 39 bpm. I would wake freezing cold, then it would race to 189 bpm and I would wake in the sweats; completely wet. I was told that there was nothing clinically wrong. My doctor found no reason to do anything further. I was very upset. I demanded copies of all my tests and .went to an endocrinologist in Medford, Oregon. We do not have one in Klamath Falls. On my third visit he said he expected to find a pituitary tumor and also began treatment for hypothyroidism. I had only slight improvement with the thyroid. I had a couple of MRI's that revealed my pituitary was about three times its normal size. At this point I was referred to Dr. David Cook at Oregon Health Sciences. I have seen or had my films reviewed by several neurosurgeons, including Dr. Charles Wilson. There are two basic opinions of the situation, one being that the gland is perforated for some unknown reason, the other that maybe a tumor has engulfed the entire gland. Although the exact cause is not agreed upon the treatment plan was: treat the hormone deficiencies. All of them! Dr. Cook did further testing showing that I was growth hormone deficient. He prescribed growth hormone. I began the growth hormone treatment in late December 1995. It did not take long for me to notice improvement.

I realized that this was going to be a life long problem and received warnings about extra stress. At this point in my life I was still running my commercial janitorial service and operating a fabric store I had opened two years previously. I had two young children, a husband and a household to care for. I was only 33 years old when this ordeal began. In order to reduce stress in my life I liquidated my fabric store. This was very disappointing and caused a huge financial loss.

I pleaded and petitioned my insurance company for coverage as GH was not yet FDA approved for adults (use for children had long been approved). They gave me a six month trial period in which they would cover my treatment at 80%. This was great news, but still I had what may have been the worse six months of my life. I had to liquidate my store or renew a two year lease and that was not an option when all was considered. My husband took a job out of town, the partners in the business left me to close the store alone (big mess, lots and lots of stress!!), and to make matters worse my stepfather died very unexpectedly. Well, now my six months was over and my check up did not go as expected. I lost 105 points in my growth hormone and showed no real improvement in body composition. I felt so much heifer compared to what I had but because the improvements that I experienced could not be measured scientifically the insurance was discontinuing coverage for the growth hormone. This was about August 7, 1996. Then I heard from my sister-in-law that Dr. Cook had heard that growth hormone for adults had just received FDA approval. With the FDA approval my insurance would continue coverage of my treatment.

My condition and improvement has been continually monitored and I have steadily improved. In May of 1997 my doctor rechecked my testosterone. I was not gaining muscle back like expected and was still on the tired side. It was found that I had no testosterone. So, that too was replaced. What a wonderful difference. I had more energy, a libido, and began to gain back muscle. Just yesterday I had a body fat analysis and I am down to 16.4% body fat. This is a huge drop from the whopping 41% measured in December of 1996. This works out to be a 40% decrease in body fat!!! When I was first tested I had lost at least 15% in bone density. I will not have this checked until December this year but I am sure that will show the same type of improvement.

It is now August of 1997. 1 have been on treatment for 20 months. I take growth hormone, estrogen, thyroid and testosterone. All these are hormones. Things are going beautifully. I feel wonderful. I only have a bad day here and there. I have gained back a lot of muscle, my mental health, my libido and my self-esteem. I do not need glasses anymore, I do not have migraines. I feel I have gained back my life and the *quality* of my life! How wonderful it is to feel human again.

This experience has not been pleasant or easy! I have no doubt that if I had not become aggressive I would not be on growth hormone or most likely any treatment. What made this experience so difficult besides the obvious illness itself was the attitudes of many of the doctors I had to visit and overcome! I do not want my statements to be deemed as "doctor bashing," but if the issue is not recognized it will certainly not improve. I was not upset that my family physician did not find the problem , but that she did not take me seriously and refer me to a specialist (endocrinologist). I had to find one in the phone book. This was not a pleasant experience. This individual was rude and indifferent. I realize that their jobs are difficult and stressful but when we go to them it is because we need them. Not only do we need them for their skill and knowledge but we need them to recognize that we the patients are often scared and feel vulnerable! We do not need to be coddled, but just given a little recognition of the whole picture.I did appreciate that when my family physician received copies of my test results showing the tumor she phoned me at my business. We had a very long discussion about how my situation was handled by her and the conclusion I drew because of it. I was very candid with her. There is no perfection in this world but we can try our best and she showed a true interest so that she herself could evaluate her attitude and handling of my case. I very much appreciated her call.

All I can say to others is this. If you know that there is something wrong, you must take charge of the situation and pursue an answer. If you will not do it for yourself do not expect someone else to do it for you. It is unfortunate that you need to have that attitude but you may not have any choice. If you can find an organization or support group for you condition you will most likely find help. This was my experience with the Pituitary Tumor Network Association. It was through this network that I received copies of the studies that I used to make my case to my insurance company and also found the names of many specialists concerning my condition. This organization has been absolutely invaluable to me!

> "Whatever you can do,
> or dream you can,
> Begin it.
> Boldness has genius,
> power and magic in it.
> BEGIN IT NOW."
> —*Goethe*

Caught in the Web - www.pituitary.com
Kathleen Wong - Patient

I have just visited your website, and wish that I had found this wonderful and comprehensive resource years and years earlier! I have been a prolactinoma patient since 1990. At the time, I was an otherwise perfectly healthy and active university student majoring in biology. I had access to a significant amount of academic research sources, including Medline and many scientific journals. As you may suspect, the results of my search were futile and frustrating. Searches for prolactinoma information returned article titles that investigated arcane scientific minutiae, but no resources that would improve my chances of obtaining competent care or to cope with the symptoms of this condition. All I could find I had already learned in an undergraduate endocrinology course.

So I gave up my search for more information and submitted to the care of my endocrinologist. When I took Bromocriptine, I came down with hives. When I took Permax, I felt depressed, suffered chronic insomnia, and drowsy for over 18 hours a day. My physician gave up and advised me to wait until the tumor became a macroadenoma large enough to merit transsphenoidal surgery. The surgery was successful, but the symptoms returned within six months. My endocrinologist recommended trying the Permax again, but I refused because it made me incapable of functioning on a daily basis. At that point, my physician got angry and frustrated, and essentially told me not to return unless I started taking the drug again. Not wishing to give up my daily activities, I never saw him again.

Though I knew about the potential for optic, endometrial, and osteoporosis problems, I essentially ignored the prolactinoma for about two years. I wound up taking the drug only when I could afford a day to lie on the couch. As you can imagine, that wasn't very often.

When I changed health plans, my new endocrinologist assured me there were better methods of handling the problem than forcing myself to take drugs with terrible side effects. And he was right, because two weeks after I saw him, Dostinex was approved by the FDA.

This drug has revolutionized the state of my health. I feel no side effects, am on the lowest dosage (0.25 mg twice a week), and my prolactin levels are normal. I now feel completely healthy for the first time in almost a decade.

I've never before been able to share this story with anyone else who has been through the same frustrating situations. I think your website is a wonderful resource, and that more endocrinologists should tell their patients about it. The site is the only place I have been able to find any medical and lifestyle information useful to pituitary patients, and the only place I have found a reference to Dostinex. And I think the subject of the sexual response of pituitary tumor patients is perfectly germane to the site. The subject should be given as much coverage as other aspects of coping with pituitary dysfunction. From what I can tell, your site is not only a clearinghouse for patient information about pituitary tumors, but a place where the far-flung and hidden population of pituitary patients can come together to share their bewildering and often frightening experiences.

I greatly appreciate the medical sophistication of the scientific articles and the candor of the personal stories, and plan to continue visiting periodically in the future.

Radiation Therapy - A Patient's Journal

Lisa Bensmihen - Patient

Tuesday January 10. 1995. Day 1

First. I had to have my mouthpiece fitted. This is the device that prevents my head from moving when my head is in the metal traction. This piece allows for no movement of my head when I am on the bed in the machine. This took approximately 1/2 hour, due to adjustments.

Then I went to Brigham and the Women's Radiation Department where I met with Marc and Jay, the technicians. They took the mouthpiece and custom fitted it to the headpiece that I will use for the next 5 weeks. First, they put putty in the back of the frame, filling in where my head meets the frame, making sure it has a snug fit.

Next, I laid down on the table and they fit my head into the "helmet." This "helmet" has 30 different coordinates; these coordinates will then be fed into the computer, matching up exactly where the machine's beam and my tumor will meet.

Before I left, Linda, the head nurse/technician, gave me a mimeographed sheet of paper, you know, the kind you fill out for an office supply order. She asked me to please sign it and return it on Thursday. I looked it over and it was a list of possible side effects ranging from common, (tiredness), to extremely rare, (death). I really didn't know what to do with this. I mean, do I sign it? I did. Already I was tired and the first treatment, we call it treatment, not radiation, was not starting until Friday.

Going about this is like a job. First go there, then come here. Walking along the corridors of this hospital, I look at the names on the doors: social services, financial this or that. Department of Cardio radio trans something. All the while looking at the people trying to figure out why they are here. Everyone definitely looks very directed. I mean they all have to get somewhere.

It's 7 a.m. and this place is buzzing. everyone clutching their Au Bon Pain (bakery) coffee cups. In the dentist's office, I see the same man I will see later in the radiation waiting room.

Thursday, January 12. 1995, Day 4

No breakfast today. It's 8 a.m. and time for the imaging of the brain. I go one floor up with Ed, (technician) to get a CT Scan. This place looks like Star Trek with all its advanced imaging machines, and a Fifth Avenue skin doctor's office, with its marble floors. First though, I get an I-V of gallein contrast. Finding a vein for this nurse was no problem, so much so that when she put the needle in, so much blood spurted out she had to change her pants, and mop the floor. So much for "bad veins." As the gallein is going through, I have a very, very warm sensation running up and down my arms.

Next. it's to the CT scan room. There is a visiting physician there: he must be 20 years older than Eddy, so I figure this is the old adage of the children teaching the adults.

So far I've seen some pretty sick people. I mean, I bop in here, wearing blue jeans, a knapsack and a Walk-Man. And then I look into this room, and there *she* is. She's so frail, the head frame is on her, even though she is not in the treatment room, she's wrapped in white blankets, and she's bald. This basement is the "Great Equalizer."

I also see Marc everyday. He was at the dentist's office the same day as me, and has been on the same course as me. We compare diagnoses, talk about his family, and all the other things to distract us from talking about the reason why we are both here now. Misery loves company.

Friday, January 13th. 1995. Day 1 Treatment
I didn't sleep last night. I'm starting today (as opposed to Monday) because Monday is Martin Luther King Day. Everything is connected. I get there at 8 a.m., and Linda takes me into "The Room". I look around, no biggy, looks like any other MRI/CT Scan room. She puts the frame and helmet on, takes the measurements, and then goes into the booth behind the wall.

I wait to waste away. I am thinking about the power of this all. Pumping in through the speakers is the Eurythmics, a somewhat funky, Euro-pop band. My mind is wandering. The machine is relatively quiet compared to an MRI. It's a constant buzz. How could this be so powerful, and I can't feel or see anything. What else is like this? I've figured it out: God, love, and radiation. A sermon can be thought of from anything.

"Well that's it, Lisa." I pop up. "Thanks Linda, see you Tuesday at 9."

Tuesday, January 17, 1995.
Lots of traveling. My mother is here with me this week. She can't deal with the illness, which is understandable, watching me sleep all day long. I'm getting used to this routine: taxi, basement, waiting room, fitting, treatment, taxi back to the hotel, breakfast, CNN, sleep.

My device does not fit, so I now must bite down on this rubber tube to stabilize the helmet. I look like Hannibal Lecter from "Silence of the Lambs." Today's music selection is "Back in the Saddle Again" - how appropriate.

I meet with Dr. Loeffler. He's very nice, and professional. He tells me I'm going to be tired (understatement of the century), and that I'll feel like I have the flu. I tell him I have my period, and I know the pituitary grows during menstruation; he says it doesn't matter because they'll radiate 4 times the size anyway. What a relief.

I tell my mom what's wrong with all the other patients here. Somehow you know everyone else's business, kinda like at work when you know what everyone else makes. She can't deal. She wants to shop and talk about cousin Linda's face-lift.

My hair fits much better in the clamps now that I got my haircut, good move. It's 10:31 a.m., and I fall asleep to CNN.

Wednesday, January 18th. 1995.
Yesterday I was very tired. I just couldn't shake it, and I really didn't want to. Today on the speakers is "When Tomorrow Comes." I think, will it ever?

Can't believe I have 22 more of these. Damn! I'm reading Tim Robbins' inspirational book. "Giant Steps." He has acromegaly like me. He's positive and made millions selling hope and inspiration. Maybe some of it will rub off.

Thursday, January 19th. 1995. Max's (my nephew's) 7th Birthday.
I'm getting into the routine, trying to deal with this in the best possible manner. I mean, I'm at the Westin hotel, having my kosher dinner delivered to me every night, clicker in hand, seeing bad movies, talking to my brothers and sisters everyday. It's four-star cancer. I really appreciate my mom being here, especially when I see how this is affecting her.

Friday, January 20th. 1995.
The minute I get up from the treatment I feel funny, a little like being stoned, seeing the world in slow motion, having no inhibitions in thought or speech. Time to get ready to travel back to NYC: always scared I'm not going to make it in time for Shabbot. On the plane, I'm out cold,

sleeping straight up: horses sleep like this, don't they?

It feels good to be back in my apartment. Shabbot is here, and so are friends, food, familiarity. I go to the Rabbi's for dinner but leave early: I have a headache the size of Montana. I take two Tylenol and sleep for 13 hours.

Saturday night I go to a friend's place for a little party. Very interesting people are there. John works in Mid-town in an ad agency, currently working on the Gillette campaign, while his wife works for the Whitney. Charlie works for the Policy Group, writing political papers on current world events, he used to be with Clinton Administration. Charlie asks me what I do. "Oh, I'm having radiation in Boston."

Monday, January 23. 1995.
Traveled on a Saab Prop Plane back to Boston and I'm a little nervous. Wouldn't be ironic to die in one of these planes, as opposed to the radiation? The plane is smaller than the Columbus Avenue bus.

Today's treatment, and all Mondays to follow, will be at 12:45 p.m., because I'm traveling. There are a lot more people in here now. I see Marc, he has headaches, and wants to talk/share. I'm not in the mood. Sometimes yon just want to do your thing and not dive into your feelings: this happens to be one of those times. Linda comes in and tells me they're running late due to technical difficulties: this is something I don't want to hear. Sounds like an airline delay due to maintenance. Today on the speakers is "This is the End of Innocence." Feeling tired, but go with it.

Tuesday, January 24. 1995.
I'm getting pretty good at this job. I never used to judge a new employee at the restaurant until they knew where the rice was. Well, I've found the rice. I met with Dr Loeffler today and I knew things were going all right when he walked in and started talking about the Cavaliers (the Cleveland basketball team). I tell him I'm tired and I want to go.

Wednesday, January 25. 1995.
Lots of O.J. and Rose Kennedy coverage. I'm learning a lot about courtroom proceedings and a Democratic American family. I had a facial yesterday, and my skin feels so much better, and so do I.

I went to the support group last night for Adults with Brain Tumors. I really enjoyed being able to talk to others like myself. I don't have to hold back or censor my thoughts. We were able to talk about my issues: expectations not being met. For example, when I have blood tests and they miss a vein, then everything comes crashing down and I realize what the hell I'm doing and going through. Also, dealing with friends' and families' reactions, doctors. Jack and Norma, the other patients, had the same story I did. Basically, it was good to share.

Today, Jay, the medical physicist. came to my treatment because the measurements seem to be off. He's going to talk to Dr. Loeffler. Today on the radio is "What's it all About." I felt very tired and weak again.

Friday, January 27. 1995.
I saw my brain on the computer yesterday. Jay explained my case to me, 3D of course. showing me how through the computer the machines' radiation will slice through the brain. The tumor will receive 80%, following concentric circles around the tumor though the rest of the brain will receive less and less damage to the cerebrum,

I told Dr. Loeffler that I'm getting headaches, so he took me in one of his offices and drew my brain on the board explaining to me that some of the nerves are getting radiation. He's such an intellectual, and he's caring. What a good combo.

Going back to NYC today, and getting used to this.

Tuesday, January 31. 1995.
I felt very strange tonight. The first time I felt like this, like my balance was way off. Told Anne, the head nurse, the following morning and received a prescription for Tylenol with codeine.

Wednesday, February 1. 1995.
Today, during my massage, I was lying on my back and felt the enormity of it all. It's easy to snap in and out of what you're doing, and this just happens to be the snap in the extreme direction.

I'm getting sick of explaining to people what I'm doing, so when asked, I now say I'm here on business. You know, when you work for the CIA and someone asks you what you do, you answer "I'm in insurance". There's no follow-up. I mean, probably one of the most boring professions. So now I'm employed by John Hancock Insurance. It's easy because they're based out of Boston.

I talked to Will, another patient, today, and he's in the hospital all day getting chemo, plus going through the radiation, so on the days he's there, I go to his room and give him a kibitz (good talk).

Friday, February 3. 1995.
I'm going back to New York City now and expecting a big snow storm. Today's selections on the radio are "Pretty Women Who Lunch", "The Sun Will Come Out Tomorrow", and "Everything's Coming up Roses." I sang this last song 20 years ago at camp when I was in the Miss Hawaii pageant. I didn't win; lost to Miss Kauai. Gosh, 20 years goes quickly.

Tuesday, February 7. 1995.
Yesterday JR. surprised me. Boy was I the happiest person in Boston - what love can do.

Today, as on every Tuesday, I meet with Dr Loeffler. First, he always asks what I do all day long. That's his way of finding out how I'm doing without directly asking. To be a good doctor you also have to be a good therapist. Then he asked me what I did before, and what I plan on doing once this is over, and he said. "Why don't you think about getting involved in the medical profession?" I must say, I was very flattered. Most doctors look at the illness first, and then if you're lucky, they remember a person. As my friend Alissa says, "I have the tumor, it doesn't have me." All those years at the Forum really paid off.

Then I went and typed a resume to work at Israel Bonds. I have the interview on Wednesday, February 15th, so hopefully I'll get this job. It sounds perfect: Jews, cash, high-powered, fun, and best of all, I'll be making a real living. What a novel idea.

I saw Will again today. The chemo is getting to him. He's tired and his stomach is hurting. There's degrees of everything. Compared to him I look like Queen Esther.

After my treatment, I went to get my coat, and this other elderly woman started talking to me. I could tell it was her first day. You could always tell rookies right away. They look around, they are all confused, they don't know the procedure of how people are called, and they have that look on their face like they really need to talk. And that's exactly what she did. I told her about the support group on Tuesday nights and she seemed interested. After my fourth week, I've become the "rookie of radiation", not a title I should really be too proud of. I mean, I've got this trip down. I don't mind lying in bed reading my beauty magazines, watching O.J. on CNN, getting facials and French manicures at Saks, and eating microwave popcorn. Maybe not such a prudent idea, since I probably use my allotted dose of radiation for the day by 9 am.

Thursday, February 9. 1995.

Michael, my brother, was here today. It was great to have him here, shopping and eating. We were in Neiman Marcus' dressing room, and he said he was 34. We both couldn't believe it. It was a day of bonding. He gave me a kiss and a hug, real heartfelt. Funny the power and unexpected ramifications of radiation.

We ate breakfast and came upstairs, and he took a nap. All that traveling and what-not can get to you. Funny, last week, Jon, my other brother, did the same thing. We went to Fanueil Hall, ate, shopped, and it felt fun to be a full-fledged tourist. Then we talked about my wedding, my future, and my health. A lot of focus on me.

I talked with Cooley (the technician) today, and asked him why I'm getting headaches. I told him I thought it had to do with the cells not regenerating, and this is what will inhibit the tumor's growth. He said. "Oh no, the reason is because were stopping the blood flow' to the brain, and your body reacts because its going through a trauma." Sometimes ignorance is bliss.

February 14, 1995. Valentine's Day.

Valentines Day is everywhere, and all I can think of is what a sham the flower, candy' and card industry pull on us. They really know how to play on peoples insecurity. I know I've been here a long time when I compliment one of the workers in the hotel on his haircut. J.R. (my brother-in-law), is here now and he's a great guest. He's very easy going, talks to taxi-cab drivers and waitresses.

I saw Dr Loeffler today and told him I'm the only girl I know who's gone through radiation and gained weight. He said that for the area they are radiating, the pituitary, this is quite normal. Then I went to Fanueil Hall with Will to grab lunch. He's so sick. He woke-up on Saturday morning with no hair. We came back to my hotel and he fell asleep on my bed before his mother came to pick him up. It's very hard to watch this because I feel like I've been dealt a much better hand. But, I must remember, everyone has their own hand, and you can't judge or compare anyones sorrow, pain, joy, or what-have-you to your own, although we constantly do it.

Wednesday, February 15. 1995.

Today is a big day. It really all started last night in "group." Basically we wound up talking about my mother and father, our relationship, and their reactions to the illness. It seems like everyone is still playing their role. I mean, reactions to events are the same: only the scene and some of the characters have changed, to protect the innocent of course.

Friday, February 17. 1995.

I've been waiting for this day for a long time now. It feels so good to have this over. As my father says, I should receive a diploma. My friend Jackie says, "enough with Boston and their striped turtlenecks." Now I just wait and see. Today I wondered if this is really gonna work, and Mark, the physicist, assured me that they gave me a big enough dose. I'll get an MRI in December and now it's back to Dr Kleinberg to start the blood work again. I can tell things are out of whack. I go to the bathroom all day long and my chest is huge. I've gained 8 pounds but I am confident that in time I'll even out. The feeling I have now is what Alissa used to say after she went out on a bad date, "ONWARD JEWISH SOLIDER".

My Name Is Phyllis Taylor

Phyllis Taylor

This letter is mainly for spouses of people with a problem like ours, but its possible that the actual patient my find some direction from my words. Friends and family around us always tell me how brave and strong we are. HA! If they could only see me curled up in my bed crying every night and every other chance I get. My mind and my brain are like JELLO. The best relief I get is when I go to work as a food service worker and we are to busy for me to think about my very stressful life. When I do have time to think about my life I just don't understand how I got to this point. In November of 1988,age 20, 1 was already a divorced mother of one. I had no special skills or talents. The only thing I was qualified to do was work in fast food. That of course left me wide open to be able to party hard with all my friends. Living from pay check to pay check was the only life I knew. I enjoyed being popular with everyone, especially the guys. How was I supposed to know that the day Doug Taylor came knocking on my door for a blind date with me, that it would change my whole life.

Doug was the kindest most gentle man I have ever met. Whenever I was with him or just talking to him on the phone he would make me feel so loved and wanted. He made me feel like I was the most important thing in his life. Naturally I fell in love with Doug, but Doug wasn't quite ready to make that final commitment. Our dating relationship went on for almost three years. A year and a half of that romance was separated by 1,000 miles and we only saw each other twice during that time. We talked on the phone almost every day. During our second visit together Doug asked me to marry him. We were married in September of 1991 and ever since then we have had marital difficulties. Immediately after starting our lives together, I noticed many changes in Doug's personality. We started marital counseling the same year we were married and now five years later we are still involved in marriage counseling. Over the years I have noticed so many changes in my husband. When I met Doug he was calm, quite, and very pleasant to be with. The day before the wedding was the first time I ever remember Doug getting angry. He was screaming and shouting at me for some kind of mistake I had made or something. I don't remember exactly what it was about. Probably because I was so shocked to see him so angry. I dismissed his anger on the account of us being in the middle of planning a very stressful wedding, and I suppose I expected that as soon as the wedding was done and over with, that Doug would return to being his normal self.

Well, I could not have been more wrong. Things just kept getting worse and Doug just kept getting more angry about everything and anything. As time went by Doug continued to get more angry and verbally abusive. We continued to go through counseling but both of us were constantly threatening to file for a divorce. We had been married exactly 4 years and 1 month when we were in our living room one day sitting through a family counseling session when a phone call came in. Three days earlier Doug's eye doctor had ordered a MRI to help find the reason that Doug was having some double vision. On the phone was the doctor reporting that Doug had a large pituitary tumor. This tumor has changed our lives forever. After having numerous tests done we have learned that this tumor caused a disorder called Acromegaly. Doug is not and probably never will be the same man I fell in love with. Acromegaly has changed not only his body size but also his heart and soul. It has caused the many personality changes that I have seen in Doug, along with frequent mood swings.This article is not being written to document medical information or to seek out information about my husband's condition.

This article is about me. My name is Phyllis Taylor and I am a person with feelings and emotions and I can only live and deal with so much This letter is directed to all the other spouses that have been cheated out of their happy marital life. I love my husband very deeply and we have certainly been through a lot together but he is not the same man I fell in love with. I want to live a normal life with the same Doug that I fell in love with. He is a very angry and violent person now. Sometimes he can be very sweet and loving but then he changes and his anger is out of control again. This disease has taken hold of not only my husband's life and body but it has also taken hold of my life and body. Now I am very angry and sometimes find myself out of control. Judging by the relationship that Doug and I had before we were married, we should have a close to perfect marriage and a very happy life together. I don't want to leave my husband, but I don't want to stay with him either. I want to continue my life with my family, but I don't want any of us to have to live this unhappy another minute. What does a person do in this situation? How do I make a decision as big as this? How do I decide what is most important to me? How can I be sure I'm making the right decision?

If your situation is anything like mine, you have thought these exact same questions. You may not want to admit that your thoughts have drifted along this direction, but they are there and if your honest with yourself you know that. Do we feel guilty for having these thoughts? Of course. Its not our spouse's fault that this happened to them. In fact, this disease could have very easily happened to me instead of my husband, and it still could happen to me or to any other spouse out there. Not only do I want to be happy again but I want my husband to be happy again. Whether we are happy together or not I don't know. So where do we go from here? Where do I turn for support and guidance? Well I personally enjoy turning to the Lord for help. I am confident that he will guide me into the right decisions. I know that he will support me and lift me up. I also know that he will support and guide my husband. This disease has destroyed the life that I had planed for my family, but I refuse to let it control my life anymore! I will be happy again. I'm not sure when, but it will happen. I'm not sure if I'll be happy with or without Doug, but I will be happy again. And I hope that one day, Doug will overcome this illness and be happy again too.

My name is Phyllis Taylor and I will be a whole person again, someday. So I guess that's how I got to this point. I still don't understand it. I don't know if there is a purpose or a reason. I feel like the worst wife in the world. I'm supposed to love my husband no matter what, for better or worse, to death do us part. I want to support him 100% right through to the end, but I don't know if I can live in this kind of relationship much longer. More importantly, do I allow my 10 year old daughter to live and grow in this kind of environment? Will it change her future? Will she hate me for not removing her from this home? I could sit and ask many more questions about my future but I have a feeling that it would not do much good. I believe that people in our situation have to do three important things...

1. You must have wonderful friends and family that will support you in every way.
2. You must live your life only one day at a time.
3. You must have faith that everything is going to work out for the best, no matter what that may be.

Sometimes I have to remind myself of these three things and sometimes I wish I had someone to talk to that is going through some of the same things that I seem to be going through. Is there anyone out there who is or has experienced these same feelings and is possibly wanting to have a friend to talk to? If your interested in a little conversation along these lines please write to....PHYLLIS TAYLOR.

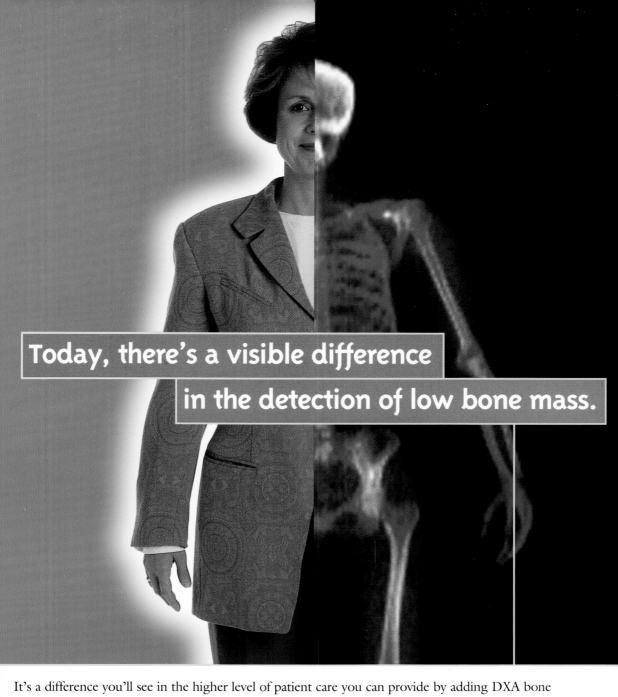

Today, there's a visible difference in the detection of low bone mass.

It's a difference you'll see in the higher level of patient care you can provide by adding DXA bone densitometry to your practice. Validated by over 1,000 studies, safe and precise DXA technology lets you assess and confirm bone loss at the hip, spine and other important skeletal sites in as little as 30 seconds.

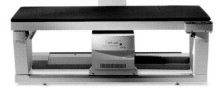

Integrate clinical bone mass measurement into your practice virtually risk free with HOLOGIC's new, flexible financing program. This shared-risk program lets you explore—with minimal investment and financial risk—the large and relatively untapped potential of a comprehensive bone disease management program in your local area. To learn more about bone densitometry and this professionally rewarding opportunity, call us at **1-800-486-4656.**

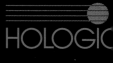

HOLOGIC

The Global Force That Simplifies Growth Hormone Therapy

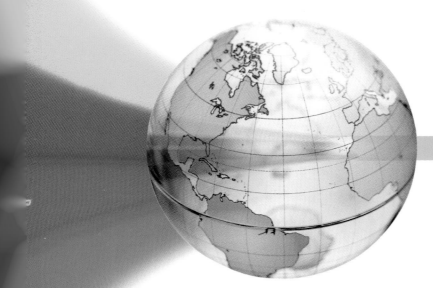

GENOTROPIN Lyophilized Powder (somatropin [rDNA origin] for injection) is indicated for the long-term treatment of children who have growth failure due to an inadequate secretion of endogenous growth hormone.

Special considerations

GENOTROPIN should not be used when there is any evidence of neoplastic activity, including intracranial lesions or tumors. Growth hormone should not be used in patients with fused epiphyses and should be used with caution in children with diabetes mellitus.

Physicians should be aware of the following precautions: intracranial hypertension (IH) has been reported in a small number of patients; a higher incidence of slipped capital femoral epiphyses (SCFE) has been reported in patients with endocrine disorders.

Please see adjacent brief prescribing information.

Pharmacia
&Upjohn

(((Genotropin™
(somatropin [rDNA origin] for injection)

Simplifies Growth Hormone Therapy

◫◫ *Genotropin*™

(somatropin [rDNA origin] for injection)

GENOTROPIN™ Lyophilized Powder
brand of somatropin [rDNA origin] for injection

INDICATIONS AND USAGE
Long-term treatment of pediatric patients who have growth failure due to inadequate secretion of endogenous growth hormone; exclude other causes of short stature.

CONTRAINDICATIONS
Do not use when there is any evidence of neoplastic activity. Institute therapy only when intracranial lesions are inactive and antitumor therapy complete. Discontinue GENOTROPIN if there is evidence of tumor growth. Do not use in pediatric patients with fused epiphyses. Use with caution in pediatric patients with diabetes mellitus.

WARNINGS
Patients with a known hypersensitivity to the preservative m-Cresol should not use the 5.8-mg and 13.8-mg presentations of GENOTROPIN. The 1.5-mg presentation is preservative free.

PRECAUTIONS
General. As with other growth hormone preparations, treatment with GENOTROPIN should be directed by physicians who are experienced in the diagnosis and management of patients with growth hormone deficiency (GHD). Properly train and instruct patients and caregivers who will administer GENOTROPIN in medically unsupervised situations. Frequently examine patients with GHD secondary to intracranial lesion for progression or recurrence of the underlying disease process. Because growth hormone may induce insulin resistance, observe patients for evidence of glucose intolerance. Concomitant glucocorticoid treatment may inhibit the growth promotion effect of growth hormone. For GHD patients with coexisting ACTH deficiency, adjust glucocorticoid replacement dose carefully to avoid an inhibitory effect on growth. Hypothyroidism may develop, and inadequate treatment of hypothyroidism may prevent an optimal response to growth hormone. Therefore, check thyroid function periodically in GHD patients, and treat with thyroid hormone when indicated. Patients with endocrine disorders, including GHD, have a higher incidence of slipped capital femoral epiphyses. Evaluate any pediatric patient at the onset of limp or complaints of hip or knee pain during growth hormone therapy. Intracranial hypertension (IH) with papilledema, visual changes, headache, nausea, or vomiting has been reported in a small number of patients treated with growth hormone products, usually within the first 8 weeks of initiating therapy. In all reported cases, IH-associated signs and symptoms resolved after terminating treatment or reducing dose. Funduscopic examination is recommended at initiation and periodically during growth hormone therapy.
Drug Interactions. Concomitant glucocorticoid treatment may inhibit the growth promotion effect of growth hormone (see PRECAUTIONS—General).
Carcinogenesis, Mutagenesis, Fertility Impairment. Carcinogenicity studies have not been conducted. No potential for mutagenicity of rhGH was revealed in a battery of tests, including induction of gene mutations in bacteria (the Ames test), gene mutations in mammalian cells grown in vitro, and chromosomal damage in intact animals. See PRECAUTIONS—Pregnancy for effect on fertility.
Pregnancy: Pregnancy Category B. Reproduction studies in rats and rabbits showed decreased maternal body weight gains but no teratogenicity. In rats, subcutaneous doses of GENOTROPIN during gametogenesis and pregnancy produced anestrus or extended estrus cycles in females and fewer and less mobile sperm in males. When given to pregnant rats (days 1 to 7 of gestation), a very slight increase in fetal deaths was observed. Perinatal and postnatal studies in rats produced growth-promoting effects in dams but not in fetuses. Young rats at the highest dose showed increased weight gain during suckling, but the effect was not apparent by 10 weeks of age. No adverse effects on gestation, morphogenesis, parturition, lactation, postnatal development, or reproductive capacity of offspring were observed. However, there are no adequate and well-controlled studies in pregnant women. Use during pregnancy only if clearly needed.
Nursing Mothers. No studies have been conducted in this population. It is not known whether this drug is excreted in human milk. Exercise caution when GENOTROPIN is administered to a nursing woman.

ADVERSE REACTIONS
As with all protein drugs, a small number of patients may develop antibodies to the protein. Growth hormone antibody with binding lower than 2 mg/L has not been associated with growth attenuation. In some cases, growth response interference has been observed when binding capacity is greater than 2 mg/L. In 419 patients evaluated in clinical studies (244 previously treated with growth hormone preparations and 175 with no previous growth hormone therapy), antibodies to growth hormone were present in six previously treated patients at baseline. Three of these six became antibody negative during the 6 to 12 months of treatment with GENOTROPIN. Of the remaining 413 patients, eight (1.9%) developed detectable antibodies to growth hormone during treatment; none had an antibody-binding capacity greater than 2 mg/L. There was no evidence that growth response to GENOTROPIN was affected in these antibody-positive patients. Antibodies to periplasmic Escherichia coli peptides are found in a small number of patients treated with GENOTROPIN, but these appear to be of no clinical significance.
In clinical studies with GENOTROPIN, the following events were reported infrequently: injection-site reactions, including injection pain or burning, fibrosis, nodules, rash, inflammation, pigmentation, or bleeding; lipoatrophy; headache; hematuria; hypothyroidism; and mild hyperglycemia. Leukemia has been reported in a small number of patients treated with growth hormone, including growth hormone of pituitary origin and recombinant somatropin. The relationship between leukemia and growth hormone therapy is uncertain.

OVERDOSAGE
There is little information on acute or chronic overdosage with GENOTROPIN. Intravenously administered growth hormone has been shown to result in acute decrease in plasma glucose with subsequent hyperglycemia. It is possible the same effect might occur on rare occasions with high doses of subcutaneously administered GENOTROPIN. Long-term overdosage may result in signs and symptoms of acromegaly consistent with overproduction of growth hormone.

DOSAGE AND ADMINISTRATION
Adjust dosage for the individual patient. Generally, a dose of 0.16 to 0.24 mg/kg/week is recommended. Divide the weekly dose into six to seven subcutaneous injections. Inject GENOTROPIN in the thigh, buttocks, or abdomen, rotating injection sites each day to help prevent lipoatrophy. **Do not inject intravenously.** When GENOTROPIN is mixed with a diluent, do not shake the cartridge to dissolve the powder; denaturation of the active ingredient may result. Inspect visually for particulate matter and discoloration prior to administration whenever solution and container permit. Do not inject contents if cloudy. Properly train and instruct patients and caregivers who will administer GENOTROPIN in medically unsupervised situations.

HOW SUPPLIED
Available in the following two-chamber cartridges: 1.5 mg (without preservative) preassembled in a GENOTROPIN INTRA-MIX™ Growth Hormone Reconstitution Device, 5.8 mg (with preservative) for use with the GENOTROPIN PEN™ 5 Growth Hormone Delivery Device and GENOTROPIN MIXER™ Growth Hormone Reconstitution Device or preassembled in a GENOTROPIN INTRA-MIX, and 13.8-mg (with preservative) for use with the GENOTROPIN PEN™ 12 Growth Hormone Delivery Device and GENOTROPIN MIXER.

Store lyophilized powder under refrigeration 36° to 46°F (2° to 8°C). Do not freeze. Protect from light. After reconstitution, the 1.5-mg cartridge may be stored under refrigeration only for up to 24 hours; use once and discard any remaining solution (no preservative). After reconstitution, the 5.8-mg and 13.8-mg cartridges may be stored under refrigeration for up to 14 days.

CAUTION: Federal law prohibits dispensing without a prescription.

Manufactured by:
Pharmacia & Upjohn AB
Stockholm, Sweden
For:
Pharmacia & Upjohn Company
Kalamazoo, MI 49001, USA

B-1-S

Pharmacia
&Upjohn

©1997 Pharmacia & Upjohn Company   September 1997   GSW 23269

Welcome to the

Pituitary Tumor Network Association

Dedicated to improving the quality of life and well-being for all patients with pituitary adenomas or afflictions, including...

Acromegaly... Cushing's Syndrome... Prolactinoma... Craniopharyngiomas... Non-functioning Tumors... Sexual and Reproductive Dysfunction... Vision Impairment... Hormonal Imbalances

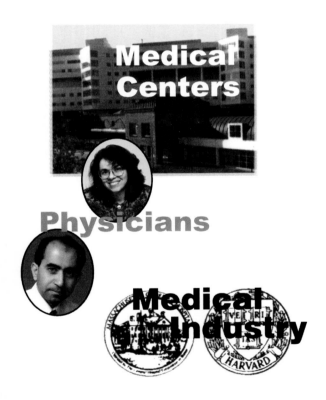

▲ The road to good health and happiness for pituitary patients can be a difficult one. It doesn't help if you can't seek directions whenever you need them. And nobody likes feeling that they are making the journey alone. That is why we created our website at *www.pituitary.com*.

▲ PTNA's website is the most authoritative website on the internet for pituitary patients. The National Institutes of Health, physicians, and hospitals often refer patients to the PTNA, and our website, as vital sources of information on pituitary disease. Loaded with information, www.pituitary.com is a 24 hour a day, 365 days a year, source of direction, empowerment, and comfort for pituitary patients.

💻 Calendar of PTNA and other pituitary related events and info.

💻 New articles from the experts and from patients who've been there.

💻 Patient chat rooms to share your experiences, and maybe learn from others.

💻 Complete current and past issues of our newsletter, *Network* , for you to download as often as you like.

💻 New articles by leading physicians you won't find anywhere else.

💻 Checklists to help you find the doctor that's right for you.

💻 Many pages of information about hospitals, medical centers, and physicians leading the fight for you.

💻 Bulletin boards to discuss the topics that are of interest to you.

💻 Full access to all bulletin board postings and discussions for the previous six months.

💻 Opportunities made available only to PTNA members.

www.pituitary.com

Section VII

Physician Listings

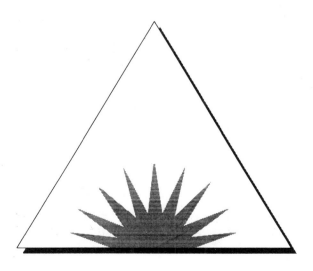

Second Edition

Endocrinologists

▲ Allweiss, Pamela, M.D.
Endocrinology and Metabolism
1401 Harrodsburg Road, B299
Lexington, KY 40504
Phone: (606) 277-8460
Fax: (606) 277-8460

Aronin, Neil, M.D.
Director, Clinical
Neuroendocrinology
University of Mass Med. Center
55 Lake Avenue North
Worcester, MA 01655
Phone: (508) 856-3239
Fax: (508) 856-6950
See display listing page 239

▲ Barkan, Ariel L., M.D.
University of Michigan
Division of Endocrinology
3920 TC, UMMC,
Ann Arbor, MI 48109-0354
Phone: (313) 936-5504
Fax: (313) 936-9240
See display listing page 240

Baum, Howard, M.D.
Dallas Diabetes & Endocrine Center
7777 Forest Ln #C-618
Dallas, TX 75230
Phone: (972) 566-7799
Fax: (972) 566-7399

Bengtsson, Bengt-Ake, M.D., Ph.D.
Associate Professor, Head, Division of
Endocrinology
Sahlgrenska University Hospital
Göteborg, Sweden
Phone: 46-31-602230
Fax: 46-31-821524

Berger, Richard E., M.D., F.A.C.P., F.A.C.E.
Dallas Endocrinology
7777 Forest Lane, Suite B-430
Dallas, TX 75230
Phone: (972) 661-7077
Fax: (972) 566-6136

▲ Besser, G.M., M.D.
Department of Medicine & Endocrinology
St. Bartholomew's Hospital
West Smitfield
London EC1A7BE U.K.
Phone: 44 171 601 8342/4
Fax: 44 171 601 8505

Blevins, Lewis, M.D.
Emory Universiy Hospital
1365 Clifton Road, N.E., Bldg. B
Atlanta, GA 30322
Phone: (404) 778-7744
Fax: (404) 778-4472
See display listing page 234

▲ **Brodie, Todd D., M.D.**
Mariposa Internal Medicine
Specialist Unlimited
2601 E. Roosevelt Street
Phoenix, AZ 85008
Phone: (602) 267-5351
Fax: (602) 267-5450

Brucker-Davis, M.D.,
Visiting Associate, NIDDK Molecular and
Cellular Endocrinology Branch
National Institutes of Health
Bethesda, Maryland

Caras, John A., M.D.
Wichita Falls Clinic
501 Midwestern Parkway
Wichita Falls, TX 76302
Phone: (817) 766-8875
Fax: (817) 766-8420

Champion, P.K. Jr., M.D., F.A.C.P., F.A.C.E.
Kelsey-Seybold Clinic, P.A.
6624 Fannin 20th Floor
Houston, TX 77030
Phone: (713) 791-8700
Fax: (713) 796-0161

▲ Christiansen, Jens Sandahl, M.D., D.Sci
Professor of Medicine
Department of Endocrinology and
Diabetes
Aarhus University Hospital
Kommunehospitalet
DK-8000 Aarhus C, Denmark
Phone:
Fax: 45-89-492010

Chertow, Bruce S., M.D., F.A.C.P.
University Physicians in
Internal Medicine
1801 Sixth Avenue
Huntington, WV 25703-1585
Phone: (304) 696-7113
Fax: (304) 696-7297

Cohen, Robert M., M.D.
University of Cincinnati College of
Medicine
231 Bethesda Avenue
Cincinnati, OH 45267-0547
Phone: (513) 558-4444
Fax: (513) 558-8581
See display listing page 232

Cook, David M., M.D.
Department of Medicine
Division of Endocrinology (L607)
Oregon Health Sciences University
3181 SW Sam Jackson Park Road
Portland, OR 97201-3098
Phone: (503) 494-3713
Fax: (503) 494-6990

Cook, Jennifer S., M.D.
Children's Health Center
1212 Pleasant St. Suite 300
Des Moines, IA 50309
Phone: (515) 241-6230
Fax: (515) 241-8728

de Herder, W. W., M.D.
Department of Internal Medicine III
and Clinical Endocrinology
University Hospital Dijkzigt
Dr Molewaterplein 40
3015 GD Rotterdam
The Netherlands
Phone: 31-10-4639222
Fax: 31-10-4633268
email: deherder@inw3.azr.nl

Ennis, Elizabeth D., M.D.
Baptist Health Systems
840 Montclar Road, Suite 317
Birmingham, AL 35213
Phone: (205) 592-5135
Fax: (205) 592-5694

▲ **Ezzat, Shereen M.D.**
Division of Endocrinology &
Metabolism
The Wellesley Hospital-University
of Toronto
160 Wellesley Street East
Room 134 Jones Bldg.
Toronto, ON M4Y 1J3, Canada
Phone: (416) 926-7000
Fax: (416) 966-5046
See display listing page 243

Fagin, James A., M.D.
University of Cincinnati College of
Medicine
231 Bethesda Avenue
Cincinnati, OH 45267-0547
Phone: (513) 558-4444
Fax: (513) 558-8581
See display listing page 232

Levoxyl®
(Levothyroxine Sodium Tablets, USP)

The Name to Remember for Quality and Cost.

At about half the cost of Synthroid®[1], it's no surprise Levoxyl® (Levothyroxine Sodium Tablets, USP) is the fastest growing brand name levothyroxine preparation on the market today. With precise dosing and consistent therapeutic effectiveness, Levoxyl® is trusted by patients, pharmacists and physicians alike.

If you are still prescribing, dispensing or taking Synthroid®, here are the facts.

You be the judge.

- *Levoxyl® is half the cost of Synthroid®[1]*
- *51st most dispensed medication in America and the second most dispensed brand name levothyroxine[2]*
- *Dependability - Levoxyl® boasts a spotless recall record*
- *Twelve strengths available for a wide range of dosing*

Jones Medical Industries, Inc.
St. Louis, MO 63146 • (800) 525-8466 • (NASDAQ: JMED)

Synthroid® is a registered trademark of Knoll Pharmaceutical Company.
[1] Cost comparison is based on Average Wholesale Price ("AWP") as published in (1997 Red Book) and may not represent actual prices to specific pharmacies or consumers.
[2] American Druggist, February 1997

Levoxyl®

(Levothyroxine Sodium Tablets, USP)

FOR ORAL ADMINISTRATION

DESCRIPTION:

Each LEVOXYL (Levothyroxine Sodium, USP) tablet contains synthetic crystalline levothyroxine sodium (L-thyroxine). L-thyroxine is the principle hormone secreted by the normal thyroid gland. Chemically, L-thyroxine is designated as L-tyrosine, 0-(4-hydroxy-3,5-diiodophenyl) - 3,5-diiodo-, monosodium salt, hydrate. The molecular formula is $C_{15}H_{10}I_4N\ NaO_4$ and the structural formula is:

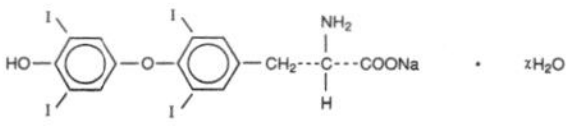

INACTIVE INGREDIENTS: lactose, microcrystalline cellulose, pre-gelatinized starch, magnesium stearate. The following are the color additives per tablet strength:

Strength (mcg)	Color Additive(s)	Strength (mcg)	Color Additive(s)
25	FD&C Yellow No. 6	125	FD&C Red No. 40 D&C Yellow No. 10
50	none	137	FD&C Blue No. 1
75	FD&C Blue No. 1 D&C Red No. 30	150	FD&C Blue No. 1 D&C Red No. 30
88	FD&C Yellow No. 6 FD&C Blue No. 1 D&C Yellow No. 10	175	FD&C Blue No. 1 D&C Yellow No. 10
100	FD&C Yellow No. 6 D&C Yellow No. 10	200	D&C Red No. 30 D&C Yellow No. 10
112	FD&C Yellow No. 6 FD&C Red No. 40 D&C Red No. 30	300	FD&C Yellow No. 6 FD&C Blue No. 1 D&C Yellow No. 10

CLINICAL PHARMACOLOGY:

The principal effect of thyroid hormones is to increase the metabolic rate of most body tissues.

The thyroid hormones are also concerned with growth and development of tissues in the young and are particularly important for the developing nervous system.

The major thyroid hormones are L-thyroxine (T_4) and L-triiodothyronine (T_3). The amounts of T_4 and T_3 released from the normally functioning thyroid gland are regulated by the amount of thyrotropin (TSH) secreted from the anterior pituitary gland. T_4 is the major component of normal thyroid gland secretions and is therefore the primary determinant of normal thyroid functions. T_4 acts as a substrate for physiologic deiodination to T_3 in the peripheral tissues. The physiologic effects of thyroid hormones are largely mediated at the cellular level primarily by T_3. LEVOXYL (L-thyroxine) tablets taken orally provide T_4 which upon absorption cannot be distinguished from T_4 secreted endogenously. Oral T_4 is absorbed in the small intestine, mainly in the jejunum and ileum; about two-thirds to three-quarters of the oral dose is actually absorbed. Absorption may be less than expected in patients with malabsorptive bowel disease, such as sprue, or with short bowel syndromes. Absorption is also affected by food and is slightly higher in the fasting state compared to when an oral dose is taken with food; the difference, however, is usually not of much clinical consequence. Certain other medications taken concomitantly by mouth can diminish absorption of T_4 from the intestinal lumen; these include aluminum hydroxide, sucralfate, ferrous sulfate, soybean-based foods (often taken for medical reasons), and binding resins used to lower serum cholesterol.

Once in the blood stream, T_4 is bound to plasma proteins, mainly to thyroxine-binding globulin (TBG); nevertheless, T_4 gains access to the tissues where it acts because the small fraction of T_4 that is not bound to plasma proteins ("free T_4") does cross cell membranes. A small fraction of circulating T_4 is also converted to circulating triiodothyronine (T_3), mainly in the liver; T_3 is also largely bound to circulating plasma proteins but not as tightly as is T_4. Once inside responsive cells, T_4 is converted to T_3 which is the major thyroid hormone acting intracellularly; circulating T_3 also gains access to the intracellular space and contributes to the action of thyroid hormone.

Circulating T_4 is gradually eliminated from the body with a plasma half-life of about seven days. Thus, an oral dose given once daily, once the dose is stabilized, results in a fairly stable level of serum T_4 over the course of the next 24 hours except for a slight rise of 10% to 15% in the few hours after the oral dose. The circulating T_3 formed from circulating T_4, on the other hand, is cleared from the blood much more rapidly with a plasma half-life of about 1 to 1 1/2 days. Thus, the oral dosing of T_4 results in a steady, stable serum level of T_4 which in turn provides an equally stable level of serum T_3. Oral T_3 given alone, on the other hand, results in a fairly rapid rise and fall in the serum T_3 level after each dose and fails to mimic the normal pattern of serum T_3.

INDICATIONS AND USAGE:

LEVOXYL (L-thyroxine) tablets are indicated as:

1. Replacement therapy for any form of diminished or absent thyroid function, e.g., as in cretinism, myxedema, or hypopituitarism, and including hypothyroidism seen in children, in pregnancy and in the elderly. The hypothyroidism may result from functional deficiency, primary atrophy, or partial or complete absence of the thyroid gland; from the effects of surgery, radiation or antithyroid agents on the thyroid gland; or from pituitary or hypothalamic disease. LEVOXYL therapy must usually be maintained continuously to control the hypothyroidism. When hypothyroidism is due to subacute or postpartum thyroiditis, it may be temporary and treatment need not be permanent.

2. A means of suppressing pituitary secretion of TSH in euthyroid patients in order to treat or prevent the recurrence of various types of goiter, including thyroid nodules, lymphocytic thyroiditis(Hashimoto's), multinodular goiter, and as part of the management of thyroid cancer. An exception is a patient with euthyroid autonomous function wherein the goiter is not under the control of pituitary TSH; T_4 therapy is not indicated in such patients (see below under CONTRAINDICATIONS).

3. A diagnostic agent in suppression tests to aid in the diagnosis of suspected mild hyperthyroidism or thyroid gland autonomy; this should be done rarely, only when clinically indicated and only when other tests such as stimulation with thyrotropin-releasing hormone (TRH) have not resolved the problem.

CONTRAINDICATIONS:

L-thyroxine therapy is contraindicated in untreated thyrotoxicosis, in other states of thyroid autonomy, acute myocardial infarction and uncorrected adrenal insufficiency.

WARNINGS:

> Drugs with thyroid hormone activity, alone or together with other therapeutic agents, have been used for the treatment of obesity. In euthyroid patients, doses within the range of daily hormonal requirements are ineffective for weight reduction. Larger doses may produce serious or even life-threatening manifestations of toxicity, particularly when given in association with sympathomimetic amines such as those used for their anorectic effects.

PRECAUTIONS:

General - Caution must be exercised in the administration of this drug to patients with cardiovascular disease. Development of chest pain or other aggravation of the cardiovascular disease may preclude its use or require a reduction of dosage in treated patients (see also DRUG INTERACTIONS). Institution of levothyroxine therapy in patients with adrenal insufficiency requires concomitant glucocorticoid therapy.

Information For The Patient-

Patients taking LEVOXYL and parents of children taking LEVOXYL should be informed that:

1. Replacement therapy is to be taken essentially for life, with the exception of cases of transient hypothyroidism, usually associated with thyroiditis, and in those patients receiving a therapeutic trial of the drug.

2. They should immediately report during the course of therapy any signs or symptoms of thyroid hormone toxicity, e.g., chest pain, increased pulse rate, palpitations, excessive sweating, heat intolerance, nervousness, or any other unusual event.

3. In case of concomitant diabetes mellitus, the daily dosage of antidiabetic medication may need readjustment as thyroid hormone replacement is achieved. If LEVOXYL is stopped, a downward readjustment of the dosage of insulin or oral hypoglycemic agent may be necessary to avoid hypoglycemia. Monitoring of urinary or blood glucose levels is mandatory in such patients during changes in thyroid medication.

4. In case of concomitant oral anticoagulant therapy, the prothrombin time should be measured frequently to determine if the dosage of oral anticoagulants is to be readjusted.

5. Patients taking LEVOXYL who then become pregnant should be monitored closely with measurements of serum TSH concentration because the requirement for T_4 usually increases during pregnancy. The daily dose of LEVOXYL may need to be increased to maintain the serum TSH concentration within the normal reference range.

6. Partial loss of hair may be experienced in the first few months of thyroid therapy, but this is usually a transient phenomenon and later recovery is the rule.

Laboratory Tests - The patient's response to thyroid replacement can be followed by laboratory tests such as serum levels of thyroxine (T_4), serum triiodothyronine (T_3), free thyroxine index and thyroid stimulating hormone (TSH). The principal test used to monitor treatment in primary hypothyroidism is the serum TSH level. In hypopituitarism, the serum TSH level is not useful and monitoring should be done with measurement of serum total or free T_4. In euthyroid goiter patients or those with thyroid cancer, the serum TSH should be suppressed below the reference range; how far below the reference range depends on the clinical goal.

Drug Interactions - In patients with diabetes mellitus, addition of oral T_4 therapy may cause an increase in the required dosage of insulin or oral hypoglycemic agents. Therefore, patients with diabetes mellitus should be observed closely for possible changes in antidiabetic drug dosage requirements.

Patients stabilized on oral anticoagulants who are found to require thyroid replacement therapy should be watched very closely when therapy is started; successful treatment with LEVOXYL in a patient who is initially hypothyroid may result in a need for a lower dose of oral anticoagulant. No special precautions appear to be necessary when oral anticoagulant therapy is begun in a patient already stabilized on maintenance LEVOXYL therapy. Cholestyramine and colestipol bind T_4 in the intestine, thus impairing its absorption. In vitro studies indicate that the binding is not easily reversed. Therefore, four to five hours should elapse between administration of cholestyramine and oral T_4. Other medications that interfere with absorption of oral T_4 from the gut include sucralfate, ferrous sulfate, aluminum hydroxide and soy-containing dietary supplements.

Estrogens tend to increase serum thyronine-binding globulin (TBG). In a patient with a non-functioning thyroid gland who is receiving thyroid replacement therapy, free thyroxine may be decreased when estrogens are started thus increasing LEVOXYL requirements. Therefore, patients without a functioning thyroid gland who are on thyroid replacement therapy may need to increase their dosage of LEVOXYL if estrogens or estrogen-containing oral contraceptives are given. This need can be assessed by measurement of the serum TSH level. Similarly, androgen therapy in hypogonadal men, or women with breast cancer, can decrease TBG; the result may be a decreased need for oral T_4 and so the dosage of LEVOXYL may need to be decreased. Again, measurement of the serum TSH level is a good method of assessing this possibility.

Drug/Laboratory Test Interactions - The following drugs or moieties are known to interfere with laboratory tests performed on patients taking thyroid hormone: androgens, corticosteroids, estrogens, oral contraceptives containing estrogens, iodine-containing preparations, and salicylates. In some instances, e.g., the use of androgens, estrogens, or oral contraceptives, patients' thyroid status may be affected and monitoring with serum TSH measurement may be indicated.

1. Pregnancy, estrogens, and estrogen-containing oral contraceptives increase TBG concentrations. TBG may also be increased during infectious hepatitis. Decreases in TBG concentrations can occur in nephrosis, acromegaly, or during androgen or corticosteroid therapy. Familial hyper- or hypo-thyroxine-binding-globulinemias have been described. The binding of thyroxine by thyroid-binding pre-albumin (TBPA) is inhibited by salicylates. In all these cases of changes in L-T_4 binding to serum proteins, the serum T_4 level may change. Measurement of the serum TSH level will determine the clinical significance of any change in serum T_4.

2. A high iodine intake interferes with radio-iodine uptake (RAIU) in normal persons but the RAIU would be low in those taking thyroxine in any case; this test has little use in patients treated with oral T_4 and the interference of a high iodine intake is of little clinical relevance.

3. Continued evidence of hypothyroidism in spite of apparently adequate dosage replacement indicates poor patient compliance, poor absorption, excessive fecal loss, interference by concomitantly ingested food, or inactivity of the preparation. Poor compliance is the most common cause but each possible cause should be considered.

Carcinogenesis, Mutagenesis, And Impairment Of Fertility - A reportedly apparent association between prolonged thyroid therapy and breast cancer has not been confirmed and patients taking LEVOXYL for established indications should not discontinue therapy. There are no data suggesting that L-T_4 is mutagenic or impairs fertility; such studies in animals over the long term have not been performed.

Pregnancy - Category A - Thyroid hormones do not readily cross the placental barrier. Clinical experience to date does not indicate any adverse effect on fetuses when thyroid hormones are administered to pregnant women. On the basis of current knowledge, LEVOXYL replacement therapy to hypothyroid women should not be discontinued during pregnancy. During pregnancy, LEVOXYL requirements may increase; dosage should be guided by periodic measurement of serum TSH concentration.

Nursing Mothers - Some thyroid hormone is excreted in human milk but this is usually insufficient for hypothyroid nursing neonates. L-T_4 taken by nursing mothers is not associated with serious adverse reactions and does not have a known tumorigenic potential; properly indicated LEVOXYL therapy should be continued.

Pediatric Use - Congenital hypothyroidism is uncommon (1:4,000) and is not prevented by the small amounts of hormone that cross the placenta. Determination of serum T_4 and/ or TSH is needed to make the diagnosis in neonates and must be done within a few days of birth to prevent the serious effects of hypothyroidism on growth and development, particularly of the brain and nervous system. Treatment should be initiated immediately upon diagnosis, and maintained for life, unless transient hypothyroidism is suspected in which case therapy may be interrupted for 2 to 8 weeks after the age of 3 years to reassess the condition. Cessation of therapy is justified in patients who have maintained a normal TSH during those 2 to 8 weeks.

ADVERSE REACTIONS:

Adverse reactions are due to overdosage and are those of induced hyperthyroidism.

OVERDOSAGE:

Excessive dosage of thyroid medication may result in symptoms of hyperthyroidism. Since, however, the effects do not appear at once, the symptoms may not appear for one to three weeks after an excessive dose is begun. The most common signs and symptoms of overdosage are weight loss, palpitation, nervousness, diarrhea or abdominal cramps, sweating, tachycardia, cardiac arrhythmias, angina pectoris, tremors, headache, insomnia, and intolerance to heat. If symptoms of overdosage appear, discontinue the medication for several days and reinstitute treatment at a lower dosage level.

Laboratory tests such as serum T_4, serum T_3 and the free thyroxine index will be elevated during the period of overdosage and the hallmark is a clearly suppressed serum TSH level. Complications as a result of the induced hypermetabolic state may include cardiac failure and death due to arrhythmia or failure.

TREATMENT OF OVERDOSAGE - Dosage should be reduced or therapy temporarily discontinued if signs and symptoms of overdosage appear. Treatment may be reinstituted at a lower dosage.

Treatment of acute massive thyroid hormone overdosage is aimed at reducing gastrointestinal absorption of the drugs and counteracting central and peripheral effects, mainly those of increased sympathetic activity. Vomiting may be induced initially if further gastrointestinal absorption can reasonably be prevented provided there are no contraindications such as coma, convulsions, or loss of the gag reflex. Treatment is mainly symptomatic and supportive. Oxygen may be administered and ventilation maintained. Cardiac glycosides may be indicated if congestive heart failure develops. Measures to control fever, hypoglycemia, or fluid loss should be instituted if needed. Antiadrenergic agents, particularly propranolol, have been used advantageously in the treatment of increased sympathetic activity. Propranolol may be administered intravenously at a dosage of 1 to 3 mg over a 10 minute period or orally, 80 to 160 mg/day, especially when no contraindications exist for its use.

DOSAGE AND ADMINISTRATION:

Primary Hypothyroidism - The goal of therapy in primary hypothyroidism should be the restoration of euthyroidism as judged by clinical response and confirmed by appropriate laboratory tests such as serum thyroxine (T_4), serum triiodothyronine (T_3), free thyroxine index and serum TSH; the principal measure in primary hypothyroidism is the serum TSH level. The age and general condition of the patient, the severity and duration of hypothyroid symptoms, and whether or not the serum TSH level remains high or has become normal determine the starting dose of LEVOXYL and the rate of incremental dosage increase leading to a final maintenance dosage.

In otherwise healthy adults with primary hypothyroidism, the recommended initial dosage of LEVOXYL is 25 to 100 mcg (0.025 to 0.1 mg) daily, while the predicted full maintenance dose of 100 to 200 mcg (0.1 to 0.2 mg) daily may be achieved in several months.

In the elderly patient with primary hypothyroidism, particularly in those with long-standing or severe primary hypothyroidism or with evidence of cardiovascular dysfunction, the initial dose of LEVOXYL may be as little as 12.5 mcg (0.0125 mg) per day; incremental increases of 25 mcg (0.025 mg) per day at 4 to 6 week intervals may be instituted depending on patient response. It is the physician's judgement of the severity of the disease and close observation of patient response and of the serum TSH level which determine the rate and extent of dosage increase.

Once the serum TSH level in those with primary hypothyroidism has fallen to the normal reference range during LEVOXYL treatment and the serum TSH concentration has been stable at this level for 4 to 8 weeks, the daily dose being taken is then the maintenance dose. To monitor the adequacy of this dose and patient compliance, periodic assessment of the serum TSH level should be done. The aim is the maintenance of the serum TSH level in the normal reference range. There are no data showing the optimum frequency of measurement of serum TSH concentration in this circumstance but common practice is 1 to 3 times per year; if there is reason to suspect poor compliance with therapy or other potential problems, the serum TSH measurement should be done more often, even when the dose of oral T_4 is unchanged.

Severe Hypothyroidism - Sometimes referred to as "myxedema coma", far-advanced hypothyroidism is an uncommon but dangerous and potentially lethal state. Often precipitated by another event, such as infection or injury, in an already hypothyroid patient and often characterized by hypothermia and somnolence or actual coma, severe hypothyroidism is a medical emergency. Other characteristics are slow pulse, electrolyte abnormalities such as hyponatremia, respiratory failure with CO_2 retention, and hypotension. The principal treatment initially is aimed at supportive therapy, treatment of infection if present, gentle warming if indicated, and correction of non-thyroid abnormalities such as abnormal electrolyte values or cardiac arrhythmias. Glucocorticoid therapy is often given, although there are no data showing clear benefit. In addition, replacement therapy with levothyroxine is essential. While oral T_4 appears to be well absorbed in such patients, there are no data showing in a controlled trial whether it is better to give the L-T_4 by mouth, by nasogastric tube, or parenterally. Nevertheless, many prefer to give the L-T_4 parenterally. Similarly, there is no clear consensus on the dose of L-T_4 to be used; some prefer to give enough to replace the entire deficiency of circulating T_4 (often 400 to 600 mcg, usually parenterally, as a single dose or given over a few hours) while other physicians prefer to begin with smaller doses, e.g., 75 to 150 mcg, (0.075-0.15 mg) given by mouth, if possible, or parenterally, if not. Further dosing of L-T_4 depends on patient response which in turn requires intensive monitoring for at least a few days. The total daily dose of L-T_4 given after the initial dose should in general not exceed the daily dose required previously by the patient or the average daily dose taken by similar patients. Clinical judgement is a major determinant of the details of treatment because laboratory results will usually not be available initially.

Secondary Hypothyroidism - Hypothyroidism due to pituitary or hypothalamic disease, or secondary hypothyroidism, is uncommon; the vast majority of hypothyroid patients have primary hypothyroidism. Secondary hypothyroidism is suspected whenever there is known hypothalamic or pituitary disease, such as pituitary tumor or diabetes insipidus; it is characterized by a low serum concentration of total T_4 or free T_4 without a clearly raised serum TSH concentration; the serum TSH level may be slightly raised, in the reference range, or low. The serum TSH level cannot be used to monitor the dosage of LEVOXYL as it is in primary hypothyroidism. The initial dose of LEVOXYL should be chosen as it is in primary hypothyroidism, observing the same guidelines and precautions (see **Primary Hypothyroidism**). Further dose increases, if any, are based on the clinical response using clinical judgement and measurement of serum total or free T_4.

Suppression of Pituitary Secretion of TSH - In selected patients with goiter, thyroid nodules, or papillary or follicular thyroid cancer, LEVOXYL can be used in an attempt to inhibit growth or prevent re-growth of the abnormal thyroid tissue; the overall management may include other therapies such as surgery or radioactive iodine. The suppressive action of LEVOXYL is based on the known ability of oral T_4 to suppress pituitary secretion of TSH even when patients are initially euthyroid (a hypothyroid person with any of the above conditions should be treated with LEVOXYL in any case for the hypothyroidism). Because most persons with these conditions are euthyroid and so have a normal serum TSH concentration, the goal of LEVOXYL therapy is to suppress the serum TSH level to below the reference range. In so doing, some patients with these conditions may have an inhibition of further growth of the abnormal thyroid tissue. Because various clinical trials have reached different conclusions on the efficacy of oral T_4 in the treatment of thyroid nodules or goiter and there are no controlled trials on its use in papillary or follicular thyroid cancer or on the degree to which the serum TSH level needs to be suppressed, the use of LEVOXYL in these conditions needs to be individualized; continued use depends on the clinical response balanced against the possibility of induced hyperthyroidism. In general, the suppression of serum TSH concentration should be to the level of 0.1 to 0.2 mU/L although some prefer to suppress the serum TSH concentration to less than 0.1 mU/L in patients with differentiated thyroid carcinoma.

Pediatric Hypothyroidism - In infants and children there is a great urgency to achieve full thyroid replacement because of the critical importance of thyroid hormone in sustaining growth and maturation as well as development of the brain and intellectual function. Despite the smaller body size, the dosage needed to sustain a full rate of growth, development and general thriving is higher in the child than in the adult. The recommended daily replacement dosage of L- thyroxine in childhood is: 0-6 months: 8-10 mcg/kg; 6-12 months: 6-8 mcg/kg; 1-5 years: 5-6 mcg/kg; 6-12 years: 4-5 mcg/kg of body weight daily.

HOW SUPPLIED:

LEVOXYL (L-thyroxine) tablets are supplied as oval, color-coded, potency marked tablets in 12 strengths:

25 mcg-Orange:
Bottles of 100,
NDC 0689-1117-01
Bottles of 1000,
NDC 0689-1117-10
Unit dose cartons of 100,
NDC 0689-1117-05

50 mcg-White:
Bottles of 100,
NDC 0689-1118-01
Bottles of 1000,
NDC 0689-1118-10
Unit dose cartons of 100,
NDC 0689-1118-05

75 mcg-Purple:
Bottles of 100,
NDC 0689-1119-01
Bottles of 1000,
NDC 0689-1119-10
Unit dose cartons of 100,
NDC 0689-1119-05

88 mcg-Olive:
Bottles of 100,
NDC 0689-1132-01
Bottles of 1000,
NDC 0689-1132-10

100 mcg-Yellow:
Bottles of 100,
NDC 0689-1110-01
Bottles of 1000,
NDC 0689-1110-10
Unit dose cartons of 100,
NDC 0689-1110-05

112 mcg-Rose:
Bottles of 100,
NDC 0689-1130-01
Bottles of 1000,
NDC 0689-1130-10

125 mcg-Brown:
Bottles of 100,
NDC 0689-1120-01
Bottles of 1000,
NDC 0689-1120-10
Unit dose cartons of 100,
NDC 0689-1120-05

137 mcg-Dark Blue:
Bottles of 100,
NDC 0689-1135-01
Bottles of 1000,
NDC 0689-1135-10

150 mcg-Blue:
Bottles of 100,
NDC 0689-1111-01
Bottles of 1000,
NDC 0689-1111-10
Unit dose cartons of 100,
NDC 0689-1111-05

175 mcg-Turquoise:
Bottles of 100,
NDC 0689-1122-01
Bottles of 1000,
NDC 0689-1122-10

200 mcg-Pink:
Bottles of 100,
NDC 0689-1112-01
Bottles of 1000,
NDC 0689-1112-10
Unit dose cartons of 100,
NDC 0689-1112-05

300 mcg-Green:
Bottles of 100,
NDC 0689-1121-01
Bottles of 1000,
NDC 0689-1121-10

Store at controlled room temperature 15°-30°C(59°-86°F) Caution: Federal (USA) law prohibits dispensing without a prescription.

JONES MEDICAL INDUSTRIES, INC.
1945 Craig Road
ST. LOUIS, MO 63146
(NASDAQ: JMED)
800-525-8466

Revised May 1996

▲ Fink, Raymond I., M.D.
Diabetes & Endocrine Associates
8851 Center Drive, Suite 603
La Mesa, CA 91942
Phone: (619) 463-1293
Fax: (619) 463-8230

▲ Friend, Keith E., M.D.
University of Texas, M.D. Anderson
Cancer Center
Section of Endocrine Neoplasia and
Hormonal Disorders
1515 Holcombe Boulevard
Houston, Texas 77030
Phone: (713) 792-2840
E-mail: friend@endocrine.mdacc.tmc.edu
See display listing page 236

▲ Frohman, Lawrence A., M.D.
University of Illinois at Chicago
840 South Wood Street
Chicago, IL 60612
Phone: (312) 996-7700
Fax: (312) 413-0342
See display listing page 231

▲ Gagel, Robert F., M.D.
Chief, Section of Endocrinology
Professor of Medicine
University of Texas, M.D. Anderson
Cancer Center
1515 Holcombe Boulevard
Houston, TX 77030
Phone: (713) 792-2840
Fax: (713) 794-4065
See display listing page 236

Glaser, Elyse W., M.D.
833 Campbell Hill Street, Suite 350
Marietta, GA 30060
Phone: (770) 425-3339
Fax: (770) 427-4467

Hart, Celeste B., M.D.
Anderson Brickler Clinic
1705 South Adams Street
Tallahassee, FL 32301
Phone: (850) 681-3653
Fax: (850) 224-5384

Hoffman, Andrew, M.D.
Stanford Health Services
Endocrine Clinic
900 Blake Wilbur Drive, Room W3045
Palo Alto, CA 94010
Phone: (415) 498-6920
Fax: (415) 725-8418

Hoffman, William H., M.D.
Medical College of Georgia
Pediatric Endocrinology
Department of Pediatrics, BG 203
Augusta, GA 30912
Phone: (706) 721-4158
Fax: (706) 721-7311

Hopwood, Nancy J., M.D.
Pediatric Endocrinology
University of Michigan Medical Center
Ann Arbor, MI 48109-0718
Phone: (313) 764-5175
Fax: (313) 763-4208
See display listing page 240

▲ Imura, Hiroo, M.D.
President
Kyoto University
53 Kawahara Cho Syogoin
Sakyo-Ku, Kyoto 606, Japan
Phone: 81-75-153-2001

▲ *Identifies a PTNA Member*

Katznelson, Larry, M.D.
Instructor in Medicine
Neuroendocrine Unit
BUL 457B
Massachusetts General Hospital
Boston, MA 02114
Phone: (617) 726-3870
Fax: (617) 726-5072
See display listing page 238

Klibanski, Anne, M.D.
Massachusetts General Hospital
Chief, Neuroendocrine Unit
15 Parkman Street. WAC7305
Boston, MA 02114
Phone: (617) 726-3870
Fax: (617) 726-5072
See display listing page 238

Koch, Michael H., M.D.
Endocrinology Associates, Inc.
2118 Rosalind Avenue SW
Roanoke, VA 24014
Phone: (540) 344—3276
Fax: (540) 342-7028

Koulianos, George T., M.D.
Director, Reproductive Endocrinology
and Infertility
Mobile Infirmary Medical Center
Clinical Assistant Professor
University of Alabama
Mobil, AL 36607

Kovacs, William J., M.D.
Division of Endocrinology
Vanderbilt University Medical Center
Office: 715 MRB II
Clinic: 2501 The Vanderbilt Clinic
Nashville, TN 37232
Office Phone: (615) 936-1653
Office Fax: (615) 936-1667
Clinic Phone: (615) 322-4752
See display listing page 244

Lechan, Ronald M., M.D., Ph.D
New England Medical Center
Professor of Medicine
Director, Neuroendocrine Clinic
750 Washington Street,
Box 268
Boston, MA 02111
Phone: (617) 636-5689
Fax: (617) 636-4719

Leidy, John W., Jr., M.D., Ph.D.
Department of Medicine
Marshall University School of Medicine
1801 6th Avenue
Huntington, WV 25703-1585
Phone: (304) 696-7113
Fax: (304) 696-7297

Marynick, Samuel P., M.D., P.A.
3707 Gaston Avenue, Suite 325
Dallas, TX 75246
Phone: (214) 828-2444
Fax: (214) 820-7620

Mastbaum, Leonard I., M.D., F.A.C.E.
Indiana Regional Medical Consultants
P.C./Endocrinology Department
7900 W. Jefferson Blvd.., Suite 201
Fort Wayne, IN 46804
Phone: (219) 432-6714
Fax: (219) 432-6388

Identifies a PTNA Member

Endocrinologists

▲ Melmed, Shlomo, M.D.
Chairman
Director, Division of Endocrinology &
Metabolism
Cedars-Sinai Medical Center
8700 Beverly Boulevard
Los Angeles, CA 90048-1869
See display listing page 229

Orth, David N., M.D., President
The Endocrine Society
5808 Beauregard Drive
Nashville, TN 37215-4805
Phone: (615) 665-1964
Fax: (615) 665-8276
e-mail: orthdn@nashville.net
See display listing page 29

Powers, Alvin C., M.D.
Division of Endocrinology
Vanderbilt University Medical Center
Office: 715 MRB II
Clinic: 2501 The Vanderbilt Clinic
Nashville, TN 37232
Office Phone: (615) 936-1653
Office Fax: (615) 936-1667
Clinic Phone: (615) 322-4752
See display listing page 244

Rice, Bernard F., M.D. F.A.C.P.
Endocrinology Mid-America, CHTD
8901 W. 74th Street, Suite 125
Shawnee Mission, KS 66204
Phone: (913) 262-9222
Fax: (913) 262-9247

Ridgeway, E. Chester, M.D.
Professor & Chief
Division of Endocrinology
University of Colorado,
Health Sciences Center
4200 E 9th Avenue, C-307
Denver, CO 80262
Phone: (303) 372-1435
Fax: (303) 372-1493
See display listing page 233

Rosecan, Marvin, M.D.
29 North 64th Street, Suite 3D
Belleville, IL 62223
Phone: (618) 398-5151

Shakir, K.M.M., M.D.
Department of Internal Medicine
Section of Endocrinology
National Naval Medical Center
Bethesda, MD 20814
Phone: (301) 295-5165

Silver, Mark A., M.D.
21616 76th Avenue W., Suite 103
Edmunds, WA 98026
Phone: (425) 774-5104
Fax: (425) 778-2620

Snyder, Peter J., M.D.
Hospital of the University of
Pennsylvania
3400 Spruce Street
Philadelphia, PA 19104
Phone: (215) 662-2300
See display listing page 241

Sobrinho, Luis G., M.D., Ph.D.
Professor of Endocrinology
Portugese Cancer Instituite
1903 Lisboa, Codex
Portugal
Phone: 351-1-726-9285

Sonino, Nicoletta, M.D.
Division of Endocrinology
Institute of Semeiotica Medica
University of Padova
Via Ospedale 105
1-35128 Padova (Italy)
Phone: 39-49-8213000
Fax: 39-49-657391

200

▲ Identifies a PTNA Member

Speiser, Phyllis W., M.D.
North Shore University Hospital
Cornell University Medical Collage
Division of Pediatric Endocrinology
300 Community Drive
Manhasset, NY 11030
Phone: (516) 562-4635
Fax: (516) 562-4029

Steiner, Ladislau, M.D.
The Neuroendocrine Center
University of Virginia
Health Sciences Center
Box 212, Private Clinics Building
Charlottesville, VA 22908
See Display Listing page 245

Stonesifer, Larry D., M.D.,F.A.C.P.
34509-9th Avenue So., #200
Federal Way, WA 98003
Phone: (253) 927-4777
Fax: (253) 927-6580

Stratakis, Constantine A., M.D.
Pediatric Endocrinology, NIH
NIH, NICHD, DEB, 10 Center Dr.
MSC1862, Build. 10, Rm. 10N262 MSC 1862
Bethesda, MD 20892
Phone: (301) 476-4686
Fax: (301) 402-0574

Tamkin, James A., M.D., FACP,FACE.
Associate Clinical Professor
of Medicine, U.C.L.A.
510 N. Prospect, Suite 208
Redondo Beach, CA 90277
Phone: (310) 376-8816
Fax: (310) 376-2091
E-mail: jimmyt@AOL.com

Thomas, Carol A., M.D.
1101 Welch Road, Suite C-5
Palo Alto, CA 94304
Phone: (415) 326-8700
Fax: (415) 853-0605

▲ **Thorner. Michael O., M.B., F.R.C.P.**
Chair, Department of Internal
Medicine
Interim Chief, Division of
Endocrinology and Metabolism
University of Virginia Health
Sciences Center
Charlottesville, VA 22908
Phone: (804) 982-3297
Fax: (804) 982-3583
See display listing page 245

Vance, Mary Lee, M.D.
The Neuroendocrine Center
Division of Endocrinology
University of Virginia
Health Sciences Center Box 601
Charlottesville, VA 22908
Phone: (804) 924-2284
Fax: (804) 982-3213
See Display Listing page 245

Varsano-Aharon, N., M.D.
222 Westchester Avenue, Suite 400
White Plains, NY 10604
Phone: (914) 682-0777
Fax: (914) 682-1921

Verbalis, Joseph G., M.D.
Division of Endocrinology
Georgetown University
4000 Reservoir Road, N.W.
Washington D.C. 20007
Phone: (202) 687-2818
Fax: (202) 687-2040

Wang, Christina, M.D.
Professor of Medicine
Harbor-UCLA Pituitary Center
21840 S. Normandie Avenue #800
Torrance, CA 90502
Phone: (310) 222-5104
Fax: (310) 320-5463
See Display Listing page 225

Endocrinologists

▲ *Identifies a PTNA Member*

Endocrinologists

Weiss, Roy, M.D.
University of Chicago
Section of Endocrinology, MC3090
5841 S. Maryland Avenue
Chicago IL 60637
See Display Listing page 231

Williams, John B., M.D., Ph.D
Division of Endocrinology
Vanderbilt University Medical Center
Office: 715 MRB II
Clinic: 2501 The Vanderbilt Clinic
Nashville, TN 37232
Office Phone: (615) 936-1653
Office Fax: (615) 936-1667
Clinic Phone: (615) 322-4752
See display listing page 244

Yue, Genevieve M., M.D.
1541 Florida Avenue, Suite 103
Modesto, CA 95350
Phone: (209) 572-1200
Fax: (209) 572-1235

"When you get into a tight place and it seems you can't go on, hold on, for that's just the place and the time that the tide will turn."

Harriet Beecher Stowe

Identifies a PTNA Member

Neurosurgeons

Allen, George S., M.D.
Neurological Surgery Department
Vanderbilt University Medical Center
Office: T-4224 MCN
Clinic: 3603 The Vanderbilt Clinic
Nashville, TN 37232
Office Phone: (615) 322-7423
Office Fax: (615) 343-8104
Clinic Phone: (615) 322-7417
Clinic Fax: (615) 343-2589
See display listing page 244

Bruce, Jeffrey, M.D.
Room 431, 710 W. 168th Street
New York, NY 10032
Phone: (212) 305-7346
Fax: (212) 305-3629

Cerullo, Leonard J., M.D.
Medical Director,
Chicago Institute of Neurosurgery
& Neuroresearch
2515 N Clark Street
Chicago, IL 60614
Phone: (800) 446-1234
See display listing page 230

Chandler, William F., M.D.
Neurosurgery - University of Michigan
1500 E. Medical Center Drive
Ann Arbor, MI 48109
Phone: (313) 936-5020
Fax: (313) 936-9294
See Display Listing page 240

▲ **Chin, Lawrence S., M.D.**
Assistant Professor,
Department of Neurosurgery
University of Maryland Medical Ct.
22 S. Green Street
Baltimore, MD 21201
Phone: (410) 328-3113
Fax: (410) 328-0756
email: lchin@surgeryl.ab.und.edu

Ciric, Ivan, M.D.
Chief, Division of Neurosurgery,
Evanston Hospital
Professor of Neurosurgery, Northwestern University Medical School
2650 Ridge Avenue
Evanston, Il 60201
Phone: (847) 570-1440
Fax: (847) 570-1442

▲ Couldwell, William T., M.D., Ph.D
Professor and Chairman
Department of Neurosurgery
New York Medical College
Westchester County Medical Center
Munger Pavilion
Valhalla, New York 10595
Phone: (914) 285-8392
Fax: (914) 594-3641
See display listing page 247

Dacey, Ralph G. Jr., M.D.
Washington University School of
Medicine
Department of Neurosurgery
660 S. Euclid, Box 8057
St. Louis, MO 63110
Phone: (314) 362-1412
Fax: (314) 362-2107

DeSalles, Antonio A.F., M.D., Ph.D.
Assistant Professor of Neurosurgery
Director, UCLA Stereotactic
Radiosurgery Program
Harbor-UCLA Pituitary Center
21840 S. Normandy Avenue, Suite 800
Torrance, CA 90502
Phone: (310) 222-5101
Fax: (310) 320-5463

▲ *Identifies a PTNA Member*

Eli Lilly

Humatrope®
(somatropin [rDNA origin]
for injection)

Pituitary hormone replacement
therapy is often prescribed
for hypopituitarism.

Did you know that growth
hormone may play an
important role in that
replacement process?

If you were diagnosed with
growth hormone deficiency
as an adult resulting from
pituitary or brain disease,
surgery, radiation, or an
accident, replacement therapy
with Humatrope,® a "man made"
growth hormone, may benefit
you.[1] See your endocrinologist
for more information.

1. Data on file, Eli Lilly and Company.

Eli Lilly and Company
Indianapolis, Indiana 46285

204

Second Edition

Humatrope®
(somatropin [rDNA origin]
for injection)

Is Humatrope® what you're missing?
Consult with your endocrinologist
and consider the following
safety information:

Humatrope® is not for everyone. Only a specialist
can decide if Humatrope® therapy is right for you.
Be sure to consult with your endocrinologist before
starting Humatrope® therapy. If you have an active tumor, you should not
take Humatrope.® If you are allergic to m-cresol or glycerin, the diluent provided
is not appropriate. Tell your physician if allergies occur. If you are on Humatrope®
and have had a previous tumor, or have a skin growth, diabetes, high blood
sugar, or are on insulin or other hormone replacement therapy,
you should be watched closely by your doctor.

**And, as with any prescription drug, Humatrope®
may cause side effects.**

While on Humatrope® therapy, patients reported most
commonly: swelling (often in the hands and feet), joint
pain, numbness or tingling sensations, pain, runny nose,
muscle pain, back pain, headache, flu syndrome, and
high blood pressure. Some symptoms tended to be
temporary or lessened with a decrease in dose.

If you're like many patients with hypopituitarism, Humatrope®
may be what's missing in your life.

**Take the first step. Call your endocrinologist.
Ask if Humatrope® may help.**

For a brief summary of prescribing information, see the following pages.

Eli Lilly

Humatrope®
somatropin (rDNA origin) for injection

The following information is a BRIEF SUMMARY of the full prescribing information. The physician should consult the full prescribing information before prescribing Humatrope.

Effects of Humatrope treatment in adults with somatotropin deficiency: Two multicenter trials in adult onset somatotropin deficiency (n=98) and two studies in childhood onset somatotropin deficiency (n=67) were designed to assess the effects of replacement therapy with Humatrope. The primary efficacy measures were body composition (lean body mass and fat mass), lipid parameters, and the Nottingham Health Profile. The Nottingham Health Profile is a general health-related quality of life questionnaire. These four studies each included a 6-month randomized, blinded, placebo-controlled phase followed by 12 months of open-label therapy for all patients. The Humatrope dosages for all studies were identical: one month of therapy at 0.00625 mg/kg/day followed by the proposed maintenance dose of 0.0125 mg/kg/day. Adult onset patients and childhood onset patients differed by diagnosis (organic versus idiopathic pituitary disease), body size (normal versus small for mean height and weight), and age (mean = 44 versus 29 years). Lean body mass was determined by bioelectrical impedance analysis (BIA), validated with potassium 40. Body fat was assessed by BIA and sum of skinfold thickness. Lipid subfractions were analyzed by standard assay methods in a central laboratory.

Humatrope-treated adult onset patients, as compared to placebo, experienced an increase in lean body mass (2.59 versus -0.22 kg, p<0.001) and a decrease in body fat (-3.27 versus 0.56 kg, p<0.001). Similar changes were seen in childhood onset somatotropin deficient patients. These significant changes in lean body mass persisted throughout the 18 month period as compared to baseline for both groups, and for fat mass in the childhood onset group. Total cholesterol decreased short term (first 3 months) although the changes did not persist. However, the low HDL cholesterol levels observed at baseline (mean = 30.1 mg/mL and 33.9 mg/mL in adult onset and childhood onset patients) normalized by the end of 18 months of therapy (a change of 13.7 and 11.1 mg/dL for the adult onset and childhood onset groups, p<0.001). Adult onset patients reported significant improvements as compared to placebo in the following 2 of 6 possible health related domains: physical mobility and social isolation (Table 1). Patients with childhood onset disease failed to demonstrate improvements in Nottingham Health Profile outcomes.

Two additional studies on the effect of Humatrope on exercise capacity were also conducted. Improved physical function was documented by increased exercise capacity (VO$_2$ max, p<0.005) and work performance (Watts, p<0.01) (J Clin Endocrinol Metab 1995; 80:552-557).

Table 1
Changes[a] in Nottingham Health Profile Scores[b]
in Adult Onset Somatotropin Deficient Patients

Outcome Measure	Placebo (6 Months)	Humatrope Therapy (6 Months)	Significance
Energy Level	-11.4	-15.5	NS
Physical Mobility	-3.1	-10.5	p <0.01
Social Isolation	0.5	-4.7	p <0.01
Emotional Reactions	-4.5	-5.4	NS
Sleep	-6.4	-3.7	NS
Pain	-2.8	-2.9	NS

[a] = An improvement in score is indicated by a more negative change in the score.
[b] = To account for multiple analyses, appropriate statistical methods were applied and the required level of significance is 0.01.

NS = not significant

Indications and Usage: *Adult Patients*—Humatrope is indicated for replacement of endogenous somatotropin in adults with somatotropin deficiency syndrome who meet both of the following two criteria:

1. Adult Onset: Patients who have somatotropin deficiency syndrome, either alone or with multiple hormone deficiencies (hypopituitarism), as a result of pituitary disease, hypothalamic disease, surgery, radiation therapy, or trauma;
or
Childhood Onset: Patients who were growth hormone-deficient during childhood who have somatotropin deficiency syndrome confirmed as an adult before replacement therapy with Humatrope is started.
and
2. Biochemical diagnosis of somatotropin deficiency syndrome, by means of a negative response to a standard growth hormone stimulation test [maximum peak < 5 ng/mL when measured by RIA (polyclonal antibody) or < 2.5 ng/mL when measured by IRMA (monoclonal antibody)].

Contraindications: Humatrope should not be used for growth promotion in pediatric patients with closed epiphyses.

Humatrope should not be used when there is any evidence of activity of a tumor. Intracranial lesions must be inactive and antitumor therapy complete prior to the institution of therapy. Humatrope should be discontinued if there is evidence of tumor growth.

Humatrope should not be reconstituted with the supplied Diluent for Humatrope by patients with a known sensitivity to either *m*-cresol or glycerin.

Warning: If sensitivity to the diluent should occur, the vials may be reconstituted with Bacteriostatic Water for Injection, USP or, Sterile Water for Injection, USP. When Humatrope is used with Bacteriostatic Water (Benzyl Alcohol preserved), the solution should be kept refrigerated at 36° to 46°F (2° to 8°C) and used within 14 days. **Benzyl alcohol as a preservative in Bacteriostatic Water for Injection, USP has been associated with toxicity in newborns.** When administering Humatrope to newborns, use the Humatrope diluent provided or if the patient is sensitive to the diluent, use Sterile Water, USP. When Humatrope is reconstituted with Sterile Water, USP in this manner, use only one dose per Humatrope vial and discard the

unused portion. If the solution is not used immediately, it must be refrigerated (36° to 46°F [2° to 8°C]) and used within 24 hours.

Precautions: Therapy with Humatrope should be directed by physicians who are experienced in the diagnosis and management of patients with growth hormone deficiency.

Patients with growth hormone deficiency secondary to an intracranial lesion should be examined frequently for progression or recurrence of the underlying disease process. In pediatric patients, clinical literature has demonstrated no relationship between somatropin replacement therapy and CNS tumor recurrence. In adults, it is unknown whether there is any relationship between somatropin replacement therapy and CNS tumor recurrence.

Patients should be monitored carefully for any malignant transformation of skin lesions.

For patients with diabetes mellitus, the insulin dose may require adjustment when somatropin therapy is instituted. Because human growth hormone may induce a state of insulin resistance, patients should be observed for evidence of glucose intolerance. Patients with diabetes or glucose intolerance should be monitored closely during somatropin therapy.

In patients with hypopituitarism (multiple hormonal deficiencies) standard hormonal replacement therapy should be monitored closely when somatropin therapy is administered. Hypothyroidism may develop during treatment with somatropin, and inadequate treatment of hypothyroidism may prevent optimal response to somatropin. Therefore, patients should have periodic thyroid function tests and be treated with thyroid hormone when indicated.

Excessive glucocorticoid therapy will inhibit the growth promoting effect of human growth hormone. Patients with coexisting ACTH deficiency should have their glucocorticoid replacement dose carefully adjusted to avoid an inhibitory effect on growth.

Pediatric patients with endocrine disorders, including growth hormone deficiency, may develop slipped capital epiphyses more frequently. Any pediatric patient with the onset of a limp during growth hormone therapy should be evaluated.

Patients with epiphyseal closure who were treated with growth hormone replacement therapy in childhood should be re-evaluated according to the criteria in *INDICATIONS AND USAGE* before continuation of somatropin therapy at the reduced dose level recommended for somatropin-deficient adults.

Intracranial hypertension (IH) with papilledema, visual changes, headache, nausea and/or vomiting has been reported in a small number of patients treated with growth hormone products. Symptoms usually occurred within the first eight (8) weeks of the initiation of growth hormone therapy. In all reported cases, IH-associated signs and symptoms resolved after termination of therapy or a reduction of the growth hormone dose. Funduscopic examination of patients is recommended at the initiation and periodically during the course of growth hormone therapy.

Experience in patients above 60 years is lacking.

Experience with prolonged treatment in adults is limited.

Growth hormone has not been shown to increase the incidence of scoliosis. Progression of scoliosis can occur in children who experience rapid growth. Because growth hormone increases growth rate, patients with a history of scoliosis who are treated with growth hormone should be monitored for progression of scoliosis.

Carcinogenesis, Mutagenesis, Impairment of Fertility— Long-term animal studies for carcinogenicity and impairment of fertility with this human growth hormone (Humatrope) have not been performed. There has been no evidence to date of Humatrope-induced mutagenicity.

Pregnancy—Pregnancy Category C—Animal reproduction studies have not been conducted with Humatrope. It is not known whether Humatrope can cause fetal harm when administered to a pregnant woman or can affect reproduction capacity. Humatrope should be given to a pregnant woman only if clearly needed.

Nursing Mothers—There have been no studies conducted with Humatrope in nursing mothers. It is not known whether this drug is excreted in human milk. Because many drugs are excreted in human milk, caution should be exercised when Humatrope is administered to a nursing woman.

Information for Patients—Patients being treated with growth hormone and/or their parents should be informed of the potential benefits and risks associated with treatment. If home use is determined to be desirable by the physician, instructions on appropriate use should be given, including a review of the contents of the patient information insert. This information is intended to aid in the safe and effective administration of the medication. It is not a disclosure of all possible adverse or intended effects.

If home use is prescribed, a puncture resistant container for the disposal of used syringes and needles should be recommended to the patient. Patients and/or parents should be thoroughly instructed in the importance of proper needle disposal and cautioned against any reuse of needles and syringes (see Information for the Patient insert).

Adverse Reactions: *Adult Patients*—In clinical studies in which high doses of Humatrope were administered to healthy adult volunteers, the following events occurred infrequently: headache, localized muscle pain, weakness, mild hyperglycemia, and glucosuria.

In the first 6 months of controlled blinded trials, adult-onset somatotropin-deficient adults experienced a statistically significant increase in edema (Humatrope 17.3% vs. placebo 4.4%, p=0.043) and peripheral edema (11.5% vs. 0% respectively, p=0.017). In patients with adult onset somatotropin deficiency syndrome, edema, muscle pain, joint pain, and joint disorder were reported early in therapy and tended to be transient or responsive to dosage titration.

Two out of 113 adult onset patients developed carpal tunnel syndrome after beginning maintenance therapy without a low dose (0.00625 mg/kg/day) lead-in phase. Symptoms abated in these patients after dosage reduction.

All treatment-emergent adverse events with ≥5% overall incidence during 12 or 18 months of replacement therapy with Humatrope are shown in Table 2 (adult onset patients) and in Table 3 (childhood onset patients).

Adult patients treated with Humatrope who had been diagnosed with growth hormone deficiency in childhood reported side effects less frequently than those with adult-onset somatotropin deficiency.

Other adverse drug events that have been reported in growth hormone-treated patients include the following: 1) Metabolic: Infrequent, mild and transient peripheral or generalized edema. 2) Musculoskeletal: Rare carpal tunnel syndrome. 3) Skin: Rare increased growth of pre-existing nevi. Patients should be monitored carefully for malignant transformation. 4) Endocrine: Rare gynecomastia. Rare Pancreatitis.

Humatrope® (somatropin, rDNA origin, for injection)

Humatrope® (somatropin, rDNA origin, for injection)

Table 2
Treatment-Emergent Adverse Events with ≥5% Overall Incidence in Adult Onset Patients Treated with Humatrope for Either 12 or 18 Months

Adverse Event	12 Months hGH Exposure (N=44)		18 Months hGH Exposure (N=52)	
	n	%	n	%
Edema	5	11.4	11	21.2
Arthralgia	6	13.6	9	17.3
Paresthesia	6	13.6	9	17.3
Myalgia	4	9.1	7	13.5
Pain	6	13.6	7	13.5
Rhinitis	5	11.4	7	13.5
Peripheral Edema	8	18.2	6	11.5
Back Pain	4	9.1	5	9.6
Headache	3	6.8	4	7.7
Hypertension	2	4.6	4	7.7
Acne	0	0	3	5.8
Joint Disorder	1	2.3	3	5.8
Surgical Procedure	1	2.3	3	5.8
Flu Syndrome	3	6.8	2	3.9

Abbreviations: hGH = Humatrope; N = number of patients receiving treatment in the period stated; n = number of patients reporting each treatment-emergent adverse event.

Table 3
Treatment-Emergent Adverse Events with ≥5% Overall Incidence in Childhood Onset Patients Treated with Humatrope for Either 12 or 18 Months

Adverse Event	12 Months hGH Exposure (N=30)		18 Months hGH Exposure (N=32)	
	n	%	n	%
Flu Syndrome	3	10.0	5	15.63
SGOT Increased	2	6.67	4	12.50
Headache	2	6.07	3	9.38
Asthenia	1	3.33	2	6.25
Cough Increased	0	0	2	6.25
Edema	3	10.00	2	6.25
Hypesthesia	0	0	2	6.25
Myalgia	2	6.67	2	6.25
Pain	3	10.00	2	6.25
Rhinitis	2	6.67	2	6.25
SGPT Increased	2	6.67	2	6.25
Respiratory Disorder	2	6.67	1	3.13
Gastritis	2	6.67	0	0
Pharyngitis	2	6.67	1	3.13

Abbreviations: hGH = Humatrope; N = number of patients receiving treatment in the period stated; n = number of patients reporting each treatment-emergent adverse event; SGOT = serum glutamic oxaloacetic transaminase, or AST; SGPT = serum glutamic pyruvic transaminase, or ALT.

Overdosage: Acute overdosage could lead initially to hypoglycemia and subsequently to hyperglycemia. Long-term overdosage could result in signs and symptoms of gigantism/acromegaly consistent with the known effects of excess human growth hormone. (See recommended and maximal dosage instructions given below.)

Dosage and Administration: *Somatotropin-deficient adult patients*—The recommended dosage at the start of therapy is not more than 0.006 mg/kg/day (0.018 IU/kg/day) given as a daily subcutaneous injection. The dose may be increased according to individual patient requirements to a maximum of 0.0125 mg/kg/day (0.0375 IU/kg/day).

During therapy, dosage should be titrated if required by the occurrence of side effects. To minimize the occurrence of adverse events in patients with increasing age or excessive body weight, dose reductions may be necessary.

Each 5-mg vial of Humatrope should be reconstituted with 1.5 to 5 mL of Diluent for Humatrope. The diluent should be injected into the vial of Humatrope by aiming the stream of liquid against the glass wall. Following reconstitution, the vial should be swirled with a GENTLE rotary motion until the contents are completely dissolved. DO NOT SHAKE. The resulting solution should be inspected for clarity. It should be clear. If the solution is cloudy or contains particulate matter, the contents MUST NOT be injected.

Before and after injection, the septum of the vial should be wiped with rubbing alcohol or an alcoholic antiseptic solution to prevent contamination of the contents by repeated needle insertions. Sterile disposable syringes and/or needles should be used for administration of Humatrope. The volume of the syringe should be small enough so that the prescribed dose can be withdrawn from the vial with reasonable accuracy.

Stability and Storage: *Before Reconstitution*—Vials of Humatrope as well as the Diluent for Humatrope are stable when refrigerated (36° to 46°F [2° to 8°C]). Avoid freezing Diluent for Humatrope. Expiration dates are stated on the labels.

After Reconstitution—Vials of Humatrope are stable for up to 14 days when reconstituted with Diluent for Humatrope and stored in a refrigerator at 36° to 46°F (2° to 8°C). Avoid freezing the reconstituted vial of Humatrope.

How Supplied:
Vials:
5 mg (No. 7335)—(6s) NDC 0002-7335-16, and 5-mL vials of Diluent for Humatrope (No. 7336)

CAUTION—Federal (USA) law prohibits dispensing without prescription.

PA 1645 AMP   [032197]

Eli Lilly and Company
Indianapolis, Indiana
46285

Humatrope® (somatropin, rDNA origin, for injection)

Frim, D., M.D.
University of Chicago
Section of Neurosurgery, MC 3026
5841 S. Maryland Avenue
Chicago, IL 60637
Phone: (773) 702-2123
Fax: (773) 702-3518
See display listing page 231

Goodman, Julius M., M.D.
Indianapolis Neurosurgical Group
1801 N. Senate Boulevard, #535
Indianapolis, IN 46202
Phone (317) 926-5411
Fax: (317) 924-8472
email: jgoodman@clarian.com

Guthikonda, Murali, M.D.
University Neurological Associates
Department of Neurological Surgery
4160 John "R", Suite 925
Detroit, MI 48201
Phone: (313) 993-8600
Fax: (313) 966-0368

Hekmatpanah, Javad, M.D.
University of Chicago
Section of Neurosurgery, MC 3026
5841 S. Maryland Avenue
Chicago, IL 60637
Phone: (773) 702-2123
Fax: (773) 702-3518
Seed display listing page 231

Helenowski, Tomasz K., M.D.
Director, Stereotactic Radiosurgery
Chicago Institute of Neurosurgery
& Neuroresearch
2515 N Clark Street
Chicago, IL 60614
Phone: (800) 446-1234
See display listing page 230

Kotapka, Mark J., M.D.
Assistant Professor of Surgery
University of Pennsylvania
3400 Spruce Street
Philadelphia, PA 19104
Phone: (215) 349-8325
Fax: (215) 349-5534
See display listing page 241

Krieger, Mark D., M.D.
USC University Hospital
Pituitary Neuroendocrine Center
USC School of Medicine
1500 San Pablo Street
Los Angeles, CA 90033
Phone: (213) 342-8500
See display listing page 228

Krisht, Ali F., M.D.
University of Arkansas for Medical
Sciences
4301 West Markham, slot 507
Little Rock, AR 72205
Phone: (501) 296-1463
Fax: (501) 686-7928
See display listing page 222

Laws, Edward R. Jr., M.D.
Director, Neuroendocrine Center
University of Virginia
Virginia Neurological Institute,
Health Sciences Center, Box 212
Charlottesville, VA 22908
Phone: (800) 650-2650
Phone: (804) 924-2650
Fax: (804) 924-5894
See display listing page 245

Lillehei, Kevin O., M.D.
Associate Professor,
Division of Neurosurgery
University of Colorado
Health Sciences Center
4200 E. 9th Avenue, C-307
Denver, CO 80262
Phone: (303) 315-5651
Fax: (303) 315-6197
See display listing page 233

Litofsky, N. Scott, M.D.
Division of Neurosurgery
University of Massachusetts
Medical Center
55 Lake Avenue North
Worcester, MA 01655
Phone: (508) 856-6354
Fax: (508) 856-5074
See display listing page 239

Macdonald, R. Loch, M.D.
University of Chicago
Section of Neurosurgery, MC 3026
5841 S. Maryland Avenue
Chicago, IL 60637
Phone: (773) 702-2123
Fax: (773) 702-3518
See display listing page 231

Maciunas, Robert J., M.D.
Neurological Surgery Department
Vanderbilt University Medical Center
Office: T-4224 MCN
Clinic: 3603 The Vanderbilt Clinic
Nashville, TN 37232
Office Phone: (615) 322-7423
Office Fax: (615) 343-8104
Clinic Phone: (615) 322-7417
Clinic Fax: (615) 343-2589
See display listing page 244

▲ Muszynski, Cheryl A., M.D.
Beth Israel Medical Center - I.N.N.
170 East End Avenue at 87th Street
New York, NY 10128
Phone: (212) 870-9600
Fax: (212) 870-9665
email: cmuszynki@bethisraelny.org
See display listing page 223

Nelson, Curtis N., M.D., Ph.D.
Neurological Surgery
300 White Spruce Boulevard
Rochester, NY 14623
Phone: (716) 272-1730
Fax: (716) 272-8361

Oyesiku, Nelson M., M.D.
Emory Universiy Hospital
1365 Clifton Road, N.E., Bldg. B
Atlanta, GA 30322
Phone: (404) 778-7744
Fax: (404) 778-4472
See display listing page 234

Rhoton, Albert L. Jr., M.D.
University of Florida
Medical Center
Department of Neurological
Surgery
1600 SW Archer Road,
P. O. Box 100265
Gainesville, FL 32610-0265
Phone: (352) 392-4331
Fax: (352)392-8413
See display listing page 235

Rosseau, Gail L., M.D.
Director, Cranial Base Surgery
Chicago Institute of Neurosurgery
& Neuroresearch
2515 N Clark Street
Chicago, IL 60614
Phone: (800) 446-1234
See display listing page 230

▲ Identifies a PTNA Member

Swearingen, Brooke, M.D.
Massachusetts General Hospital, ACC 331
15 Parkman Street
Boston, MA 02114
Phone: (617) 726-3910
Fax: (617) 726-7546
See display listing page 238

Tew, John M., M.D.
Department of Neurosurgery
University of Cincinnati College of
Medicine
231 Bethesda Avenue,
P.O. Box 670515
Cincinnati, OH 45267-0515
Phone: (513) 558-3563
Fax: (513) 558-7702
See display listing page 232

▲ Weiss, Martin, M.D., Director
Professor and Chairman of
Neurosurgery
USC University Hospital
Pituitary Neuroendocrine Center
USC School of Medicine
1500 San Pablo Street
Los Angeles, CA 90033
Phone: (213) 342-8500
See display listing page 228

White, William L., M.D.
Neurosurgical Associates, LTD
2910 N. Third Avenue
Phoenix, AZ 85013
Phone: (602) 406-3466
Fax: (602) 406-6117

Weir, Bryce, M.D.
University of Chicago
Section of Neurosurgery, MC 3026
5841 S. Maryland Avenue
Chicago, IL 60637
Phone: (773) 702-2123
Fax: (773) 702-3518
See display listing page 231

▲ Wilson, Charles B., M.D.
University of California,
San Francisco (UCSF)
U-126 Box 0350
San Francisco, CA 94143-0350
Phone: (415) 476-1911
Fax: (415) 502-4276
See display listing page 227

Zervas, Nicholas T., M.D.
Massachusetts General Hospital
55 Fruit Street
Boston, MA 02114
Phone: (617) 726-8581
Fax: (617) 726-6789
See display listing page 238

▲ Identifies a PTNA Member

Radiation Oncologists

Creasy, Jeffrey L., M.D.
Department of Radiology &
Radiological Sciences
Sterotactic Radiosurgery Center
Vanderbilt Center for Radiation
Oncology
Office: 907 Vanderbilt Hospital
Nashville, TN 37232
Phone: (615) 343-1187
Phone: (615) 343-0890
Fax: (615) 322-3764
See display listing page 244

Eisert, Donald, M.D.
Department of Radiology &
Radiological Sciences
Sterotactic Radiosurgery Center
Vanderbilt Center for Radiation
Oncology
B902 The Vanderbilt Clinic
Nashville, TN 37232
Phone: (615) 322-2555
Fax: (615) 343-0161
See display listing page 244

Epstein, Barry E., M.D.
Department of Radiology &
Radiological Sciences
Sterotactic Radiosurgery Center
Vanderbilt Center for Radiation
Oncology
B902 The Vanderbilt Clinic
Nashville, TN 37232
Phone: (615) 322-2555
Fax: (615) 343-0161
See display listing page 244

Maciunas, Robert J., M.D.
Neurological Surgery Department
Vanderbilt University Medical Center
Office: T-4224 MCN
Clinic: 3603 The Vanderbilt Clinic
Nashville, TN 37232
Office Phone: (615) 322-7423
Office Fax: (615) 343-8104
Clinic Phone: (615) 322-7417
Clinic Fax: (615) 343-2589
See display listing page 244

Rheaume, Dorianne E., M.D., F.R.C.P.C
British Columbia Cancer Agency
Vancouver Center, 600 West 10th Ave.
Vancouver, BC V52 4E6
Phone: (604) 877-6000

Psychosocial Oncology

Weitzner, Michael A., M.D.
Psychosocial Oncology Program
H. Lee Moffitt Cancer Center
12902 Magnolia Drive
Tampa, FL 33612-9497
Phone: (813) 979-3856
Fax: (813) 979 -3906

Dentistry

Sung, Eric C., D.D.S.
UCLA School of Dentistry CHS AO-156
10833 Le Conte Avenue
Los Angeles, CA 90095-1668
Phone: (310) 825-5059
Fax: (310) 206-4201

Gastroenterologist

Strom, Carey B., M.D.
Assistant Professor of
Clinical Medicine
UCLA School of Medicine
8631 W. 3rd Street Suite 540E
Los Angeles, CA
Phone: (310) 657-7779

Pathology

▲ Asa, Sylvia L., M.D., Ph.D.
Associate Professor of Pathology
Department of Pathology &
Laboratory Medicine
Mount Sinai Hospital
Department of Laboratory Medicine &
Pathobiology
University of Toronto
600 University Avenue
Toronto, Ontario
Canada MSG 1X5
See display listing page 242, 243

Psychotherapists

Hotchkiss, Sandy, L.C.S.W.
Board Certified Diplomat,
Clinical Social Work
745 S. Marengo Avenue
Pasadena, CA 91106
Phone: (818) 795-8576

▲ *Identifies a PTNA Member*

Other Physicians

Section VIII

Endocrinology Groups

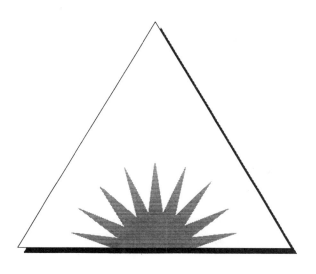

Second Edition

**Endocrinology & Diabetes
Consultants, P.C.
Rojeski, Maria T., M.D.
Tennyson, Gregory E., M.D.
3200 Eagle Park Drive N.E.
#103
Grand Rapids, MI 49505
Phone: (616) 956-6900
Fax: (616) 956-3212**

The Lawson Wilkins Pediatric
Endocrine Society
Lippe, Barbara, M.D.
Secretary C/O Onyx
6100 Wilshire Blvd., Suite 1150
Los Angeles, CA 90048
Phone: (213) 938-5128
Fax: (213) 938-8326
See Display Below

Massachusetts General Hospital
Neuroendocrine Clinical Center
Klibanski, Anne, M.D.
Chief, Neuroendocrine Unit
15 Parkman Street, WAC 730S
Boston, MA 02114-3139
Phone: (617) 726-3872
Fax: (617) 726-5905
See Display Listing page 238

Vanderbilt University Medical Center
Division of Endocrinology
Department of Medicine
715 MRB II
Nashville, TN 37232-6303
Office: (615) 936-1653
Clinic: (615) 322-4752
Fax: (615) 936-1667
See display listing page 244

The Lawson Wilkins Pediatric Endocrine Society

is a professional organization of pediatric endocrinologists dedicated to promote acquisition and dissemination of knowledge of endocrine and metabolic disease of the young from conception through adolescence.

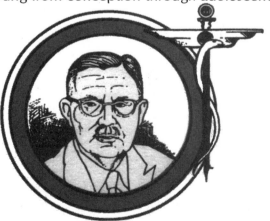

Lawson Wilkins Pediatric Endocrine Society (LWPES)
Secretarial Address: Barbara Lippe, M.D., Department of Pediatrics,
UCLA Medical Center
10833 Le Conte Avenue, Los Angeles, CA 90024-1752
Phone: (310) 825-6389 Fax: (310) 206-5843

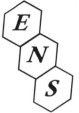

"You may have to fight a battle more than once to win it."
Margaret Thatcher

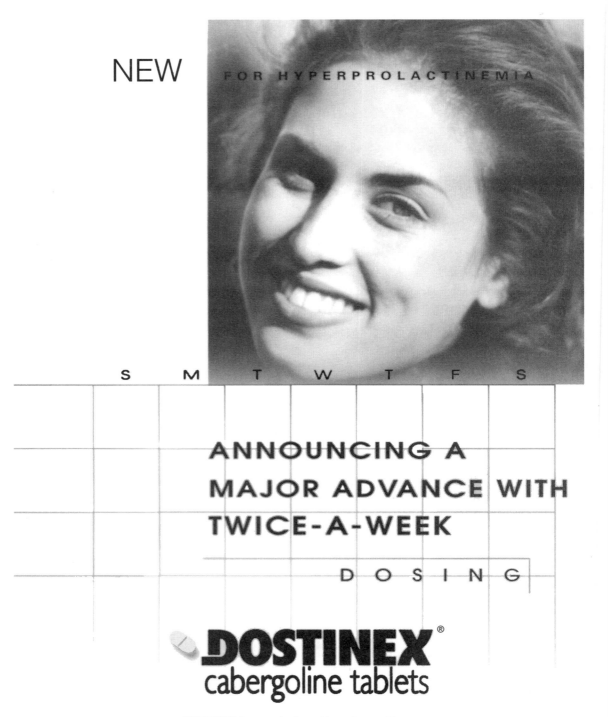

NEW

FOR HYPERPROLACTINEMIA

S M T W T F S

ANNOUNCING A
MAJOR ADVANCE WITH
TWICE-A-WEEK
DOSING

DOSTINEX®
cabergoline tablets

DOSTINEX is contraindicated in patients with uncontrolled
hypertension or known hypersensitivity to ergot derivatives.

Second Edition

DOSTINEX® Tablets
brand of cabergoline tablets

INDICATIONS AND USAGE Treatment of hyperprolactinemic disorders, either idiopathic or due to pituitary adenomas

CONTRAINDICATIONS Patients with uncontrolled hypertension or known hypersensitivity to ergot derivatives

WARNINGS

In general, do not use dopamine agonists in patients with pregnancy-induced hypertension, for example, preeclampsia and eclampsia, unless the potential benefit is judged to outweigh the possible risk.

PRECAUTIONS General: Initial doses higher than 1 mg may produce orthostatic hypotension. Exercise care when administering DOSTINEX with other medications known to lower blood pressure.

Postpartum Lactation Inhibition or Suppression: DOSTINEX is not indicated for inhibition or suppression of physiologic lactation. Use of bromocriptine, another dopamine agonist for this purpose, has been associated with cases of hypertension, stroke, and seizures.

Patients With Hepatic Impairment: Since cabergoline is extensively metabolized by the liver, use caution and exercise careful monitoring when administering DOSTINEX to patients with hepatic impairment.

Information for Patients: Instruct a patient to notify her physician if she suspects she is pregnant, becomes pregnant, or intends to become pregnant during therapy. A pregnancy test should be done if there is any suspicion of pregnancy and treatment continuation should be discussed with her physician.

Drug Interactions: Do not administer DOSTINEX concurrently with D_2-antagonists, such as phenothiazines, butyrophenones, thioxanthines, or metoclopramide.

Carcinogenesis, Mutagenesis, Impairment of Fertility: Carcinogenicity studies were conducted in mice and rats with cabergoline in doses that were calculated on a body surface area basis to be seven times and four times the maximum recommended human dose, respectively. There was a slight increase in the incidence of cervical and uterine leiomyomas and of uterine leiomyosarcomas in mice. In rats, there was a slight increase in malignant tumors in the cervix and uterus and in interstitial cell adenomas. The occurrence of tumors in female rodents may be related to the prolonged suppression of prolactin secretion because prolactin is needed in rodents for corpus luteum maintenance. In the absence of prolactin, the estrogen/progesterone ratio is increased, thereby increasing the risk for uterine tumors. In male rodents, the decrease in serum prolactin levels was associated with an increase in serum luteinizing hormone, which is likely a compensatory effect to maintain testicular steroid synthesis. These hormonal mechanisms are thought to be species-specific, and the relevance of these tumors to humans is not known. Cabergoline was not mutagenic in a battery of in vitro tests: the bacterial mutation (Ames) test with *Salmonella typhimurium,* the gene mutation assay with *Schizosaccharomyces pombe* P_1 and V79 Chinese hamster cells, DNA damage and repair in *Saccharomyces cerevisiae* D_4, and chromosomal aberrations in human lymphocytes. Cabergoline was also negative in the bone marrow micronucleus test in the mouse. In female rats, a daily dose of 0.003 mg/kg (approximately 1/28 the maximum recommended human dose) for 2 weeks prior to mating and throughout the mating period inhibited conception.

Pregnancy: Teratogenic Effects: Category B. There were maternotoxic effects but no teratogenic effects in mice given cabergoline at doses up to 8 mg/kg/day (approximately 55 times the maximum recommended human dose) during the period of organogenesis. A dose of 0.012 mg/kg/day (approximately 1/7 the maximum recommended human dose) during the period of organogenesis in rats caused an increase in postimplantation embryofetal losses. At daily doses of 0.5 mg/kg/day (approximately 19 times the maximum recommended human dose) during the period of organogenesis in the rabbit, cabergoline caused maternotoxicity characterized by a loss of body weight and decreased food consumption. Doses of 4 mg/kg/day (approximately 150 times the maximum recommended human dose) during the period of organogenesis in the rabbit caused an increased occurrence of various malformations. However, in another study in rabbits, no treatment-related malformations or embryofetotoxicity were observed at doses up to 8 mg/kg/day (approximately 300 times the maximum recommended human dose). In rats, doses higher than 0.003 mg/kg/day (approximately 1/28 the maximum recommended human dose) from 6 days before parturition and throughout the lactation period inhibited growth and caused death of offspring due to decreased milk secretion. There are, however, no adequate and well-controlled studies in pregnant women. Because animal reproduction studies are not always predictive of human response, this drug should be used during pregnancy only if clearly needed.

Nursing Mothers: It is not known whether this drug is excreted in human milk. Because many drugs are excreted in human milk and there is the potential for serious adverse reactions in nursing infants from cabergoline, decide whether to discontinue nursing or to discontinue the drug, taking into account the importance of the drug to the mother. Use of DOSTINEX for inhibition or suppression of physiologic lactation is not recommended. Because the prolactin-lowering action of cabergoline suggests that it will interfere with lactation, do not give DOSTINEX to women postpartum who are breast-feeding or who plan to breast-feed.

Pediatric Use: Safety and effectiveness have not been established.

ADVERSE REACTIONS The safety of DOSTINEX Tablets has been evaluated in more than 900 patients with hyperprolactinemic disorders. Most adverse events were mild or moderate in severity.

Four-week, double-blind, placebo-controlled study: Treatment consisted of placebo or cabergoline at fixed doses of 0.125, 0.5, 0.75, or 1.0 mg twice weekly (doses halved during the first week). A possible dose-related effect was observed for nausea only, so the four cabergoline groups are combined; the most common adverse events reported for cabergoline (n=168) and placebo (n=20) were as follows: Gastrointestinal: nausea (27% and 20% for DOSTINEX and placebo, respectively), constipation (10% and 0%), abdominal pain (5% and 5%), dyspepsia (2% and 0%), and vomiting (2% and 0%); Central and Peripheral Nervous System: headache (26% and 25%), dizziness (15% and 5%), paresthesia (1% and 0%), and vertigo (1% and 0%); Body as a Whole: asthenia (9% and 10%), fatigue (7% and 0%), and hot flashes (1% and 5%); Psychiatric: somnolence (5% and 5%), depression (3% and 5%), and nervousness (2% and 0%); Autonomic Nervous System: postural hypotension (4% and 0%); Reproductive–Female: breast pain (1% and 0%) and dysmenorrhea (1% and 0%); and Vision: abnormal vision (1% and 0%).

Eight-week, double-blind period of a comparative trial with bromocriptine: DOSTINEX (0.5 mg twice weekly) was discontinued because of an adverse event in 2% of 221 patients, while bromocriptine (2.5 mg twice a day) was discontinued in 6% of 231 patients. The most common reasons for discontinuation from DOSTINEX were headache, nausea, and vomiting (3, 2, and 2 patients, respectively); the most common reasons for discontinuation from bromocriptine were nausea, vomiting, headache, and dizziness or vertigo (10, 3, 3, and 3 patients, respectively). The incidence of the most common adverse events is presented in the following table:

Incidence of Reported Adverse Events During the 8-Week, Double-Blind Period of the Comparative Trial With Bromocriptine

Adverse Event*	Cabergoline (n=221)	Bromocriptine (n=231)
	Number (percent)	
Gastrointestinal		
Nausea	63 (29)	100 (43)
Constipation	15 (7)	21 (9)
Abdominal pain	12 (5)	19 (8)
Dyspepsia	11 (5)	16 (7)
Vomiting	9 (4)	16 (7)
Dry mouth	5 (2)	2 (1)
Diarrhea	4 (2)	7 (3)
Flatulence	4 (2)	3 (1)
Throat irritation	2 (1)	0
Toothache	2 (1)	0
Central and Peripheral Nervous System		
Headache	58 (26)	62 (27)
Dizziness	38 (17)	42 (18)
Vertigo	9 (4)	10 (4)
Paresthesia	5 (2)	6 (3)
Body as a Whole		
Asthenia	13 (6)	15 (6)
Fatigue	10 (5)	18 (8)
Syncope	3 (1)	3 (1)
Influenza-like symptoms	2 (1)	0
Malaise	2 (1)	0
Periorbital edema	2 (1)	2 (1)
Peripheral edema	2 (1)	1
Psychiatric		
Depression	7 (3)	5 (2)
Somnolence	5 (2)	5 (2)
Anorexia	3 (1)	3 (1)
Anxiety	3 (1)	3 (1)
Insomnia	3 (1)	2 (1)
Impaired concentration	2 (1)	1
Nervousness	2 (1)	5 (2)
Cardiovascular		
Hot flashes	6 (3)	3 (1)
Hypotension	3 (1)	4 (2)
Dependent edema	2 (1)	1
Palpitation	2 (1)	5 (2)
Reproductive - Female		
Breast pain	5 (2)	8 (3)
Dysmenorrhea	2 (1)	1
Skin and Appendages		
Acne	3 (1)	0
Pruritus	2 (1)	1
Musculoskeletal		
Pain	4 (2)	6 (3)
Arthralgia	2 (1)	0
Respiratory		
Rhinitis	2 (1)	9 (4)
Vision		
Abnormal vision	2 (1)	2 (1)

*Reported at ≥1% for cabergoline.

Other adverse events reported at an incidence of <1% in the overall clinical studies follow. Body as a Whole: facial edema, influenza-like syndrome, and malaise. Cardiovascular: hypotension, syncope, and palpitations. Digestive: dry mouth, flatulence, diarrhea, and anorexia. Metabolic/Nutritional: weight loss and weight gain. Nervous System: somnolence, nervousness, paresthesia, insomnia, and anxiety. Respiratory: nasal stuffiness and epistaxis. Skin and Appendages: acne and pruritus. Special Senses: abnormal vision. Urogenital: dysmenorrhea and increased libido.

The safety of cabergoline has been evaluated in more than 1,200 patients with Parkinson's disease in controlled and uncontrolled studies at dosages of up to 11.5 mg/day, which greatly exceeds the maximum recommended dosage of cabergoline for hyperprolactinemic disorders. In addition to the adverse events that occurred in the patients with hyperprolactinemic disorders, the most common adverse events in patients with Parkinson's disease were dyskinesia, hallucinations, confusion, and peripheral edema. Heart failure, pleural effusion, pulmonary fibrosis, and gastric or duodenal ulcer occurred rarely. One case of constrictive pericarditis has been reported.

OVERDOSAGE Expect nasal congestion, syncope, or hallucinations. Take measures to support blood pressure if necessary.

DOSAGE AND ADMINISTRATION The recommended initial dosage of DOSTINEX Tablets is 0.25 mg twice a week. Dosage may be increased by 0.25 mg twice weekly up to a dosage of 1 mg twice a week, according to the patient's serum prolactin level. Do not increase dosage more rapidly than every 4 weeks, so that the patient's response to each dosage level can be assessed. If the patient does not respond adequately, and no additional benefit is observed with higher doses, use the lowest dose that achieved maximal response, and consider other therapeutic approaches. After a normal serum prolactin level has been maintained for 6 months, DOSTINEX may be discontinued, with periodic monitoring of the serum prolactin level to determine whether or when treatment with DOSTINEX should be reinstituted. The durability of efficacy beyond 24 months of therapy with DOSTINEX has not been established.

HOW SUPPLIED Bottles of eight tablets, NDC 0013-7001-12; white, scored, capsule-shaped tablets containing 0.5 mg cabergoline. Store at controlled room temperature, 20° to 25° C (68° to 77° F) [see USP].

CAUTION: Federal law prohibits dispensing without a prescription.

Manufactured by:
Pharmacia S.p.A.
Milan, Italy

For:
Pharmacia & Upjohn Company
Kalamazoo, MI 49001

B-1-S

Pharmacia &Upjohn

COMMITTED TO WOMEN'S HEALTH

USJ 7984.00

May 1997

Quest Diagnostics

Quest Diagnostics offers a wide range of valuable diagnostic services and products. Our routine testing facilities, supported by an extensive service infrastructure, integrate with the specialty testing services of Nichols Institute, Quest's Center for Diagnostic Innovation.

Nichols Institute endocrinology testing is focused in the areas of:

- pituitary
- diabetes
- thyroid
- steroids
- infertility
- calcium metabolism

Ask your doctor about Quest Diagnostics at Nichols Institute.

For Technical Information Call: 1.800.NICHOLS
1.800.642.4657

Integrating Nichols Institute as
Quest's Center for Diagnostic Innovation

Section IX

Pituitary Tumor Centers, Hospitals & Clinics

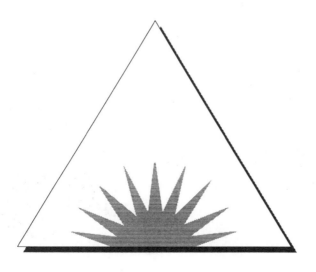

Second Edition

University of Alabama
Division of Neurosurgery
701 20th Street South, Suite 1370
Birmingham, AL 35294-0113
Phone: (205) 934-2918
Fax: (205) 975-5791
See display listing page 221

University of Arkansas
NeuroEndocrine Clinic
4301 W. Markham
Little Rock, AR   72205
Phone: (501) 296-1463
See display listing page 222

Beth Israel Medical Center
170 East End Avenue
New York, NY 10128
Phone: (212) 870-9600
Fax: (212) 870-9665
See display listing page 223

University of California Los Angeles
UCLA Medical Plaza, 300 Building
Los Angeles, CA 90095
Phone: (310) 794-1222
See display listing page 224

Harbor-UCLA Medical Foundation Inc.
21840 S. Normandy Avenue Suite 800
Torrance, CA 90502
Phone: (310) 222-5101
Fax: (310) 320-5463
See display listing page 225

University of California San Francisco
Parnassus at Third Avenue
San Francisco, CA 94143-0350
Phone: (415) 476-1911
Fax: (415) 476-7965
See display listing page 227

University of Southern California
Richard K. Eamer Medical Plaza
Weiss, Martin, M.D., Director
Professor and Chairman
Department of Neurosurgery
USC School of Medicine
1500 San Pablo Street
Los Angeles, CA 90033
Phone: (231) 342-8500
See display listing page 228

Cedars Sinai Medical Center
8700 Beverly Blvd.
Becker Building 131
Los Angeles, CA 90048
Office: (310) 855-4774
Fax: (310) 967-0119
See display listing page 229

UAB PITUITARY DISORDER CLINIC

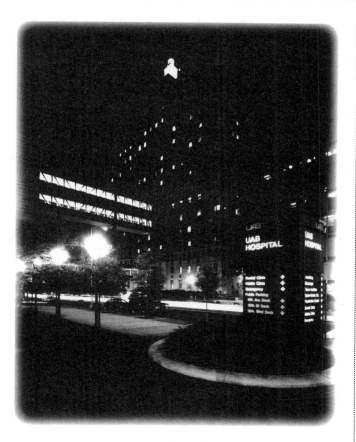

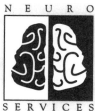

NEURO
SERVICES

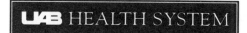

UAB HEALTH SYSTEM

UAB Neuroscience Services

The Division of Neuroscience Services at the University of Alabama at Birmingham (UAB) has earned national and world attention for successfully blending modern medicine and groundbreaking research with excellent patient care. Housed in UAB Hospital and The Kirklin Clinic at UAB, two facilities containing advanced diagnostic and treatment centers, UAB Neuroscience Services is staffed by experienced and skilled specialists, including several listed in the book *The Best Doctors in America*.

UAB Pituitary Disorder Clinic

• The UAB Pituitary Disorder Clinic provides comprehensive diagnosis and treatment for patients with pituitary tumors, pituitary hormone abnormalities, problems of growth and development, and related disorders.

• Individualized care is coordinated through a multispecialty approach involving experts in endocrinology, neuroimaging, and neurosurgery. For more information, please call (205) 934-2918. Or write

UAB Division of Neurosurgery
1813 6th Avenue South
MEB 512
Birmingham, Alabama
35294-3295

E-mail: self@cans.uab.edu

Pituitary Tumor Centers, Hospitals & Clinics

221

NeuroEndocrine Clinic

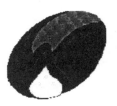

University of Arkansas for Medical Sciences, 4301 W. Markham, Little Rock, Arkansas 72205

Staff: **Ali F. Krisht, M.D., Neurosurgery (Director)**
Fred Faas, M.D., Endocrinology
Michael Vaphiades, M.D., Neuro-ophthalmology
Eddie J. Angtuaco, M.D., Neuro- radiology
Ronalda Williams, Secretary and Administrative Coordinator

The Neuroendocrine clinic was established in September 1994 with the goal of providing a multi-disciplinary approach to the management of patients with disorders of the pituitary gland. The clinic is supported by an endocrinologist, a neuro-ophthalmologist and a neuro-radiologist and directed by a neurosurgeon. Referrals are received regionally, nationally and internationally

For inquiries and appointments:
(501) 296-1463

Chicago Institute of Neurosurgery
and Neuroresearch
Cerullo, Leonard J. , M.D.
Medical Director,
Helenowski, Tomasz K., M.D.
Director, Stereotactic Radiosurgery
Rosseau, Gail L., M.D.
Director, Cranial Base Surgery
2515 N. Clark St.
Chicago, IL 60614
Phone: (800) 446-1234
See display listing page 230

The University of Chicago Hospitals
5841 S. Maryland Avenue (MC 3026)
Chicago, IL 60637
Phone: (773) 702-2123
See display listing page 231

University of Illinois at Chicago
840 S. Wood Street (M/C 787)
Chicago, IL 60612
Phone: (312) 996-7700
Fax: (312) 413-0342
See display listing page 231

University of Cincinnati
221 Piedmont
Cincinnati, OH 45267
Phone: (513) 558-8889
Fax: (513) 558-3755
See display listing page 232

University of Colorado
Health Sciences Center
4200 E. 9th Avenue, Campus Box C-307
Denver, CO 80262
Phone: (303) 315-5651
Fax: (303) 315-6197
See display listing page 233

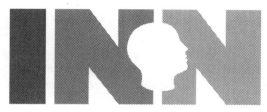

**Institute for Neurology and Neurosurgery
Beth Israel Medical Center**

PITUITARY ENDOCRINE SERVICES

170 East End Avenue, New York, NY 10128
Tel: 212-870-9600
Fax: 212-870-9665

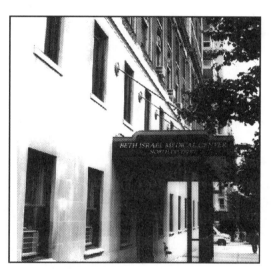

The Pituitary Endocrine Services at the
Institute for Neurology and Neurosurgery
(INN) at Beth Israel Medical Center
provides multidisciplinary diagnosis and
treatment of pituitary / hypothalamic
tumors and disease for children and adults.

http://www.bethisraelny.org

PATIENT SERVICES

**Neurosurgery
(Adult and Pediatric)**
Fred J Epstein, M.D.
Rick Abbott, M.D.
Cheryl Muszynski, M.D.
Eric Elowitz, M.D.
Tania Shiminski-Maher, M.D.

Endovascular Surgery
Alex Berenstein, M.D.
Avi Setton, M.D.

Neuro-Oncology
Jeffrey S. Allen, M.D.
Joao Siffert, M.D.

Pediatric Neurology
Walter Molofsky, M.D.

Neuro-Endocrinology
Brenda Kohn, M.D.
Bonnie Franklin, M.D.

Neuro-Ophthalmology
Jay Wisnicki, M.D.
Mark Kuppersmith, M.D.

Neuroradiology
Richard Pinto, M.D.
Dan Lefton, M.D.
Francisco DeLara, M.D.

Radiation Oncology
Susan Kim, M.D.

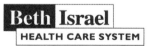

**Beth Israel Medical Center is the Manhattan Campus for the
Albert Einstein College of Medicine**

Second Edition

The UCLA Pituitary Program
UCLA Medical Plaza, 300 Building
Los Angeles, California 90095

The UCLA Pituitary Center provides *comprehensive evaluation* and treatment for patients with pituitary tumors and related disorders. Individualized *state of the art* care is coordinated through a *multi-specialty approach* involving specialists in **endocrinology, neurosurgery, stereotactic radiosurgery neuro-ophthalmology, neuro-imaging** and **neuropathology**. Complete outpatient evaluations are provided by full-time UCLA faculty members at the UCLA Medical Plaza. Patients needing hospitalization for additional testing or neurosurgical treatment are admitted to UCLA Medical Center. The Pituitary Center will also be pleased to provide second opinions and preoperative or follow-up evaluations for patients receiving treatment at other facilities.

Co-Directors
Donald P. Becker, M.D., Professor and Chief, Division of Neurosurgery
Daniel F. Kelly, M.D. Assistant Professor, Division of Neurosurgery
Stanley G. Korenman, M.D., Professor and Chief, Division of Endocrinology, UCLA Medical Center
Ronald S. Swerdloff, M.D., Professor and Chief, Division of Endocrinology, Department of Medicine

Faculty
Neurosurgery
Marvin Bergsneider, M.D., Assistant Professor - *Neuroendoscopy*
John Frazee, M.D., Associate Clinical Professor - *Neuroendoscopy*
Antonio A. F. DeSalles, M.D., Assistant Professor - *Radiosurgery*
Neurosurgical Colleague and Program Coordinator
Lisa Ianniello, M.N., R.N., N.P

Endocrinology
Inder J. Chopra, M.D., Professor of Medicine, UCLA Division of Endocrinology
Andre J. Van Herle, M.D., Professor of Medicine, UCLA Division of Endocrinology
Christina C. L. Wang, M.D., Professor of Medicine, Harbor - UCLA Division of Endocrinology

Neuro-Ophthalmology
Anthony C. Arnold, M.D., Professor and Chief, Division of Neuro-Ophthalmology, Dept. of Ophthalmology
Howard R. Krauss, M.D., Associate Clinical Professor of Ophthalmology

Neuroradiology
John R. Bentson, M.D., Professor and Section Chief of Neuroradiology, Department of Radiology

Neuropathology
Harry V. Vinters, M.D., Professor of Pathology, Chief of Neuropathology
Cynthia Welsh, M.D., Assistant Professor of Pathology

For an appointment or further information, call the Division of Neurosurgery at 310-794-1222 or:
Donald P. Becker, M.D., Chief, Division of Neurosurgery
Phone: 310-794-1222; Fax: 310-794-2147
e-mail: becker@neurosurg.medsch.ucla.edu

Daniel F. Kelly, M.D., Division of Neurosurgery
Phone: 310-206-4100; Fax: 310-794-2147
e-mail: dfkelly@ucla.edu

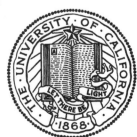

The Harbor-UCLA Pituitary Center

Harbor-UCLA Medical Foundation Inc.
21840 S. Normandy Ave., Suite 800
Torrance, CA 90502
phone   310-222-5101
fax: 310-320-5463

The Pituitary Center, established in 1994, provides *comprehensive evaluation* and treatment for patients with pituitary tumors and related neuro-endocrine disorders, including infertility and reproductive hormone problems. Individualized care is coordinated through a *multi-specialty approach* involving specialists in **endocrinology**, **neurosurgery**, **neuro-ophthalmology**, **neuro-imaging** and **neuropathology**. **Stereotactic radiosurgery** services are also available at UCLA Medical Center. Complete outpatient evaluations are provided by full-time UCLA faculty members at the Harbor-UCLA Professional Office Building. Patients needing hospitalization for additional testing or neurosurgical treatment are admitted to a specialized endocrine evaluation unit at Harbor-UCLA Medical Center. The Pituitary Center will also be pleased to provide second opinions and preoperative or follow-up evaluations for patients receiving treatment at other facilities.

Co-Directors
Ronald S. Swerdloff, M.D., Professor and Chief, Division of Endocrinology, Department of Medicine
Daniel F. Kelly, M.D. Assistant Professor, Division of Neurosurgery

Endocrinology
Christina C. L. Wang, M.D., Professor of Medicine and Program Director, Clinical Study Center
Wael Salameh, M.D. Assistant Professor, Division of Endocrinology, Department of Medicine

Neuro-Endoscopy
Marvin Bergsneider, M.D., Assistant Professor of Neurosurgery

Radiosurgery
Antonio A.F. DeSalles, M.D., Ph.D., Assistant Professor of Neurosurgery; Director, UCLA Stereotactic Radiosurgery Program

Neuro-Ophthalmology
John R. Heckenlively, M.D., Professor and Assistant Chief, Division of Ophthalmology

Neuroradiology
Mark Mehringer, M.D., Professor and Acting Chairman, Dept. of Radiology, Chief of Neuroradiology

Neuropathology
Marcia E. Cornford, M.D., Assistant Professor of Pathology, Head of Neuropathology

For an appointment or further information please call The Pituitary Clinic (310-222-5101) or:

Ronald S. Swerdloff, M.D., Division of Endocrinology
phone: 310-222-1867
fax: 310-533-0627
e-mail: swerdloff@harbor2.humc.edu

Daniel F. Kelly, M.D., Division of Neurosurgery
phone: 310-222-2754
fax: 310-618-8157
e-mail: dfkelly@ucla.edu

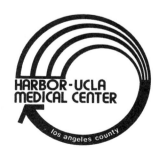

Emory University Hospital
1365 Clifton Road, N.E., Bldg. B
Atlanta, GA 30322
Phone: (404) 778-7744
Fax: (404) 778-4472
See display listing page 234

University of Florida Medical Center
P.O. Box 100265
Gainesville, FL 32610-0265
Phone: (352) 392-4331
Fax: (352) 392-8413
See display listing page 235

Hospital of the Good Samaritan
637 South Lucas Avenue Suite 501
Los Angeles, CA 90017
Phone: (800) 762-1692
See display listing page 236

M.D. Anderson Cancer Center
1515 Holcombe Boulevard
Houston, TX 77030
See display listing page 236

Mount Sinai Medical Center
5 East 98th Street
New York, NY 10029
See display listing page 240

SUNY Health Science Center
750 E. Adams Street
Syracuse, NY 13210
Phone: (315) 464-4470
Fax: (315) 464-4415
See display listing page 237

Massachusetts General Hospital
Neuroendocrine Clinical Center
Klibanski, Anne, M.D.
Chief, Neuroendocrine Unit
15 Parkman Street, WAC 730S
Boston, MA 02114-3139
Phone: (617) 726-3872
Fax: (617) 726-5905
See display listing page 238

University of Massachusetts
Medical Center
55 Lake Avenue North
Worcester MA 01655
Phone: (508) 856-3239
Fax: (508) 856-6950
See display listing page 239

University of Michigan Medical Center
1500 East Medical Center Drive
Ann Arbor, MI 48109
Phone: (313) 936-5020
Fax: (313) 936-9294
See display listing page 240

University of Pennsylvania Medical
Center
3400 Spruce Street
Philadelphia, PA 19104
Phone: (215) 349-8325
Fax: (215) 349-5534
See display listing page 241

Toronto Hospital Pituitary Clinic
399 Bathurst Street
Toronto, Ontario M5 2S8
Phone: (416) 603-6454
Fax: (416) 603-7378
See display listing page 242

Pituitary Treatment Center

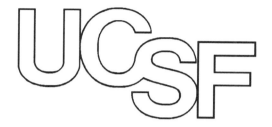

...A Health Sciences Campus

University of California, San Francisco
Parnassus at Third Avenue
San Francisco, CA
94143-0350
Tel: 415/476-1911
Fax: 415/476-7965

The University of California, San Francisco (UCSF), one of the nation's most prestigious medical institutions in both medical care and basic research, has been a major center for the diagnosis and treatment of all types of pituitary disorders for more than 50 years. UCSF offers comprehensive specialization in each aspect of the diagnosis and therapy of pituitary adenomas and other disorders of the pituitary and hypothalamus.

During the past 20 years, more than 2,700 patients with pituitary tumors have been treated surgically at UCSF, and many more have been treated with medical or radiation therapy. Our faculty are consistently ranked among the top five in the country in surveys such as the U.S. News and World Report's, and many are listed in The Best Doctors in America. UCSF provides state of the art diagnostic expertise in all aspects of endocrinology and neuroradiology, and comprehensive therapy of these disorders with expertise in neurosurgery, radiation therapy and medical therapy

Patient Services
Neurosurgery
Pituitary Adenomas/Surgery
Charles B. Wilson, M.D.
Stereotactic(GammaKnife)Radiourgery
Michael W. McDermott, M.D.
Endocrinology
Pituitary Adenomas/Neuroedocrinogy
J. Blake Tyrrell, M.D.
Pediatric Endocrinology
Felix A. Conte, M.D.
Reproductive Endocrinology
Robert B. Jaffee, M.D.
Fertility
Mary C. Martin, M.D.
Radiology
Neuroradiology
William P. Dillon, M.D.
Neurointerventional Radiology
Van Halbach, M.D.
Ophthalmology
Neuro-Ophthalmology
William F. Hoyt, M.D.
Johathan C. Horton, M.D., Ph.D.
Radiation Oncology
Conventional Radiation Therapy
Stereotactic (GammaKnife)Radiosurgery
David A. Larson, M.D., Ph.D.
Neuro-Oncology
Michael D. Prados, M.D.
Susan M. Chang, M.D.
Neuropathology
Richard L. Davis, M.D.

Pituitary Endocrine Center, USC University Hospital

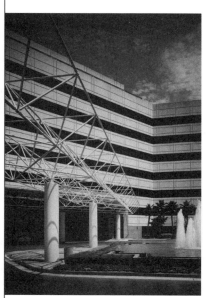

USC UNIVERSITY HOSPITAL *is a 284-bed tertiary care facility on the Health Sciences Campus of the University of Southern California. This private teaching hospital opened in May, 1991 and offers to its patients medical expertise and sophisticated technology combined with a personalized approach to health care in a comfortable, caring environment.*

PATIENT SERVICES
Neurosurgery
Comprehensive Neuroendocrinology
Neuro-ophthalmology
Reproductive Endocrinology
Endovascular Surgery
Sophisticated Imaging

Martin Weiss, M.D., Director
Professor and Chairman
Department of Neurosurgery
USC School of Medicine

To make an appointment
or for further information,
please call **1-800-USC-CARE**.

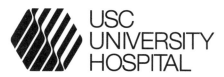

Richard K. Eamer Medical Plaza
1500 San Pablo Street
Los Angeles, California 90033   www.uscuh.com

CEDARS-SINAI MEDICAL CENTER.

The Pituitary Center

The Pituitary Center is under the co-leadership of Dr. Shlomo Melmed and Dr. Hrayr Shahinian. Dr. Melmed is internationally known in the field of pituitary management and directs both the clinical and research activities of the Division of Endocrinology and Metabolism. Dr. Shahinian is well known as an expert in Pediatric Craniofacial and Pituitary Surgery.

The Pituitary Center at Cedars-Sinai Medical Center is exclusively dedicated to the diagnosis and treatment of pituitary disorders.

The Center's faculty presently cares for several hundred patients with pituitary disorders.

We are currently the leading center on the West Coast conducting clinical trials for pre-operative and post-operative medical management of pituitary disorders.

Patient Services

- Neuroendocrinology
- Skull Base Surgery
- Endocrine Diagnostic Testing Unit
- Comprehensive Cancer Center
- Functional Stereotactic Neurosurgery

- Magnetic Resonance & SPECT Imaging
- Neuroradiology
- Patient Support Groups
- Radiotherapy
- Neuro-ophthalmology

All services are provided at one location for your convenience and comfort.

Faculty

Shlomo Melmed, M.D., Co-Director
Director, Division of Endocrinology
Professor of Medicine,
UCLA School of Medicine

Hrayr Shahinian, M.D., Co-Director
Director, Division of Skull Base Surgery

Glenn Braunstein, M.D.
Chairman, Department of Medicine
Professor of Medicine,
UCLA School of Medicine

Vivien Bonert, M.D.
Staff Endocrinologist
Assistant Professor of Medicine,
UCLA School of Medicine

Ted Friedman, M.D., Ph.D.
Staff Endocrinologist
Assistant Professor of Medicine
UCLA School of Medicine

We Offer Comprehensive Clinical Services Available In One Center For Pituitary Disorders
World Renowned Specialists In The Comprehensive Diagnosis And Treatment Of Pituitary Disorders

8700 Beverly Blvd.
Becker Building 131
Los Angeles, CA
90048

Office: (310) 855-4774   Fax: (310) 967-0119

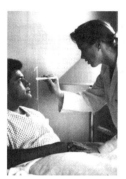
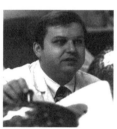

Pituitary Tumor Centers, Hospitals & Clinics

The Multidisciplinary Pituitary Center At The University of Cincinnati

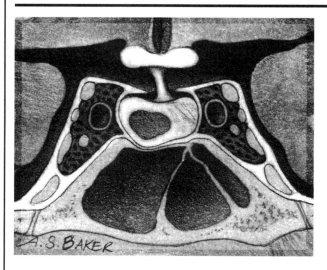

University of Cincinnati Medical Associates

University Hospital Cincinnati, Ohio

Part of The Health Alliance of Greater Cincinnati

Members of The University of Cincinnati Multidisciplinary Pituitary Center Team:

John M. Tew, Jr, MD
Neurosurgery
Robert E. Albright, Jr, MD
Neuro-Oncology
Harry van Loveren, MD
Neurosurgery
John C. Breneman, MD
Radiation-Oncology
Mary F. Gaskill-Shipley, MD
Neuroradiology
Robert M. Cohen, MD, FACP
Endocrinology
M. Gregory Balko, MD
Neuropathology
Nancee Splitt, RN, BSN
Nurse Clinician
Nancy McMahon, RN, BSN
Nurse Clinician

University Hospital and the physicians and surgeons of the Mayfield Clinic and University of Cincinnati Medical Associates have created a neurosciences center that treats patients from all over the world. Our physicians are pioneers in developing and utilizing new methods to diagnose, treat, and rehabilitate such major neurological disorders as pituitary tumors, brain and spinal cord tumors, stroke, epilepsy, and aneurysms.

Leading-edge medical advances are available first from physicians who teach and practice medicine at major national academic health centers–like the physicians of Mayfield Clinic, University of Cincinnati Medical Associates and University Hospital.

And while they have access to the latest and best medical technology and research, what sets our physicians apart is their commitment to providing each patient with personalized attention and compassionate care.

You or your physician can access this dynamic neuroscience resource by calling the University of Cincinnati Multidisciplinary Pituitary Center. Our physicians make it a priority to evaluate every case to determine how each patient may benefit from this unique program.

To learn more about the University of Cincinnati's Multidisciplinary Pituitary Center, please call:

Mayfield Clinic
1 (800) 325-7787
University Hospital Physician Referral
(513) 475-8701
or toll-free, outside Cincinnati,
1 (888) 640-CARE
e-mail: pituitary@healthall.com

PITUITARY ENDOCRINE CENTER

University Hospital

University of Colorado

Offering a multidisciplinary approach to neuroendocrine disorders including pituitary region tumors.

University of Colorado Health Sciences Center

4200 East Ninth Avenue
Denver, CO 80262

Outside Colorado: (800) 621-5857

Inside Colorado: (800) 621-7621

PATIENT SERVICES

- Microneurosurgery
- Comprehensive Endocrinology
- Reproductive Endocrinology
- Diagnostic Neuroradiology
- Multidisciplinary Patient Management Conference
- Stereotactic Radiosurgery

PROGRAM DIRECTORS

Kevin O. Lillehei, M.D.
Associate Professor
Division of Neurosurgery

E. Chester Ridgway, M.D.
Professor & Chief
Division of Endocrinology

University of Toronto
See display listing page 243

Vanderbilt University Medical Center
Division of Endocrinology
715 MRB II
Nashville, TN 37232-6303
Phone: (615) 936-1653
See display listing page 244

University of Virginia Health
Science Center
Box 212 Private Clinics Building
Charlottesville, VA 22908
Toll Free: (800) 650-2650
Phone: (804) 924-2650
See display listing page 245

University of Washington
Seattle, WA
See display listing page 246

Westchester County Medical Center
Valhalla, NY 10595
Phone: (914) 285-7000
Fax: (914) 285-7607
See display listing page 247

Pituitary Tumor Centers, Hospitals & Clinics

233

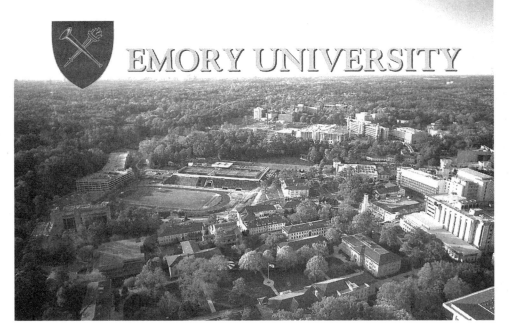

The Emory Clinic and its affiliated hospitals are leaders in today's competitive healthcare environment committed to:
- high quality, cost-effective patient care
- clinical and financial support for teaching and research
- the mission of the Emory University System of Health Care (EUSHC)
- partnership with the community to promote wellness

Emory University Hospital
1365 Clifton Road, N.E., Bldg. B
Atlanta, GA 30322
Phone: (404) 778-7744
Fax: (404) 778-4472

To Make an appointment or for further information, please call the Emory Health Connection at **(404) 778-7744**

Patient Services

Endocrinology:
Diane Biskobing, M.D.
Lewis Blevins, M.D.
James H. Christy, M.D.
Imad El-Kebbi, M.D.
Suzanne S.P. Gebhardt, M.D.
Lawrence S. Phillips, M.D.
David G. Robertson, M.D.
Nelson B. Watts, M.D.

Neurology & Neuro-Opthalmology:
Nancy J. Newman, M.D.

Neurosurgery:
Nelson M. Oyesiku, M.D., Ph.D.

Psychiatry/Psychology:
Nadine J. Kaslow, M.D.
Dominique Musselman, M.D.

Radiation Oncology:
Ian Richard Crocker, M.D.

Reproductive Medicine
Anne B. Namnoun, M.D.

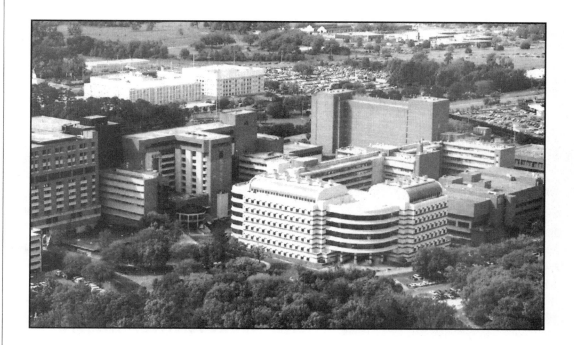

UNIVERSITY OF FLORIDA MEDICAL CENTER

SHANDS HOSPITAL

The University of Florida Medical Center and the Shands Hospital at the University of Florida offer a broad range of services for patients with pituitary tumors and associated disorders. Dr. Albert L. Rhoton, fit, Chairman of the Department of Neurological Surgery, directs the program for the treatment of pituitary tumors. He has experience with more than 1,000 pituitary surgery patients. He has also developed a number of surgical instruments commonly used for pituitary operations and has written one book and numerous papers about the pituitary and sellar region.

Please contact us for our booklet for patients regarding the surgical treatment of pituitary tumors.

PITUITARY SERVICES
Pituitary Tumor Microsurgery
Stereotactic Unidose and Fractionated
  (LINAC) Radiosurgery
Pediatric and Adult Endocrinology
Reproductive Endocrinology & Fertility
Neuroradiology
Neurointerventional Radiology
Neuro-ophthalmology
Conventional Radiation Therapy
Neuro-oncology
Neurology
Neuroanesthesia
Neuropathology

For information, contact:

Albert L. Rhoton, Jr., M.D.
R.D. Keene Family Professor and Chairman
Department of Neurological Surgery
University of Florida Medical Center
P.O. Box 100265
Gainesville, Florida 326 10-0265
Telephone: *(352) 392-4331*
Fax: *(352) 392-8413*

UF Consultation Center:
Physician Referral Line: 1-800-633-2122

Pituitary Tumor Centers, Hospitals & Clinics

235

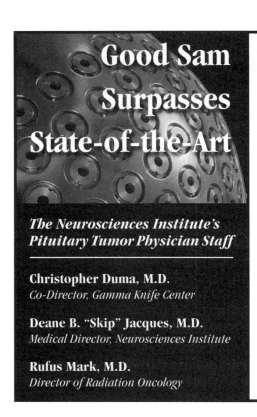
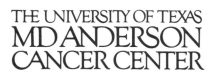
Second Edition

Pituitary Tumor Center

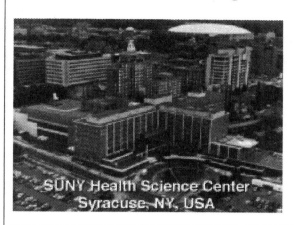

SUNY Health Science Center
Syracuse, NY, USA

**University Hospital
750 E. Adams St.
Syracuse, NY 13210**

**tel: 01-315-464-4470
1-800-255-5011
fax: 01-315-464-4415
email: rodziewg@vax.cs.hscsyr.edu
web page: www.neuro.hscsyr.edu**

Services
Evaluation and consultation for all pituitary disorders
Clinical Research testing unit for pituitary endocrine diagnosis
Infertility diagnosis and treatment
Access to the latest medication and treatments for pituitary disorders
Endoscopic surgery of the pituitary gland
Stereotactic radiosurgery for lesions in and around the pituitary gland
Active research programs for diagnosis and treatment of pituitary
disorders

Members

Endocrinology
B.L. Feuerstein, MD
R.E. Izquierdo, MD
K.F. Kartun, MD
P. Knudson, MD
A. Moses, MD
D. Streeten, MD
R. Weinstock, MD, Ph.D

Neuroradiology
L. Hochhauser, MD, FRCPC
J.J. Wasenko, MD

Reproductive Endocrinology
S. Badawy, MD
M. Singh, MD

Neurosurgery
G. Rodziewicz, MD, FACS
M.V. Smith, MD

Neuro-ophthalmology
D. Friedman, MD

Radiation Therapy
G. King, MD

Neuroendocrine Clinical Center

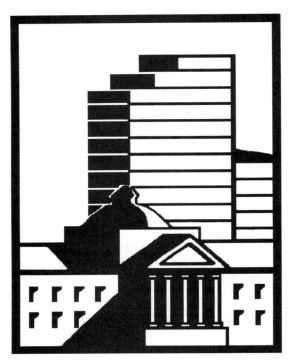

The Massachusetts General Hospital is the largest Hospital of Harvard Medical School. The Neuroendocrine Clinical Center at MGH is a multi - disciplinary service founded in 1984 offering innovative therapies, technologic advances and dedicated care to patients with pituitary disorders and other neuroendocrine diseases.

MASSACHUSETTS GENERAL HOSPITAL
HARVARD MEDICAL SCHOOL

15 Parkman Street, WAG 730S
Wang Ambulatory Care Center
Boston, MA 021 14-3139
Telephone: (617) 726-3872
Fax:(617) 726-5905

PATIENT SERVICES

Endocrinology:
Anne Klibanski, MD.
Chief Neuroendocrine Unit
Beverly M.K. Biller, M.D.
Steven K. Grinspoon, MD.
Larry Katznelson, M.D.
Kristin E. Baker, RN.

Neurology:
Peter Riskind, M.D., Ph.d

Neurosurgery:
Nicholas T. Zervas, M.D.
Chief, Neurosurgical Service
Brooke Swearingen, M.D.

Radiation Medicine:
Allan F. Thornton, M.D.

To make an appointment or for further information, please call
(617) 726-3872

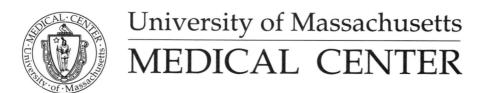

University of Massachusetts
MEDICAL CENTER

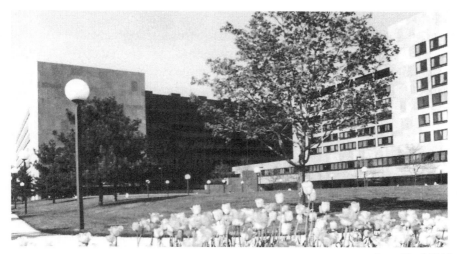

photo: Chuck Kidd

The Clinical Neuroendocrinology Unit

The Clinical Neuroendocrinology Unit at the University of Massachusetts Medical Center offers care for patients with pituitary tumors, medical problems involving pituitary hormones, altered growth and development in children, and reproductive endocrine problems and infertility related to the pituitary. A multidisciplinary team of specialists provides individualized diagnosis and treatment for each patient.

SPECIALISTS

Neil Aronin, M.D.
Director, Clinical Neuroendocrinology
Pituitary Tumors/Clinical Neuroendocrinology

Rosalind Brown, M.D.
Chief, Pediatric Endocrinology
Growth and Development

T.J. Fitzgerald, M.D.
Chief, Radiation Oncology
3-dimensional conformal radiotherapy

John W. Gittinger, Jr., M.D.
Chair, Ophthalmology
Neuro-ophthalmology

N. Scott Litofsky, M.D.
Neurosurgery
Pituitary Tumors/Surgery

Veronica Ravnikar, M.D.
Chief, Reproductive Endocrinology
Reproductive Endocrinology and Fertility

Lawrence D. Recht, M.D.
Neuro-oncology
Tumors of the Central Nervous System

For appointments and information, please call (508) 856-3239

Pituitary Tumor Centers, Hospitals & Clinics

239

Second Edition

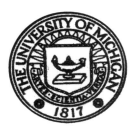

Pituitary and Neuroendocrine Center
University of Michigan Medical Center

Dedicated to comprehensive diagnosis and treatment
of patients with pituitary disease

Patient Services
- Comprehensive clinical evaluation
- Endocrine diagnostic unit
- State-of-the-art neuroradiology, including petrosal sinus sampling
- Surgery of all pituitary and parapituitary lesions
- Radiotherapy, including stereotactic radiosurgery
- Pharmacologic and replacement therapy
- Access to research trials of new medications

Co-Directors

Ariel Barkan, M.D.
Professor, Endocrinology

William F. Chandler, M.D.
Professor, Neurosurgery

1500 East Medical Center Drive, Ann Arbor, MI 48109
Phone: 313-936-5020 Fax: 313-936-9294
Email: wchndlr@umich.edu

Pituitary Tumor Program

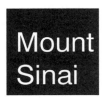

Mount Sinai Medical Center
5 East 98th Street
New York, NY 10029

Patient Services
- Neurosurgery, Adult and Pediatric
- Endocrinology, Adult and Pediatric
- Neuroradiology
- Neuro-Oncology
- Magnetic Resonance and SPECT Imaging
- Functional Stereotactic Neurosurgery
- Radiosurgery
- Radiotherapy

Program Directors
Kalmon D. Post, M.D., Chairman of Neurosurgery, directs the neuroendocrine surgery and has experience with over 1,000 pituitary surgery patients. Dr. Alice Levine and Dr. Gillian Katz direct clinical and research aspects of endocrinology, and Dr. Linda Mandel directs the Radiosurgery Program

For more information, please contact:
Dr. Kalmon D. Post   (212) 241-0933

The Pituitary Tumor Program

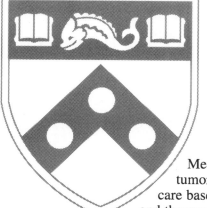

**University of Pennsylvania
Medical Center
3400 Spruce Street
Philadelphia, PA 19104
Telephone: 215-349-8325
Fax: 215-349-5534**

The University of Pennsylvania Medical Center offers patients with tumors of the pituitary gland comprehensive care based on the most advanced diagnostic and therapeutic techniques available.

All patients are evaluated by board certified specialists in neurosurgery, endocrinology, otorhinolaryngology and neuro-ophthalmology. These specialists have dedicated themselves to delivering state-of-the-art care to patients with pituitary tumors.

An individualized treatment plan is devised for each patient, which may include advanced techniques such as minimally invasive endoscopic surgery, intraoperative real-time image guidance systems, and linear accelerator radiosurgery. The plan of treatment for each patient optimizes safety along with the removal of tumor tissue.

Patients or their physicians may contact any of the following members of the Pituitary Tumor Program to schedule an appointment or consultation.

Neurosurgery
Mark J. Kotapka, MD
Eugene S. Flamm, MD

Endocrinology
Peter Snyder, MD
Susan Mandel, MD

Otorhinolaryngology
Donald Lanza, MD

Neuro-ophthalmology
Steven Galetta, MD
Nicholas Volpe, MD
Grant Liu, MD

Neuroradiology
Robert Grossman, MD

Radiation Oncology
James Ruffer, MD

U.S. News and World Report ranks Penn's neurology care higher than any other in Pennsylvania, New Jersey and Delaware and lists the program in its top ten nationally.

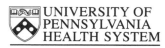

**UNIVERSITY OF
PENNSYLVANIA
HEALTH SYSTEM**
The future of medicine®

THE TORONTO HOSPITAL PITUITARY PROGRAM

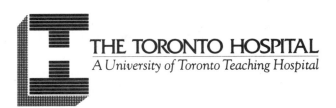

THE TORONTO HOSPITAL
A University of Toronto Teaching Hospital

A major teaching hospital of the University of Toronto, The Toronto Hospital offers a full program for the diagnosis and management of adult patients with pituitary disorders.

Our pituitary team consists of specialists in endocrinology neurosurgery, neuro radiology, neuro-ophthalmology, endocrine and neuropathology and radiation oncology who are able to deliver comprehensive care in all aspects of pituitary disease or dysfunction.

Patients may be referred for assessment to the combined endocrine-neurosurgical pituitary clinic at the Western Division of The Toronto hospital

The Toronto Hospital
Pituitary Clinic
399 Bathurst Street
Toronto, Ontario
41ST 258
Phone: (416) 603-6454
Fax: (416) 603-7378

SPECIALISTS

Endocrinology
G.L.A. From, MD, FRCPC
S.R. George, MD, FRCPC

Neurosurgery
F Gentili, MD, MSc., FRCSC
J.F.R. Fleming, MD, MS, FRCSC

Neuroradiology
W. Kucharczyk, MD, FRCPC
W. Montanera, MD, FRCPC

Otolaryngology
P.J. Gullane, MD, FRCSC
J.A. Rutka, MD, FRCSC

Pathology
S. Nag, MD, FRCPC
S.L. Asa, MD, Ph.D., FRCPC

Radiation Oncology
R.W.C. Tsang, MD, *FRCPC*
J.D. Brierley, MB, FRCR, FRCPC

The University of Toronto
Pituitary Program

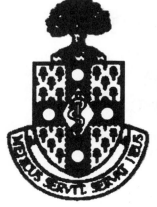

Faculty of Medicine
University of Toronto

The University of Toronto has been the site of major advances in the understanding of pituitary disease since the 1970's. We now have a group of world renowned experts who offer a full spectrum of expert diagnosis, quality patient management, and advances in research in the setting of a high caliber teaching institute.

All pituitary patients are seen initially by a pituitary Endocrinologist, Dr. Shereen Ezzat, who performs a comprehensive examination and is responsible for all medical treatment. Dr. Harley Smyth has over the last 20 years performed more than 1000 surgeries and consults on all patients who will require surgical management. All surgically resected tumors are carefully examined by an expert pituitary pathologist, providing a multidisciplinary integrated team approach to the management of patients with pituitary disorders

Medical and Research Staff

Endocrinologists:
Dr. Shereen Ezzat
Phone: (416) 926-7000
Fax: (416) 966-5046

Neurosurgeon:
Dr. Harley S. Smith
Phone: (416) 926-7792
Fax: (416) 966-5046

Pathologist:
Dr. Sylvia L. Asa
Phone: (416) 586-8445
Fax: (416) 586-8589

Pituitary Tumor Centers, Hospitals & Clinics

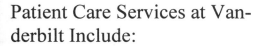

Vanderbilt
University
Medical Center

Patient Care Services at Vanderbilt Include:

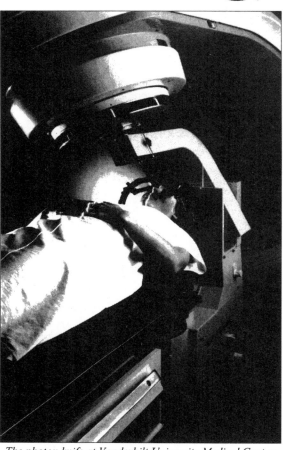

The photon knife at Vanderbilt University Medical Center

- Endocrinology, Adult and Pediatric
- Neurosurgery
- Radiology
- Radiation Oncology
- Magnetic Resonance
- Imaging
- Computerized Tomography
- Stereotactic Radiosurgery utilizing the Photon Knife
- Transphenoidal and Craniotomy Microsurgery
- Treatment modalities for patients with recurrent or

From the photon knife, used to treat otherwise inoperable tumors, to artificial intelligence based software programs to assist with microsurgical techniques, Vanderbilt University Medical Center has a technologically advanced facility for the treatment of patients with pituitary tumors.

Its technical capabilities, an interdisciplinary team approach to patient care and a patient-friendly environment make Vanderbilt a premier health care center.

For More information on the above Vanderbilt University Medical Center Services please contact:

Vanderbilt University Medical Center
Division of Endocrinology
715 MRB II
Nashville, TN 37232-6303
(615) 936-1653

NEUROENDOCRINE CENTER AT UVA

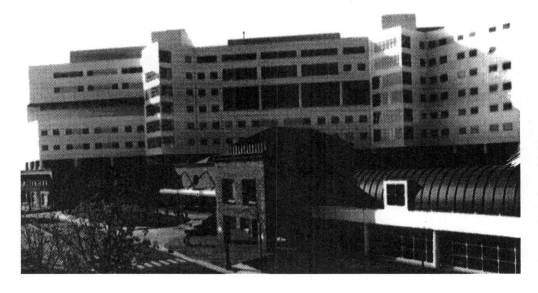

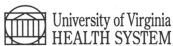 University of Virginia
HEALTH SYSTEM

The University of Virginia is an academic teaching institution equipped with state-of-the-art facilities and equipment and well-known physicians. The Neuroendocrine Center is run by four outstanding physicians known nationally and internationally.

Dr. Edward Laws directs neuroendocrine surgery and has experience with some 2,900 pituitary surgery patients.
Dr. Michael Thorner and Dr. Mary Lee Vance direct clinical and research aspects of endocrinology and Dr. Ladislau Steiner directs the Gamma Knife Radiosurgery Program.

For more information, please contact The Neuroendocrine Center at the University of Virginia. 1(800) 650-2650, (804) 924-2650.

The Neuroendocrine Center

Box 212, Private Clinics Building
Charlottesville, VA 22908
(800) 650-2650, (804) 924-2650

PATIENT SERVICES

- Neurosurgery
  Adult and Pediatric
- Endocrinology
  Adult and Pediatric
- Neuroradiology
- Neuro-Oncology
- Magnetic Resonance and
  SPECT Imaging
- Computerized Tomography
- Functional Stereotactic
  Neurosurgery
- Gamma Knife Radiosurgery
- Radiotherapy

Neuroendocrine Treatment Center

- NEUROLOGICAL SURGERY
  H. Richard Winn, M.D.
  Marc R. Mayberg, M.D.
  Daniel Silbergeld, M.D.

- PEDIATRIC NEUROLOGICAL SURGERY
  Richard Ellenbogan, M.D.
  Theodore Roberts, M.D.

- STEREOTACTIC RADIOSURGERY
  Marc R. Mayberg, M.D.
  H. Richard Winn, M.D.
  Daniel Silbergeld, M.D.
  Keith Stelzer, M.D.
  Mark Phillips, Ph.D.

- ENDOCRINOLOGY
  Alan Chait, M.D.
  Wil Fujimoto, M.D.
  George R. Merriam, M.D.
  David D'Alessio, M.D.
  Michael Schwartz, M.D.
  Jonathan Purnell, M.D.

- PEDIATRIC ENDOCRINOLOGY
  C. Patrick Mahoney, M.D.
  Gad B. Kletter, M.D.
  Catherine Pihoker, M.D.

- NEURO-OPHTHALMOLOGY
  Richard Mills, M.D.
  James Orcutt, M.D.
  Avery Weiss,, M.D. (Pediatrics)

- RADIATION ONCOLOGY
  Keith Stelzer, M.D., Ph.D.

- NEURO-ONCOLOGY
  Alex Spence, M.D.
  Russ Geyer, M. D. (Pediatrics)

- INTERVENTIONAL & NEURORADIOLOGY
  Joseph Eskridge, M.D.
  Kenneth Maravilla, M.D.
  Robert Dalley, M.D.
  David Haynor, M.D.

- OTOLARYNGOLOGY, HEAD & NECK SURGERY
  Ernest Weymuller, M.D.
  Larry Duckert, M.D.
  George Gates, M.D.
  Eric Pinczower, M.D.
  Robert Stanley, M.D.

- TUMOR MOLECULAR BIOLOGY RESEARCH
  Richard Morrison, Ph.D.

The University of Washington Affiliated Medical Centers in Seattle, Washington, offer comprehensive care to pituitary tumor and neuroendocrine patients.

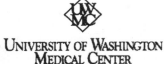
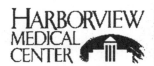

Neuroendocrine Clinic - Multi-specialty evaluation of complex pituitary problems.

Microsurgery - Microsurgical treatment of pituitary and parasellar tumors.

Linac Scalpel Stereotactic Radiosurgery - Outpatient therapy for pituitary and parasellar tumors.

Neuro-oncology Tumor Board - Weekly review of cases by a multidisciplinary panel of specialists.

Interventional Neuroradiology - Including petrosal vein sampling, embolization of tumors and carotid test occlusion.

Frameless Stereotactic Intraoperative Navigation - Allows precise localization during surgery.

Skull Base Surgery Team - Optimal treatment of this region determined by a multidisciplinary team.

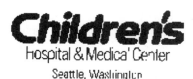

Pediatric Endocrinology/Neurosurgery-Multidisciplinary evaluation/management of pituitary tumor and neuroendocrine problems in children.

Patient Contacts
UWMC Neuroendocrine Clinic, (206) 548-5068
HMC Pituitary Clinical Specialist, (206) 521-1848
UWMC Pituitary Clinical Specialist, (206) 543-3572
Children's Hospital Endocrinology, (206) 528-2616
Children's Hospital Neurological Surgery, (206) 526-2544
Children's Hospital Brain Tumor Clinic (206) 527-3997
Visit our web site: http://www.neurosurgery.washington.edu

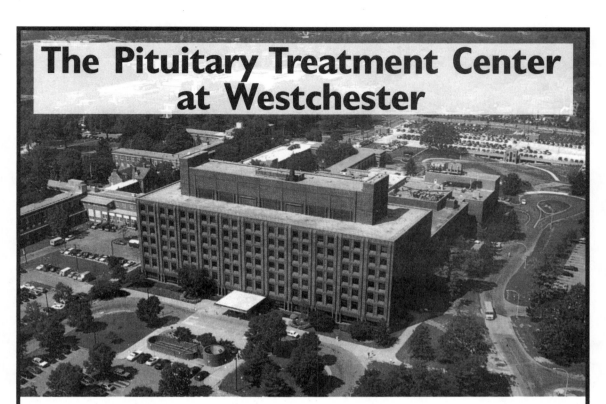
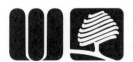
Second Edition

"Alone we can do so little;
together we can do
so much."

Helen Keller

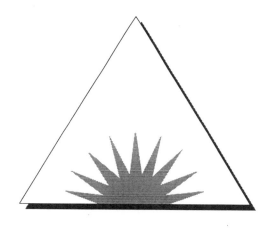

Section X

Index of
Listings

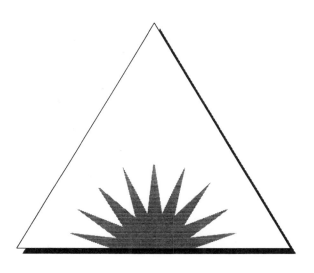

Second Edition

Endocrinologists Alphabetically

Endocrinologists Alphabetically

Index of Listings

Endocrinologists Alphabetically

Endocrinologists by State

Index of Listings

Endocrinologists by State

Endocrinologists by State

Endocrinologists by State

Second Edition

Neurosurgeons Alphabetically

Index of Listings

259

Pituitary Tumor Centers, Hospitals & Clinics

Pituitary Tumor Centers, Hospitals & Clinics

Endocrinology Groups by State

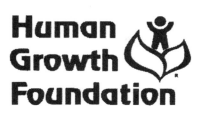

Human Growth Foundation
7777 Leesburg Pike, Suite 202 South
Falls Church, VA 22043

Telephone: **(800) 451-6434** • (703) 883-1773
Fax: (703) 883-1776

Patient Services
Family and Health Professional Education,
Public Awareness
Medical and Psychological Research Grants
30 Local Chapters, Nationwide

Contact:
Kim Frye, Executive Director
e-mail: hgfound@erols.com

The Human Growth Foundation helps individuals with growth related disorders, their families, and health care professionals through education, research, and advocacy.

National Organization for Rare Disorders

The National Organization for Rare Disorders (NORD) is the federation of voluntary health organizations dedicated to helping people with rare (orphan) diseases and assisting the organization that serve then. NORD is committed to the identification, treatment, and cure of rare disorders through programs of education, advocacy, research, and service.

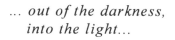

... out of the darkness, into the light...

National Organization for Rare Disorders (NORD)
P.O. Box 8923, New Fairfield, CT 06812-8923 •
(800) 999 NORD • (203) 746-6518

Section XI

Additional Help & Resources

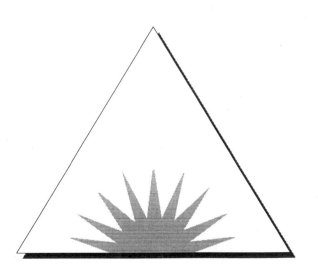

Second Edition

How Do I Find The Best Doctor for Me?

As of now, few criteria exist for evaluation of physicians and their experiences with pituitary issues in general and tumors in particular. The PTNA, with the help of doctors and patients experienced with pituitary diseases and tumors, has compiled this list of simple, straightforward questions.

Ask these questions of your current physician to help confirm your comfort level with him/her. Take a copy of this list when looking for a new doctor to treat you. Decide what answers you will accept and which ones are automatic red flags. If at all possible, bring your spouse or friend to keep notes and help you stay focused on the medical interview(s). Remember, you are in charge of your own care. You have the final vote. Take care of yourself first.

The following two questions should be answered before you visit the doctor. The information is available from you state's Medical Association.

1. Is the doctor board certified in his/her field of specialty?
2. Where did he/she receive training?

For the Endocrinologist:

Do you have many patients with my type of problem? How Many?
Since there are many types or varieties of pituitary tumors, no specific answer can be expected. If the physician has seen many patients with this problem then that is a positive sign. However, it gives no insight into the quality of their experience.

Do you specialize in pituitary tumors and disease?
There are many areas of endocrinology. You want a pituitary specialist.

Do you have a neurosurgical colleague that you routinely refer patients to?
It is generally encouraged that an endocrinologist would develop a relationship with one or several neurosurgeons that would be able to discuss the evaluation, decision making and post operative treatment.

Do your neurosurgical colleagues routinely refer pituitary patients to you for pre- and post-operative management?
It is highly desirable that a neurosurgeon work with an endocrinologist before and after surgery to assure the intervention decision is correct, that the patient is well prepared for surgery, and that the patient has post-operative endocrine assessment which helps ensure proper post-operative treatment. In general, it is recommended that endocrinologists handle the long term follow-up of a patient with pituitary disease.

How do you usually treat patients with my problem?
Does the doctor treat with medication first before resorting to surgery or radiation, or does he/she use combined approaches?

How will my hormone levels influence your decision on treatment of my pituitary tumor?
No patient with a pituitary adenoma should go to surgery without a pituitary hormone level baseline test being done and a decision made as to whether medical or surgical treatment would be most appropriate. Decision would be based upon the individual circumstances. In general, however, there is an increasing trend to treat these tumors with drugs to shrink the tumor mass. In many instances this is used as primary treatment, with surgery only after drug therapy fails to bring about the desired tumor shrinkage.

Second Edition

For the Neurosurgeon:

Do you specialize in pituitary surgery?
How many pituitary surgeries do you perform every week/month/year?
There is reason to believe that 2 - 5 operations per month are the minimum for a neurosurgeon to perform to maintain a high degree of surgical competency.

Do you always treat patients with prolactin secreting macroadenomas with surgery?
No patient with a pituitary adenoma should go to surgery without a pituitary hormone level baseline test being done and a decision made as to whether medical or surgical treatment would be most appropriate. Decisions would be based upon the individual circumstances. In general, however, there is an increasing trend to treat these tumors with drugs to shrink the tumor mass. In many instances this is used as primary treatment, with surgery only after drug therapy fails to bring about the desired tumor shrinkage.

To whom do you refer patients for pre and post-operative management?
It is highly desirable that a neurosugeon work with an endocrinologist especially before and after surgery to assure that the intervention decision is correct, that the patients is well prepared for surgery, and that the patient has post-operative endocrine assessment which helps ensure proper post-operative treatment.

On an annual basis, what are the outcomes of your surgeries?
Morbidity? (Complications)
Outcome? (Chemical cure/total resection, remission, etc.)

Questions for any Physician, Endocrinologist or Neurosurgeon:

What written information do you provide to patients with my problem?

Where do you refer them for additional information?

Are there new approaches to treatment of my pituitary problem? How did you hear about them?
Is the doctor keeping up on things? There may or may not be new approaches, but the response can give you a comfort level that the doctor is keeping up. Ideally, his/her information would come from literature or medical meetings, not from a pharmaceutical company representative alone.

May I speak to some of your other patients with similar problems?
He/she should have patients willing to talk about their experiences and results.

What is the best scan to see a pituitary tumor?
It is generally acknowledged that an MRI is much more effective in assessing a pituitary mass lesion than a CT scan. A physician that is not aware of that would not be experienced in dealing with pituitary tumors.

Where and under what circumstances do you refer patients for radiology?

Psychological counseling?

Other specialists?

PTNA believes that patient care must include interdisciplinary management of the patient's problems.

ALZA PHARMACEUTICALS,
MAKERS OF INNOVATIVE TRANSDERMAL
DRUG DELIVERY SYSTEMS, IS COMMITTED TO
THE CARE OF THE PITUITARY PATIENT

FOR MORE INFORMATION CALL
1 - 8 0 0 - 6 3 4 - 8 9 7 7

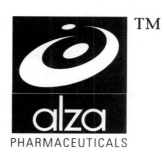

A division of ALZA Corporation

Alza

Government & Patient Organizations

Acoustic Neuroma Association
P.O. Box 12402
Atlanta, GA 30355
Phone: (404) 237-8023
Fax: (404)237-2704

American Brain Tumor Association
2720 River Road, Ste. 146
Des Plaines, IL 60018
Phone: (847) 827-9910
Fax: (847) 827-9910
Toll Free: (800) 886-2282

Australian Pituitary Foundation
P.O. Box 126
Yagoona 2199
NSW Australia
Phone: (612) 630-7209
Fax: (612) 790-4055

The Brain Tumor Society
84 Seattle Street
Boston, MA 02134
Phone (800) 770-8287
Fax: (617) 783-9712

Brain Tumor Foundation of Canada
111 Waterloo Street, Suite 600
London, Ontario N6B 2M4, Canada
Phone: (519) 642-7755
Fax: (519) 642-7192

Children's Brain Tumor Foundation
274 Madison Ave. Suite 1301
New York, NY 10016
Phone: (212) 448-9494
Fax: (212) 448-1022

Diabetes Insipidus Foundation
4533 Ridge Drive
Baltimore, MD 21229
Phone: (410) 247-3953

**Diabetes Insipidus and
Related Disorders**
235 North Hibiscus Drive
Miami Beach, FL 33139
Phone: (305) 538-3904
Fax: (305) 532-7399

Human Growth Foundation
7777 Leesburg Pike, Suite 202 South
Falls Church, VA 22043
Phone: (703) 883-1773
Toll free: (800) 451-6434
Fax: (703) 883-1776

**The Magic Foundation for
Children's Growth**
1327 N. Harlem Ave.
Oak Park, IL 60302
Phone: (708) 383-0808
Fax: (708) 383-0899
Toll free: (800): 3 MAGIC 3
www.magicfoundation.org

National Graves Disease Foundation
2 Tsitsi Court
Brevard, NC 28712
Phone: (704) 877-5251

National Brain Tumor Foundation
785 Market Street, Suite 1600
San Francisco, CA 94103
Phone: (800) 934-CURE
Fax: (405) 284-0209
E-mail: nbtf@braintumor.org
Web site: www.braintumor.org

National Health Directory
Aspen Publishers, Inc.
200 Orchard Ridge Drive
Gaithersburg, MD 20808
Phone: (800) 638-8437
*A comprehensive listing of organizations
relating to health services.*

National Health Information Center
P.O. Box 1133
Washington D.C. 20013-1133
Phone: (800) 336-4797
*Referral services for national organizations
relating to health issues.*

National Institutes of Health
Clinical Center
National Institute of Child Health and
Human Development (NICHD) and
National Institute of Diabetes and
Digestive and Kidney Disease (NIDDK)
Patient Referral Center
Phone: (800) 411-1222
http://www.cc.nih.gov/nihstudies/

**National Organization for
Rare Disorders (NORD)**
P.O. Box 8923, New Fairfield, CT
06812-8923
Toll free: (800) 999-NORD
(203) 746-6518

**The Paget Foundation for
Paget's Disease of Bone and
Related Disorders**
120 Wall Street, Suite 1602
New York, NY 10005
Phone: (212) 509-5335
Fax: (212) 509-8492
e-mail; pagetfdn@aol.com

The Pituitary Foundation
17/18 The Courtyard, Woodlands
Almondsbury, Bristol
BS12 4NQ, U.K.
Phone: 44 (454) 616046
Fax: 44 (454) 616071

Pituitary Tumor Network Association
16350 Ventura Blvd., Suite 231
Encino, CA 91436
Phone: (805) 499-2262
Fax: (805) 499-1523
e-mail: ptna@pituitary.com

**Turner's Syndrome Society
of the United States**
1313 5th St. S.E. - Suite 327
Minneapolis, MN 55414
Phone: (612)379-3607
www.turner-syndrome-us.org

United Way
There is no national hotline number. Please
check your local telephone directory for
nearest chapter.

Government & Patient Organizations

269

NIDDK Directory of Organizations for Endocrine and Metabolic Diseases

The following are nonprofit service/support, education, and advocacy groups. Inquiries from the public are welcome.

American Porphyria Foundation

P.O. Box 22712
Houston, TX 77227
(713) 266-9617
Desiree Lyon, Executive Director

Purpose: Provides financial support for researchers in porphyria; improves the diagnosis and treatment of porphyria through educational programs; serves as a network for porphyria patients. Also sponsors support groups, political action, seminars and fund-raising projects.

Publications: General brochure; Diet and Nutrition in Porphyria; Porphyria Cutanea Tarda; (AIP) Acute Intermittent Porphyria; (EEP) Erytbropoietic Protoporphyria; The Prophyrias--An Overview; 1-lematin; and Newsletter. These brochures are all available with membership. Bulk orders are available upon request.

✉

American Thyroid Association

Montefiore Medical Center
111 East 210th Street
Room 311
Bronx, NY 10467
(718) 882-6047
Diane Miller, Administrator

Purpose: A professional organization of physicians and scientists dedicated to scientific research on the thyroid. The association refers the public to member physicians in their geographic area on request.

Publications: Newsletter (quarterly); information pamphlets.

✉

Association for Glycogen Storage Disease

P.O. Box 896
Durant, IA 52747
(319) 785-6038

Purpose: Acts as a forum for the discussion of glycogen storage disease (GSD), its treatment, and the problems faced by parents raising children with GSD. Disseminates medical information; fosters communication between the families of GSD patients and health care professionals. Helps obtain equipment necessary for home care of GSD patients.

Disorder: GSD is a hereditary condition characterized by a lack of or deficiency in any of the enzymes used by the body to break down glycogen. Glycogen storage diseases include: von Gierke's disease, Pompe's disease, McArdle's disease, Forbes' disease, and Andersen's disease.

Publications: The Ray (periodic newsletter); Parent Handbook and other brochures.

Association for Neuro-Metabolic Disorders
5223 Brookfield Lane
Sylvania, OH 43560
(419) 885-1497
Cheryl Volk, Parent Representative

Purpose: A member organization of families with children who have metabolic disorders that affect the brain. The organization provides support through personal awareness, family understanding and participation, and professional health care intervention.

Disorder: Neuro-metabolic disorders include many different, often inherited, diseases such as maple syrup urine disease, galactosemia, and biotinidase deficiency. These diseases affect body chemistry, but the organ damaged is the brain.

Publications: Newsletter (3 times a year).

Cushing's Support and Research Foundation, Inc.
65 East India Row 22B
Boston, MA 02110
(617) 723-3824 or (617) 723-3674
Louise L. Pace, Founder and President

Purpose: Provides information and support for patients along with expert medical advice from physicians. Facilitates correspondence between members and maintains a referral listing of hospitals, endocrinologists and surgeons.

Cystic Fibrosis Foundation
6931 Arlington Road
Bethesda, MD 20814
(301) 951-4422 or 1-800-FIGHT CF
Robert Beall, President

Purpose: Supports medical research, professional education, and a nationwide network of care centers to benefit patients with cystic fibrosis (CE). Supports services for young adults with CF.

Publications: Information brochures.

H.E.L.P., The Institute for Body Chemistry
P.O. Box 1338
Bryn Mawr, PA 19010
(610) 525-1225
Edward A. Krimmel and Patricia T. Krimmel Co-directors

Purpose: Promotes medical/scientific research concerning the relationship between food chemistry and body chemistry specifically related to hypoglycemia. Disseminates information on body chemistry.

Hemochromatosis Research Foundation

P.O. Box 8569
Albany, NY 12208
(518) 489-0972
Margaret A. Krikker, M.D., President

Purpose: Seeks to increase public and professional awareness of hereditary hemochromatosis (HI-I) and the hazards of supplemental iron. Encourages routine use of screening tests by physicians. Assists public, patients, families, and physicians with Hill diagnosis, treatment, and genetic counseling and in forming regional support networks. Provides telephone referral service to patients requesting names of physicians and research centers concerned with HI-I.

Disorder: Hereditary hemochromatosis is a disorder of iron metabolism in which dietary iron absorption exceeds body needs. If not diagnosed and treated, the accumulating iron may result in one or more complications such as liver enlargement, heart irregularities and failure, diabetes and other hormonal deficiencies, and arthritis.

Publications: Hemochromatosis Awareness (quarterly newsletter); information booklets and videotapes.

Human Growth Foundation

7777 Leesburg Pike
Suite 202 South
Falls Church, VA 22043
(703) 883-1773 or 1-800-451-6434
Kimberly Frye, Executive Director

Purpose: A member organization of families of children with physical growth problems and interested persons united to help medical science better understand the process of growth. Distributes funds for basic and clinical growth research.

Publications: Fourth Friday (monthly newsletter); Growth Series (brochures).

Hypoglycemia Support Foundation, Inc.

3822 NW 122nd Terrace
Sunrise, FL 33323
(954) 742-3098
Roberta Ruggiero, President

Purpose: Seeks to inform, support, and encourage people with hypoglycemia about diet and hypoglycemia.

Publications: The Hypoglycemia Support Foundation Newsletter (quarterly); The Do's & Don'ts of Low Blood Sugar (book).

NIDDK Directory of Organizations

Iron Overload Diseases Association, Inc.
433 Westwind Drive
N. Palm Beach, FL 33408-5 123
(561) 840-8512
Roberta Crawford, President

Purpose: Serves and counsels hemochromatosis patients and families and offers doctor referral, as well as patient advocacy with insurance, Medicare, blood banks, and the FDA; encourages research and public information; emphasizes early diagnosis and encourages research.

Publications: Ironic Blood: Information on hon Overload (bimonthly newsletter); Overload: An Ironic Disease (booklet); Iron Overload Alert (information brochure).

March of Dimes
1275 Mamaroneck Avenue
White Plains, NY 10605
(914) 428-7100
Jennifer Howe, Ph.D., President

Purpose: Promotes education and research on genetic and environmental causes of birth defects.

Publications: Information pamphlets.

Metabolic Information Network
P.O. Box 670847
Dallas, TX 75367-0847
(214) 696-2188 or 1-800-945-2188
Susan G. Mize, Project Director

Purpose: Provides a system for sharing reported data on inborn errors of metabolism that may be useful to professionals caring for patients, to research investigators, and to patients seeking access to treatment.

Disorders: The 10 groups of disorders in MIN's working database of inborn errors of metabolism are: biotin defects, galactosemias, glycogen storage diseases, hereditary tyrosine disorders, homocystinurias, hyperphenyla- laninemias, maple syrup urine diseases, mucopolysaccharidoses, organic acidurias, and urea cycle disorders.

National Adrenal Diseases Foundation
505 Northern Boulevard, Suite 200
Great Neck, NY 11021
(516) 487-4992
Joyce Mullen, Executive Director

Purpose: Provides a national self-help network for educational and emotional support for patients and their families.

Publications: NADE Newsletter (periodic); educational materials.

National Center for the Study of Wilson's Disease
432 West 58th Street
Suite 614
New York, NY 10091
(212) 523-8717
I.Herbert Scheinberg, M.D., President

Purpose: Encourages and supports research concerning hereditary diseases of copper metabolism (Wilson's disease and Menkes' disease). Seeks to increase doctors' awareness of these diseases; and sponsors a diagnostic and treatment center for Wilson's disease.

Disorder: Wilson's disease is a genetic disorder in which excessive amounts of copper collect in the liver, brain, and kidneys. Menkes' disease is the reverse of Wilson's disease and is characterized by a defect in intestinal absorption of copper that leads to copper deficiency.

Publications: Information brochures.

National Graves' Disease Foundation
2 Tsitsi Court
Brevard, NC 28712
(704) 877-5251
Nancy Patterson, Ph.D., Executive Director

Purpose: Provides medical information, referral, and resource information to patients; aids in the development of support groups; provides professional education through lectures and forums; and sponsors, develops, participates in, and supports research on Graves' disease.

Publications: Newsletter (quarterly); information brochures.

National MPS Society, Inc.
17 Kraemer Street
Hicksville, NY 11801
(516) 931-6338
Marie Capobianco, President

Purpose: Acts as a support group for families of children with MIPS (mucopolysaccharidoses) and ML (mucolipidoses); increases professional and public awareness; facilitates diagnosis and treatment through referrals to doctors and hospitals; and raises funds to further research on MIPS and ML.

Disorders: MIPS and ML are rare hereditary disorders caused by the body's inability to produce certain enzymes, resulting in an abnormal deposit of complex sugars in tissues and cells. This causes progressive damage that can range in severity from bone and joint involvement to massive complications in all organ systems.

Publications: Courage (quarterly newsletter); information booklets.

National Organization for Rare Disorders
P.O. Box 8923
New Fairfield, CT 068 12-8923
(203) 746-6518
Abbey S. Meyers, Executive Director

Purpose: Acts as a clearinghouse for information about orphan diseases and as a network for families with similar disorders; encourages and promotes increased scientific research on the cause, control and ultimate cure of rare disorders, including inherited metabolic diseases; accumulates and disseminates information about orphan drugs and devices; and educates the general public and medical profession about the existence, diagnosis, and treatment of rare disorders.

Publications: Orphan Disease Update (quarterly newsletter).

National Osteoporosis Foundation
1150 17th Street, N.W.
Suite 500
Washington, DC 20036
(202) 223-2226
Sandra C. Raymond, Executive Director

Purpose: Increases public awareness and knowledge about osteoporosis; provides information to patients and their families; educates physicians and allied health professionals; and supports basic biomedical, epidemiological, clinical, behavioral, and social research and research training.

Publications: Osteoporosis Report (quarterly newsletter); Osteoporosis: A Woman's Guide, and Boning Up on Osteoporosis: A Guide to Prevention and Treatment; information brochures and other educational materials.

Organic Acidemia Association, Inc.
2287 Cypress Avenue
San Pablo, CA 94806
(510) 724-0297
Carol Barton, President

Purpose: Fosters communication among parents and professionals; acts as a support group. Members include dietitians, researchers, and geneticists; clinics; parents and relatives of children with organic acidemia disorders.

Disorder: Organic acidemia is the collective name for a class of genetic metabolic disorders that lead to enzyme deficiencies and require protein-restricted diets. Organic acidemia disorders include: propionic acidemia, arginino succinic aciduria, isovaleric acidemia, and methylmalonic aciduna.

Publications: Organic Acidemia Association Newsletter (quarterly).

The Oxalosis and Hyperoxaluria Foundation
P.O. Box 1632
Kent, WA 98035
(508) 461-0614
Ann Dayton, Director

Purpose: Informs patients, their families, physicians, and medical professionals about hyperoxaluria and related conditions, oxalosis and calcium oxalate kidney stones. Provides support network to patients and supports and encourages research efforts to find the cure for hyperoxaluria.

Disorder: Primary hyperoxaluria is an inherited disorder characterized by a missing enzyme from the liver that causes calcium oxalate crystals to form, which leads to kidney failure.

Publications: In Touch (quarterly newsletter); Understanding Oxalosis and Hyperoxaluria and information on low oxalate diet.

The Paget Foundation for Paget's Disease of Bone and Related Disorders
200 Varick Street, Suite 1004
New York, NY 10014-4810
(212) 229-1582 or 1-800-23-PAGET
Charlene Waldman, Executive Director

Purpose: Serves patients with Paget's disease of bone, primary hyperparathyroidism, and other related disorders; and assists the medical conimunity that treats these patients.

Publications: Newsletter (quarterly); Primary Hyperparathyroidism (patient education-brochure).

Pituitary Tumor Network Association
16350 Ventura Boulevard
Suite 231
Encino, CA 91436
Tel: (805) 499-2262 Fax: (805) 499-1523
Robert Knutzen, Chairman, CEO

Purpose: Promotes early diagnosis; encourages research and pursues the cure of diseases caused by pituitary tumors; serves patients with diseases caused by pituitary tumors; and provides a telephone network of people with pituitary tumors in all age groups.

Publications: Network (bi monthly newsletter); information pamphlets. The Pituitary Patient Resource Guide; for pituitary patients, their families, physicians and all health care providers.

The Thyroid Foundation of America, Inc.
Room 350, Ruth Sleeper Hall
40 Parkman Street
Boston, MA 02114-2698
(617) 726-8500 or 1-800-832-8321
Ilia Stacy, Executive Director

Pituitary Patient Resource Guide

Purpose: Provides public education programs, patient information, and support. Refers patients to qualified endocrinologists. Please send a business sized self-addressed stamped envelope.

Publications: The Bridge (quarterly newsletter); information brochures.

✉

Thyroid Society for Education and Research
7515 South Main Street, Suite 545
Houston, TX 77030
(713) 799-9909 or 1-800-THYROID
Kathy Kobos, Executive Director

Purpose: Pursues the prevention, treatment, and cure of thyroid disease. Participates in and raises funds for patient and community education programs, professional education, and scientific research.

Publications: Patient education brochures.

✉

United Leukodystrophy Foundation
2304 Highland Drive
Sycamore, IL 60178
(815) 895-3211
Paula Braazeal, President

Purpose: Acts as a support group for parents and families of patients with various forms of inherited leukodystrophy.

Disorder: The leukodystrophies are a group of genetically determined neurologic disorders in which progressive degeneration occurs, primarily affecting white matter. The leukodystrophies include: Krabbe's leukodystrophy (globoid cell leukodystrophy or GLD), metachromatic leukodystrophy (MILD), adrenoleukodystrophy, Pelizaeus-Merzbacher disease, spongy degeneration of the brain, and Alexander's disease.

✉

Wilson's Disease Association
4 Navaho Drive
Brookfield, CT 06804
800-399-0266
H. Ascher Sellner, President

Purpose: Promotes and sponsors research concerning the cause, treatment, and cure of Wilson's and Menkes' diseases; stresses the importance of public awareness, early diagnosis, and treatment; provides financial aid and moral support to needy individuals and organizations sharing the association's goals; collects and disseminates information to members and the public concerning developments, current research, and legislation; and acts as a clearinghouse.

Publications: The Wilson's Disease Association publishes brochures on Wilson's disease. Serial publication: Wilson's Disease Association Newsletter, quarterly--tips for patients and reports about current research and legislation.

Internet Resources for Pituitary Tumor Patients

- Pituitary Tumor Network Association
  www.pituitary.com
- National Institute of Diabetes and Digestive and Kidney Diseases (NIDDK)
  www.niddk.nih.gov
- NIDDK's Directory of Organizations for Endocrine and Metabolic Diseases
  www.nih.gov/EndoOrg/endoorg.htm
- National Center for Research Resources (NCRR)
  www.ncrr.nih.gov/
- National Human Genome Research Institute (NHGRI)
  www.nhgri.nih.gov/
- National Institute of Child Health and Human Development (NICHD)
  www.nih.gov/nichd/
- National Cancer Institute (NCI)
  www.nci.nih.gov/
- NCI's Rare Diseases Database
  www.rarediseases. info.nih.gov/
- National Institute of Neurological Disorders and Stroke (NINDS)
  www.ninds.nih.gov/
- National Library of Medicine (NLM)
  www.nlm.nih.gov/
- NLM's Internet Grateful Med (Medline)
  www.igm.nlm.nih.gov/
- NLM's PubMed
  www.ncbi.nlrn.gov/BubMecl/
- NIH's Clinical Center (CC)
  www.cc.nih.gov/
- NIH's Computer Retrieval of Information on Scientific Projects
  www.nih.gov/grants/award/crisp.htm
- Cushing's Support and Research Foundation, Inc.
  www.world.std.comUCSRF/
- Alliance of Genetic Support Groups
  medhelp.org/www/agsg.htm
- National Adrenal Diseases Foundation
  medhelp.org/www/nadf.htm
- Endocrine Society
  www.endo-society.org/index.htm
- American Association of Clinical Endocrinologists
  www.aace.com
- National Organization for Rare Disorders
  www.pbs.org/pov/more/nord.html
- American Society of Human Genetics
  www.faseb.org/genetics
- The Thyroid Foundation of America, Inc.
  www.clark.net/pub/tfa/brochures.html

Second Edition

Pharmaceutical Reimbursement Hotlines

Alza Corp:
- Testoderm   **800-634-8977**

Eli Lilly & Company:
- Humatrope   **800-847-6988**

Genentech:
- Nutropin & Protropin   **800-879-4747**

Novartis:
- Sandostatin   **800-772-7556**
- Parlodel   **888-669-6682**

Pharmacia & Upjohn:
- Genotropin   **800-645-1280**
- Dostinex

Serono:
- Saizen   **800-582-7989**

SmithKline Beecham:
- Androderm   **888-454-2401**

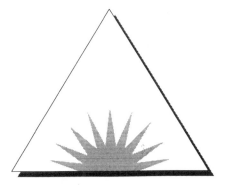

Second Edition

SmithKline Beecham

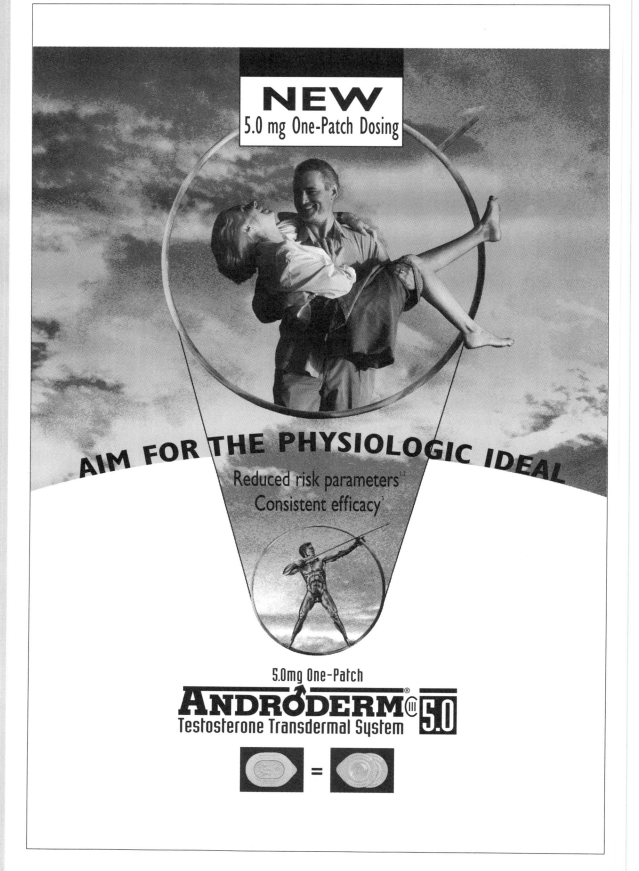

NEW
5.0 mg One-Patch Dosing

AIM FOR THE PHYSIOLOGIC IDEAL

Reduced risk parameters[1,2]
Consistent efficacy[3]

5.0mg One-Patch
ANDRODERM®[III] 5.0
Testosterone Transdermal System

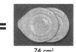
References:
1. Arver S, Meikle AW, Dobs AS, et al. Hypogonadal men treated with the Androderm® Testosterone Transdermal System had fewer abnormal hematocrit elevations than those treated with testosterone enanthate injections. In: *Program and Abstracts of the 79th Annual Meeting of The Endocrine Society;* June 1997; Minneapolis, Minn. Abstract P1-327. **2.** Meikle AW, Arver S, Dobs AS, et al. Prostate size in hypogonadal men treated with a nonscrotal permeation-enhanced testosterone transdermal system. *Urology.* 1997;49:191-196. **3.** Data on file, SmithKline Beecham Pharmaceuticals. **4.** Wilson DE, Kaidbey K, Boike SC, et al. Use of topical corticosteroid cream in the pretreatment of skin reactions associated with Androderm® Testosterone Transdermal System. In: *Program and Abstracts of the 79th Annual Meeting of The Endocrine Society;* June 1997; Minneapolis, Minn. Abstract P1-323.

Why Join the PTNA?

We'd like to share something called *Lessons from the Geese.* It seems that in a study of geese, there are some characteristics they can teach us in our own relationships...

Fact 1: As each goose flaps its wings, it creates an uplift for the birds that follow. By flying in a "V" formation, the whole flock adds 71% greater flying range than if each bird flew alone.

Lesson: People who share a common direction and sense of community can get where they are going quicker and easier because they are traveling on the thrust of one another.

Fact 2: When a goose falls out of formation, it suddenly feels the drag and resistance of flying alone. It quickly moves back into formation to take advantage of the lifting power of the bird immediately in front of it.

Lesson: If we have as much sense as a goose, we stay in formation with those headed where we want to go. We are willing to accept their help and give our help to others.

Fact 3: When the lead goose tires, it rotates back into the formation to take advantage of the lifting power of the bird immediately in front of it.

Lesson: It pays to take turns doing the hard tasks and sharing leadership. As with geese, people are interdependent on each others skills, capabilities and unique arrangements of gifts, talents, or resources.

Fact 4: The geese flying in formation honk to encourage those up front to keep up their speed.

Lesson: We need to make sure our honking is encouraging. In groups where there is encouragement, the production is much greater. The power of encouragement (to stand by ones heart or core values, encourage the heart and core of others) is the quality of honking we seek.

Fact 5: When one goose gets sick, wounded or shot down, two geese drop out of formation and follow it down to help and protect it. They stay with it until it dies or is able to fly again. Then, they launch out with another formation or catch up with the flock.

Lesson: If we have as much sense as geese, we will stand by each other in difficult times as well as when we are strong.

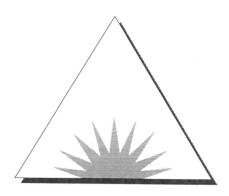

About the PTNA

The Pituitary Tumor Network Association (PTNA) is an international non-profit organization for patients with pituitary tumors and disorders, their families, loved ones, and the physicians and health care providers who treat them.

PTNA was founded in 1992 by a group of acromegalic patients in order to communicate and share their experiences and concerns. PTNA has rapidly grown to become the world's largest and fastest growing patient volunteer organization devoted to the treatment and cure of pituitary disorders.

PTNA is supported by an international network of the world's finest physicians and surgeons. Our goal is to reach every patient who may be forgotten, abandoned, or worse yet, undiagnosed after many years of suffering. We are doing this in three ways: (1) By providing public awareness programs and educational seminars, (2) By assisting the medical community in developing uniform standards for early diagnosis, surgery, radiation, pharmacological treatment and follow-up, and (3) by having an interactive website and referral program at *www.pituitary.com*.

How the PTNA Helps

♦   In the brief time since its inception, PTNA has served more than 46,000 pituitary tumor patients, and lectured to more than 3,500 doctors, nurses, and other professionals on three continents.

♦   PTNA distributes timely and pertinent information regarding new testing procedures, medications, and treatment to thousands of members and interested individuals, via its Newsletter. *Network*, keeps you up to date on what's happening in regard to pituitary issues. The latest breakthroughs in treatment, medications, and other information too recent to be included in the latest edition of the Pituitary Patient Resource Guide will all be brought to you here. Updates on conferences and happenings around the corner and around the world. Articles on pituitary issues by some of the world's leading physicians and specialists in their fields.

♦   PTNA's web site at *www.pituitary.com* is the most authoritative pituitary web site for patients on the Internet. Listings of physicians and medical centers, as well as articles and a wealth of other information make this an invaluable source of information.

♦   The PTNA, and the subject of acromegaly, were featured in a half-hour segment on Lifetime Television's *Physician's Journal Update*. A one hour video titled The Experts Discuss Pituitary Tumors was released in 1997.

♦   Three patient/physician educational conferences were launched in 1995, and the first International Pituitary Awareness Planning Conference was held in December, 1996.

♦   In 1998 the PTNA plans to publish the first European edition of the Pituitary Patient Resource Guide, to be followed by Asian Pacific, and Cental/South American editions.

How You Can Help

The PTNA is funded solely by membership contributions, corporate sponsorship, private donations and volunteer support. We are a legal, non-profit 501(c)(3) organization exempt from income tax. Your gift is tax deductible to you and will help make our ongoing work possible.

With your contribution, you will receive our newsletter *Network*, access to our web sites, discounts on our books and videos, notices about upcoming conventions, new and existing medications, new support group meetings, and other pertinent information.

It is our desire to make contributing to the PTNA as easy as possible for you. Listed below are some of the ways in which you can help the PTNA. Simply complete the applicable section(s) on the membership form as indicated.

- Direct donations may be made to the PTNA by filling out the included membership form.

- Many companies offer easy weekly, bi-monthly, or monthly payroll deductions to donate through an agency such as the United Way.

- To sign up for this simple process, contact your company's human resources department to obtain the necessary paperwork, fill out the attached membership form and complete Sections A & B.

- Ask your company if they have a Matching Fund Program. With this program, whatever amount you donate to the PTNA, your company matches your donation. This is a wonderful way to double your gift to the PTNA!

- You can direct your donation to the PTNA through the United Way or other agency on a donor card. Contact the agency directly for the appropriate paperwork, and fill out the included membership form.

- A Memorial Gift to the PTNA is a lasting tribute to a loved one. A message advising of your gift (without reference to the amount) will be sent to those you indicate.

In addition to monetary gifts, we welcome any other type of support you may be willing to give. Your time is an invaluable gift to our organization. If you would like to volunteer your services to our organization, please call us at (805) 499-2262, e-mail us at ptna@pituitary.com, or let us know through our Web Site at www.pituitary.com. We greatly appreciate any help you can give.

Check us out online!
www.pituitary.com

Second Edition

Section XII

Glossary

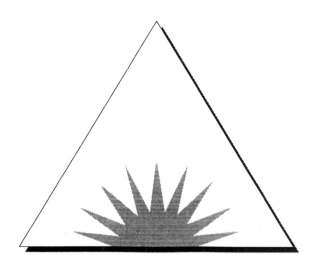

Second Edition

Glossary

A

accessible
(ak ses' sah bul) Refers to tumors that can be approached by a surgical procedure; tumors that are not deep in the brain or beneath vital structures. Inaccessible tumors cannot be approached by standard surgical techniques.

acromegaly
(ak row meg' ah lee) A disease caused by the overproduction of growth hormone by the pituitary gland. It is relatively rare and affects both men and women. In almost all cases, acromegaly is not inherited and cannot be passed on to children.

acuity
(ah ku' ib tee) Refers to clarity or distinctness of hearing or sight.

adjuvant
(ad' ju vant) A therapy used in addition to or accompanying another treatment.

adrenal glands
A pair of endocrine glands which produce small quantities of sex hormone.

alopecia
(al 0 pee' she ah) Loss of hair; baldness in areas where hair is usually present. A common side effect of radiation therapy to the brain and some chemical therapies.

amenorrhoea
The failure of a woman to menstruate.

analgesic
(an al gee' zik) A medicine used to reduce pain.

anaplasia
(an ah play' zee ah) Characteristics of a cell that make it identifiable as a cancer cell. Malignant.

angiogenesis
(an' gee o jen' ih sis) The growth of new blood vessels from surrounding tissue into growing tissue.

angiogram
(an' gee 0 gram) A diagnostic procedure done in the x-ray department to visualize blood vessels following introduction

anorexia
(an 0 rek' see ah) Loss of appetite.

anosmia
(an oz' me ah) Absence of the sense of smell. Symptom common to tumors of the frontal lobe of the cerebral hemispheres.

articulation
(ar tik U lay' shun) Speech.

artifact
(ar' tih fakt) Something artificial, a distortion that does not reflect normal anatomy or pathology, not usually found in the body. For example, in radiology, the appearance on an x-ray of a surgical metal clip that obscures the clear view of an anatomical structure.

autologous
(aw tol' 0 gus) Coming from the same individual, as opposed to being donated by another individual.

autosomes(adj. autosomal)
Those chromosomes which are not the sex chromosomes.

autosomal Kallmann's syndrome
A form of inherited Kallmann's syndrome which affects both men and women, because the sex chromosomes are unaffected.

B
benign
(be nine') Not malignant, not cancerous.

biological response modifier
(bi 0 loj' ih cul   re sponse'   mod' ih fi ur) A substance used in adjuvant therapy that takes advantage of the body's own natural defense mechanisms to inhibit the growth of a tumor.

biopsy
(bi' op see) Examination of a small amount of tissue taken from the patient's body to make a diagnosis.

bone density measurement
A procedure (bone scan) used to assess the strength and "age" of a bone by measuring its density.

bromocriptine
(bro mo krip teen) An example of a dopamine agonist.

C
calcification (v. to calcify)
The strengthening and hardening of a bone in areas where calcium has been deposited.

cancer
(kan' sur) Malignant tissue that is invasive, destroys healthy tissue, and tends to spread to distant locations.

carcinoma
(car sih no' mah) A malignant tumor that arises from epithelium found in skin or, more commonly, the lining of body organs, for example, breast, prostate, lung, stomach or bowel. Carcinomas tend to infiltrate into adjacent tissue and spread (metastasize) to distant organs, for example, to bone, liver, lung or the brain.

catheter
(kath' ih tur) A flexible, tubular surgical instrument. Used in body cavities or vessels for the removal or insertion of fluids.

cell
(sel) The basic living unit of body tissue. It contains a nucleus surrounded by cytoplasm and is enclosed by a membrane.

central nervous system (CNS)
(sen' tral   nur' vus   sis' tem) Pertaining to the brain, cranial nerves and spinal cord. It does not include muscles or peripheral nerves.

cerebral
(ser e' brul) Referring to the cerebrum.

cerebrospinal fluid
(ser e bro spi' nal . flu' id) The clear fluid made in the ventricular cavities of the brain that bathes the brain and spinal cord. It circulates through the ventricles and the subarachnoid space.

cerebrum
(ser e' brum) The largest area of the brain, the cerebrum occupies the uppermost part of the skull. It consists of two halves called hemispheres. Each half of the cerebrum is further divided into four lobes: frontal, temporal, parietal and occipital.

chemotherapy

(ke mo ther' ah pee) The use of chemical agents to treat brain tumors.

circumscribed

(sir' come skribd) Having a border, localized. Often associated with a capsule and benign tumors of the brain. for example, meningiomas, pituitary adenomas and acoustic neuromas. See diffuse.

clinical

(klin' ih kul) That which can be observed in patients. Research that uses patients to test new treatments. as opposed to laboratory testing or research in animals.

clinical cooperative group

(klin' ih kul   Co op' ur ah tiv   groop) A group of medical institutions cooperating to perform clinical research.

CNS

See central nervous system.

colonoscope

(kuh lahn oh skope) An instrument which allows visualization of the inside of the colon.

congenital

(con jen' ih tul) Existing before or at birth.

cranial cavity

(kra' nee ul . kav' vih tee) The skull.

craniectomy

(kra nee ek' toe me) Surgery performed on the skull where pieces of bone are removed to gain access to the brain. and the bone pieces are not replaced.

craniotomy

(kra ne ot' o me) Surgery performed on the skull where a portion of bone is removed to gain access to the brain, and the bone is put back in its place.

CSF

See cerebrospinal fluid.

CT or CAT scan

Computerized Axial Tomography.

An x-ray device linked to a computer that produces an image of a predetermined cross-section of the brain. A special dye material may be injected into the patient's vein prior to the scan to help make any abnormal tissue more evident.

cytotoxic

(sigh toe tok' sic) Capable of killing cells.

D

debulk

(dee bulk') A surgical procedure to decrease mass effect by removing a portion of a tumor or dead tissue. See mass effect.

Decadron®

(Dek' ah dron) Dexamethasone. A glucocorticosteroid medication used to reduce brain tissue swelling.

decompressive

(dee kom pres' sive) Refers to a surgical procedure during which bone, tissue, or tumor is removed to lessen intracranial pressure.

dedifferentiate

(dee dif' fur en she ate) A mature cell returning to a less mature state. See differentiate, undifferentiated.

delivery

(dee liv' ur ee) See drug delivery.

density

(den' sih tee) The amount of darkness or light in an area of a scan reflects the compactness and density of tissue. Differences in tissue density are the basis for CT and MR scans.

diabetes insipidus

(di ah be' tez e in sip' id us) A problem with water balance in the body causing excess urine production and great thirst, due to pituitary-hypothalamic damage. Diabetes mellitus, which has the same symptoms, is due to insufficient insulin production by the pancreas.

differentiate

(dif fur en' she ate) The process cells undergo as they mature into normal cells. Differentiated cells have distinctive characteristics, perform specific functions, and are less likely to divide. See dedifferentiate, undifferentiated.

diffuse

(dif fuse') Lacking a distinct border, not localized, spread out. See circumscribed.

diplopia

(dih plo' pee ah) Double vision.

dopamine agonists

(dope ah meen . ag oh nists) Medications with predominant effects on pituitary cells that harbor receptors for the chemical transmitter dopamine.

drug delivery

(drug de liv' ur ee) The method and route used to provide medication.

duramater

(du' rah . ma' tur) The outermost, toughest, and most fibrous of the three membranes (meninges) that cover the brain and spinal cord.

dysarthria

(dis ar' three ah) Impairment of speech (articulation), caused by damage or disorder of the tongue or speech muscles. Symptom may indicate pressure on the brain stem (medulla oblongata) or elsewhere in the posterior fossa.

dysfunctional

(dis funk' shun al) Working improperly or abnormally.

dysphagia

(dis fay' gee ah) Difficulty in swallowing or inability to swallow. Symptom usually indicates tumors involving the lower brain stem.

E

edema

(eh dee' mah) Swelling due to an excess of water.

emesis

(em' ih sis) Vomiting.

encapsulated

(en kap' sue la ted) Refers to a tumor that is wholly confined to a specific area, surrounded by a capsule. Localized.

endocrine glands

Those parts of the body which produce and secrete (release) hormones.

endocrinologist

A doctor who specialises in diseases of the endocrine glands and their hormones.

endocrinology

The study of the endocrine glands and their hormones.

epidemiology

(ep ih dee me ol' 0 gee) The study of the distribution of disease and its impact upon a population, using such measures as incidence, prevalence, or mortality.

etiology

(e tee ol' 0 gee) The study of the cause of a disease.

F

focal

(foe' kal) Limited to one specific area.

FSH

The Follicle Stimulating Hormone; a gonadotrophin secreted by the pituitary gland, the hormone promotes fertility in men and helps to regulate the menstrual cycle in women.

G

GH

The Growth Hormone, secreted by the pituitary gland; one of the hormones responsible for normal bone development and teenage growth.

GnRH

The Gonadotrophin Releasing Hormone, secreted by the hypothalamus; GnRH stimulates the release of LH and FSH from the pituitary gland.

GnRH pulsatile therapy

A form of treatment which uses a portable, battery-driven pump to replace the missing GnRH by releasing it in pulses at regular intervals, typically every 90 minutes.

generic

(je ner' ik) A drug not protected by a trademark. Also, the scientific name as opposed to the proprietary, brand name.

genesis

(jen' ih sis) The beginning of a process.

genetic engineering

A laboratory technique sometimes used to identify a defective gene in an unborn child which may cause a particular disease.

gland

(gland) An organ of the body that produces materials (hormones) released into the bloodstream, such as the pituitary or pineal gland. Hormones influence metabolism and other body functions.

glucagon test

An alternative to the insulin tolerance test; used to test for normal function of the hypothalamus and pituitary gland; glucagon increases blood sugar levels, causing a number of hormones to be released in response.

glucose

A type of sugar found in the blood; an important source of energy in the body.

glucocorticosteroids

(glu ko kor tih ko stair' oids) Medications used to decrease swelling around tumors. Medication to duplicate the effects of cortisol.

gonadotrophin

A hormone which regulates the function of the gonads; the two main gonadotrophins are LH and FSH, both released from the pituitary gland.

growth factor

(growth   fak' tur) A naturally occurring protein chemical that stimulates cell division and proliferation. It is produced by normal cells during embryonic development, tissue growth, and wound healing. Tumors, however, produce large amounts of growth factors.

gynaecomastia
A usually harmless female-like enlargement of one or both breasts; a characteristic of some hypogonadal males.

H

hCG
The Human Chorionic Gonadotrophin; a hormone which behaves like LH; made by the placenta, hCH may be extracted and used together with hMG to treat hypogonadism.

hMG
The Human Menopausal Gonadotrophin; derived from the urine of post-menopausal women, hMG not only contains LH but also FSH.

hCG/hMG therapy
A type of treatment on offer to hypogonadal patients who wish to become fertile.

hemianopsia
(hem e an op' see ah) Loss of one half of the field of vision (the area that can be seen by each eye when staring straight ahead).

hereditary
(heh red' ih tair e) Transferred via genes from parent to child. Also called genetic.

herniation
(her nee a' shun) Bulging of tissue through an opening in a membrane, muscle or bone.

heterogeneous
(het er 0 gee' nee us) Composed of varied cell types.

homogeneous
(ho mo gee' nee us) Composed of identical cell types.

hormone (adj. hormonal)
A chemical "messenger" which is made and secreted by an endocrine gland and which targets one or more parts of the body, modifying its structure or changing the way it works.

Hormone Replacement Therapy
The name given to a form of treatment in which missing or deficient hormones can be replaced, the body being encouraged to behave normally as if it were making the hormones naturally.

hydrocephalus
(hi dro sef' ah lus) Hydro = water, cephalo = head. Excess water in the brain due to blockage of cerebrospinal fluid flow, increased production. or decreased absorption.

hyperfractionation
(hi per frak shun a' shun) An increased number of smaller dosage treatments of radiation therapy.

hypogonadism (adj. hypogonadal)
The inability of the gonads to function normally.

hypogonadotrophic hypogonadism
The inability of the gonads to function normally because of subnormal levels of the gonadotrophins LH and FSH.

hypophysis
(hi pof' ih sis) Pituitary gland.

hypothalamic-pituitary-gonadal axis
The name given to the "team" of endocrine glands which is responsible for regulating sexual development.

hypothalamus

A thumbnail-sized endocrine gland located in the brain just above the pituitary gland to which it is connected; the hypothalamus normally contains cells which make and release GnRH.

hypotonicity

(hi P0 toe nis' ih tee) Diminished muscle tone; limp muscles.

I

ICP

Intracranial pressure, harmful when increased.

IICP

Increased intracranial pressure.

immunotherapy

(im mu no ther' ah pee) Use of the body's immune system to fight tumors. See biological response modifier.

inaccessible

(in ak ses' sab bul) See accessible.

infiltrating

(in' fil tray ting) Refers to a tumor that penetrates the normal, surrounding tissue.

informed consent

(informed kon sent') The right to have
information explained to you so that you fully understand and agree to the nature of the proposed treatment.

interstitial radiation therapy

(in ter stish' al e ray dee a' shun ~ther' ah pee) The implantation of radioactive seeds directly into a tumor.

intestinal polyps

(in tes' ten al . pah' lips) Small growths in the bowel with the potential for further growth. May transform from a benign to a malignant state.

intracranial

(in trah kra' nee al) Within the skull.

intramuscular

(in trah mus' ku lar) Into a muscle.

intratumoral

(in trah tu mor' al) Into a tumor (usually performed during surgery).

intravenous

(in trah vee' nus) Into a vein.

intraventricular

(in trah ven trik' u lar) Into a ventricle.

invasive

(in vay' siv) Refers to a tumor that invades healthy tissues. The opposite of encapsulated. Also called diffuse or infiltrating.

irradiation

(ih ray dee a' shun) Treatment by ionizing radiation, such as x-rays, or radioactive sources such as radioactive iodine seeds. See radiation therapy.

L

LH

The Luteinizing Hormone; a gonadotrophin secreted by the pituitary gland, the hormone promotes masculinity in men and helps to regulate the menstrual cycle in women in conjunction with FSH.

LHRH
The Luteinizing Hormone Releasing Hormone; another name for GnRH.

laser
(lay' zur) An acronym of light amplification by stimulated emission of radiation. A surgical tool that creates intense heat and power when focused at close range, destroying cells by vaporizing them.

lethargy
(leth' ar gee) Sluggishness, drowsiness, indifference.

local
(lo' kal) In the area of the tumor; confined to one specific area.

lumbar puncture
(lum' bar ~ punk' tur) Spinal tap. Needle penetration into the subarachnoid space of the lumbar spine. Used to withdraw a sample of spinal fluid for examination. Also used to inject a dye into the spine prior to a myelogram.

M

MRI scan
Magnetic Resonance Imaging. MRI is a scanning device that uses a magnetic field, radio waves, and a computer. Signals emitted by normal and diseased tissue during the scan are assembled into a image.

malignant
(mah hg' nant) Cancerous or life-threatening, tending to become progressively worse.

mass effect
(mas . ef fekt') Damage to the brain due to the bulk of a tumor, the blockage of fluid, or excess accumulation of fluid within the skull.

median survival
(me' de an ~ sur vi' val) Median means the middle value. An equal number of people live longer as die earlier than the median.

medroxyprogesterone actetate
A semi-synthetic medication which is close in structure and function to the naturally occuring female sex hormone, progesterone.

membrane
(mem' brain) Thin layer of tissue covering a surface, lining a body cavity, or dividing a space or organ.

monoclonal antibodies (MAB)
(mon 0 klon' al ~ an' te bod eze) A biological response modifier with unique 'homing device" properties. Chemicals or radiation tagged to the MAB may be delivered directly to tumor cells. Or, the MAB itself may be capable of tumor cell destruction.

mutate
(mu tate') Change in the genetic material (DNA) inside the cell.

N

neoplasm
(nee' 0 plazm) A tumor, either benign or malignant.

neuron
(new' ron) Nerve cell; conducts electrical signals.

nervous system
(nur vus ~ sis' tem) The entire integrated system of nerve tissue in the body: the brain, brain

stem, spinal cord, nerves and ganglia.

nucleus
(noo' klee us) The center of the cell containing the genetic information (genes and chromosomes, DNA, etc.). The appearance of the nucleus is used as a criterion to determine the malignant potential of a cell or tissue.

O

olfactory cells
Specialized cells found at the top of the nasal cavity which converts a smell detected by the olfactory hairs into tiny electrical signals.

olfactory bulb
One of two structures connected to the olfactory tracts to which the olfactory cells are anchored.

olfactory tract
One of two structures containing neurons which carry the "smell" from the olfactory cells, where it has been converted into an electical signal, to the area of the brain where the smell can be identified.

osteoporosis (adj. osteoporotic)
A condition characterised by weakened and brittle bones, arising from an hormonal imbalance; also known as brittle bone disease.

P

palliative care
(pal' e ah tiv . kare) Caring for a patient by maintaining the best quality of remaining life. Also offering support and guidance to the patient and family.

palsy
(pawl' zee) Loss of function.

panhypopituitarism
(pan high P0 pih to ih ta rizm) Loss of all pituitary hormones.

papilledema
(pap il eh dee' mah) Swelling of the optic nerve. Indicates increased intracranial pressure on the optic nerve. Also called choked disk.

paralysis
(pah ral' ih sis) Loss of muscle function due to injury or disease of the nervous system.

paresis
(par ree' sis) Weakness.

paresthesia
(par Cs: thee' ze ah) Abnormal sensations, such as burning, prickling.

PET scan
Positron Emission Tomography. A scanning device which uses low-dose radioactive sugar to measure brain activity. this is a limited-use diagnostic tool.

Phenobarbitol®
(Fee no bar' bih tol) A sedating medication used to control seizures.

pituitary gland
(pih to ih terry . glan' d) A small oval endocrine gland attached to the brain. This gland plays a central role in the regulation of secretion from many other hormone-secreting glands of the body.

pituitary stalk
A tiny structure which connects the hypothalamus to the pituitary gland.

primary amenorrhoea

The inability to menstruate, caused by a failure of sexual maturation and function.

primary brain tumor

(pri' mar ee brane tu' mor) Original source of tumor in the brain rather than other areas of the body.

primitive

(prim' ih tiv) Undeveloped or in early stages of development, undifferentiated.

progesterone

A sex hormone which is made in the ovaries and during pregnancy, by the placenta as well; helps to build up the endometrium during the menstrual cycle.

prognosis

(prog no' sis) A forecast as to probable outcome.

protocol

(pro' toe kol) An outline of care; a treatment plan.

Q

quality of life

(kwol' ih tee ov life) Refers to the level of comfort, enjoyment, ability to pursue daily activities. Often used in discussions of treatment options.

R

radiation therapy

(ray dee a' shun . ther' ah pee) The use of radiation energy to interfere with tumor growth. See irradiation.

radioresistant

(ray dee o ree zis' tant) Resistant to ra.diation therapy.

radiosensitive

(ray dee o sen' sih tiv) Responsive to radiation therapy.

radiosurgery

See stereotactic radiosurgery.

recurrence

(ree kur' ens) The return of symptoms or the tumor itself, as opposed to a remission.

rehabilitation

(ree hah bil ih tay' shun) the return of function after illness or injury, often with the assistance of specialized medical professionals.

remission

(ree mish' shun) The disappearance of symptoms; the disappearance of the tumor.

resection

(ree sek' shun) Surgical removal of a tumor.

residual

(ree zid' yu al) Remaining tumor.

respiration

(res pur a' shun) Breathing. To inhale and exhale.

S

seizure

(see' zhur) Convulsions. Epilepsy. Due to temporary disruption in electrical activity of the brain.

spasticity

(spas tis' ih tee) Increased involuntary muscle contraction (the opposite of hypotonicity).

spinal fluid

(spy′ nal **e** flu′ id) See cerebrospinal fluid.

stalk

(stawk) A stem. Usually refers to the pituitary stalk that connects the pituitary gland to the hypothalamus.

stereotactic

(steh ree 0 tak′ tik) Precise postioning in three dimensional space. Refers to surgery or radiation therapy directed by various scanning devices.

stereotactic radiosurgery

(steh ree o tak′ tik ra′ deco sir′juree) A radiation therapy technique that uses a large number of narrow, precisely aimed, highly focused beams of ionizing radiation. The beams are aimed from many directions circling the head, and meet at a specific point.

steroids

(stair′ oids) See glucocorticosteroids.

subcutaneous

(sub cue tay′ nec us) Beneath the skin.

systemic

(sis tem′ ik) Circulating throughout the body.

T

testosterone

The main male sex hormone, its production encouraged by LH from the pituitary gland; small amounts also present in women.

tissue

(tish′ yu) A group of similar cells united to perform a specific function.

transsphenoidal surgery

(trans sfee noy dull . serj′ e re) A surgical procedure through the sphcnoid sinus permitting access to the pituitary gland.

tumor

(tu′ mor) An abnormal growth. Tumors may be benign or malignant by cell type, or life-threatening by their location.

tumor marker

(tu′ mor mar′ kur) Substances found in blood or other fluids that identify the presence of a tumor, and/or the tumor type.

U

ultrasound

(ul′ trah sownd) Visualization of structures in the body by recording the reflections of sound waves directed into tissues. May be used during surgery.

undifferentiated

(un′ dif fur en′ she a ted) An immature, embryonic, or primitive cell. It has a nonspecific appearance with multiple nonspecific activities and functions poorly. See differentiatc, dedifferentiate.

V

vascular

(vas′ cue lur) Relating to blood vessels.

vascularity

(vas ku lair′ ih tee) The blood supply of a tumor.

Section XIII

Tear Outs
&
Order Forms

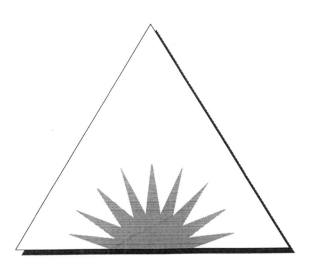

Second Edition

Prescription For Knowledge

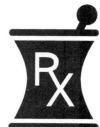

The Truro Group &
The Pituitary Tumor Network Association
A Professional Information Alliance Present

The Experts Discuss Pituitary Tumors

Recommended Dosage: View as needed for increased knowledge.

Warning: Our Educational Materials may be habit forming!

Possible Side Effects: A better understanding of your own medical needs, and heightened ability to work with your doctor in your treatment by taking charge of your life.

Contents: Words of wisdom and experience from:

Sylvia L. Asa, M.D., Ph.D

P. Michael Conn, Ph.D

William T. Couldwell, M.D., Ph.D.

Shereen Ezzat, M.D., F.R.C.P., F.A.C.P.

Delbert A. Fisher, M.D.

Daniel F. Kelly, M.D.

Nelson M. Oyesiku, M.D.

Brooke Swearingen. M.D.

Ronald Swerdloff. M.D.

Christina Wang, M.D.

Ian E. McCutcheon, M.D., F.R.C.S.

Howard R. Krauss, M.D.

$24.95 each

2 videos for $44.95

Quantity Ordered _____

Please include $6.95 for shipping and handling on all orders of $ 75.00 or less. Postage and handling rates are subject to change and may vary on orders shipped out of the United States and on orders totaling more than $75.00. California residents please add 7.25% sales tax.

Mail or fax order to: PTNA
P.O Box 1958
Thousand Oaks, Ca. 91358
Tel: 805-499-2262   Fax: 805-499-1523

Your Name:	
Ship To:	
Address:	
Payment Information:	☐ Visa/MasterCard	☐ Check payable to PTNA
Cardholder:	
Card #:	Exp. Date:
Signature:	

Second Edition

Pituitary Patient Resource Guide

The Women's Assessment Calendar

Name: _____

Age: _____ Month/Year: _____

Symptom Rating Scale:

1-Mild – does not interfere with normal activities.
2-Moderate – interferes with normal activities.
3-Severe – unable to perform normal activities.

Instruction: Find today's date column and fill in your rating for each symptom.
Rate all of the symptoms daily during the month at about the same time of each day.

Calendar Date:	1	2	3	4	5	6	7	8	9	10	11	12	13	14	15
Acne															
Bloatedness															
Breast fullness															
Breast tenderness															
Dry skin															
Fatigue															
Hot flashes															
Joint aches & pain															
Night sweats															
Palpitations															
Vaginal dryness															
Violent															
Waking up tired															
Weight gain															
Weight loss															
Crying															
Depressions															
Hyper-sensitivity															
Irritability															
Mood swings															
Nervousness															
Paranoid															
Poor self-esteem															
Tension															
Avoiding socializing															
Fear losing control															
Feel like another person															
Forgetful															
Inability to concentrate															
Need to escape															
Wish to be alone															
Alcohol consumption															
Craving salty foods															
Craving sweet foods															
Menses ("X" at onset)															

Hormone:	1	2	3	4	5	6	7	8	9	10	11	12	13	14	15
Growth hormone															
Prednisone															
DDAVP															
Estrogen															
Progesterone															
Thyroid															
Testosterone															

Second Edition

The Women's Assessment Calendar

Name: _____

Age: _____ Month/Year: _____

Symptom Rating Scale:
1-Mild – does not interfere with normal activities.
2-Moderate – interferes with normal activities.
3-Severe – unable to perform normal activities.
Instruction: Find today's date column and fill in your rating for each symptom.
Rate all of the symptoms daily during the month at about the same time of each day.

Calendar Date:	16	17	18	19	20	21	22	23	24	25	26	27	28	29	30	31
Acne																
Bloatedness																
Breast fullness																
Breast tenderness																
Dry skin																
Fatigue																
Hot flashes																
Joint aches & pain																
Night sweats																
Palpitations																
Vaginal dryness																
Violent																
Waking up tired																
Weight gain																
Weight loss																
Crying																
Depressions																
Hyper-sensitivity																
Irritability																
Mood swings																
Nervousness																
Paranoid																
Poor self-esteem																
Tension																
Avoiding socializing																
Fear of losing control																
Feel like another person																
Forgetful																
Inability to concentrate																
Need to escape																
Wish to be alone																
Alcohol consumption																
Craving salty foods																
Craving sweet foods																
Menses ("X" at onset)																

Hormone:	16	17	18	19	20	21	22	23	24	25	26	27	28	29	30	31
Growth hormone																
Prednisone																
DDAVP																
Estrogen																
Progesterone																
Thyroid																
Testosterone																

The Womens Assessment Calendar

300

Second Edition

Membership

Please print or type

MEMBERSHIP LEVEL

❏ $500 Lifetime Member   ❏ $10,000 Akhenaton's Council

❏ $100 Sponsor   ❏ $ 5,000 Lifetime Corporate

❏ $ 50 Patron   ❏ $ 500 Corporate Member

❏ $ 30 Active Member   ❏ $ 1,000 Lifetime Professional

❏ $ 35 Active Non U.S.   ❏ $ 100 Professional Member

PAYROLL DEDUCTION OR UNITED WAY/AGENCY DONATION

On your company contribution form or agency donor card, please designate the following:

Recipient:	Pituitary Tumor Network Association
Address:	16350 Ventura Boulevard, #231
	Encino, CA 91436
Phone:	805-499-2262 Employer ID# 33-0530465

Check the appropriate box below and mail this form with a copy of your contribution form to the PTNA to expedite your membership process.

I have donated to the PTNA through:

❏ A Company Payroll Deduction   ❏ United Way/Agency Donation

MEMORY GIFT

Amount: _____   In Memory/Honor of: _____

Send a gift notice to: _____

Name: _____

Address: _____

From: _____

PAYMENT INFORMATION

Cardholder: _____

Card #: _____

Expiration Date: _____

Signature: _____

Membership

Please print or type

Name:

Affiliation/Organization:

Street Address:

City/State/Postal Code:

Country: Tel:

Signature: Work Tel:

SS#   Fax:

Occupation: Date:

E-mail Address:

Website Address:

SURVEY

This survey is intended for internal use only. All information is strictly confidential. Our intent is to use this data to disseminate pertinent information regarding new treatments, medications, etc. to those who would benefit most. (Attach additional page if needed)

Date of birth: Male ❑   Female ❑

Date of diagnosis: Estimated age at onset:

Diagnosing physician:

Current physician:

Number of surgeries:

Where treated now:

Types of treatment and
surgery (include dates):

Medications/Hormone
replacement therapy:

Have you volunteered for
any clinical trials? Which?

Other patients in family?

Child genders & ages:

To List In Upcoming Worldwide Editions

To better reach pituitary patients around the world, the Pituitary Patient Resource Guide will now be published in geographically specific editions. The first of these will be the European, Asian-Pacific, and Central-South American editions.

For information on how to be listed in one or more of these editions of the Resource Guide, please fill out the following form and fax or mail it to us at the address listed below. Or you can visit our website at *www.pituitary.com* and e-mail the form to us. You can find it in the Publications section of the website.

Name: _____ Title: _____

Company/
Institution: _____

Address: _____

City: _____ State/Province: _____

Phone: _____ Postal Code: _____

Fax: _____ Country: _____

E-Mail: _____ Website: _____

What edition(s) would you like information about? _____

To order additional copies of the second
edition Pituitary Patients Resource Guide, Please fill out
and return this form to:

Pituitary Tumor Network Association
P.O. Box 1958
Thousand Oaks, Ca. 91358
Tel: (805) 499-2262   Fax: (805) 499-1523

Please include $6.95 for shipping and handling on all order of $75.00 or less. Postage and handling rates are subject to change and may vary on orders shipped out of the United States and on orders totaling more than $75.00. California residents please add 7.25% sales tax.

PTNA Members: $29.95 ea   2 books for $25.50 ea   3 to 10 books for $19.95 ea   Quantity: _____

Non-members: $39.95 ea   Non-members pay $29.95 when order is accompanied by a membership form & payment.

Your Name: _____ Phone: _____

Ship To: _____

Address: _____

Payment Information: ☐ Visa/MasterCard   ☐ Check payable to PTNA

Cardholder: _____

Card #: _____ Exp. Date: _____

Signature: _____

Second Edition

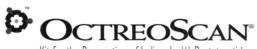

OCTREOSCAN®

Kit for the Preparation of Indium In-III Pentetreotide

BRIEF SUMMARY OF PRESCRIBING INFORMATION

DESCRIPTION

OctreoScan® is a kit for the preparation of indium In-111 pentetreotide, a diagnostic radio-pharmaceutical. It is a kit consisting of two components:
1) A 10-mL OctreoScan Reaction Vial which contains a lyophilized mixture of 10 μg pentetreotide.
2) A 10-mL vial of Indium In-111 Chloride Sterile Solution.
Indium In-111 pentetreotide is prepared by combining the two kit components.

INDICATIONS AND USAGE

Indium In-111 pentetreotide is an agent for the scintigraphic localization of primary and metastatic neuroendocrine tumors bearing somatostatin receptors.

CONTRAINDICATIONS

None known.

WARNINGS

DO NOT ADMINISTER IN TOTAL PARENTERAL NUTRITION (TPN) ADMIXTURES OR INJECT INTO TPN INTRAVENOUS ADMINISTRATION LINES; IN THESE SOLUTIONS, A COMPLEX GLYCOSYL OCTREOTIDE CONJUGATE MAY FORM.

The sensitivity of scintigraphy with indium In-111 pentetreotide may be reduced in patients concurrently receiving therapeutic doses of octreotide acetate. Consideration should be given to temporarily suspending octreotide acetate therapy before the administration of indium In-111 pentetreotide and to monitoring the patient for any signs of withdrawal.

PRECAUTIONS

General

1. Therapy with octreotide acetate can produce severe hypoglycemia in patients with insulinomas. Since pentetreotide is an analog of octreotide, an intravenous line is recommended in any patient suspected of having an insulinoma. An intravenous solution containing glucose should be administered just before and during administration of indium In-111 pentetreotide.

2. The contents of the two vials supplied with the kit are intended only for use in the preparation of indium In-111 pentetreotide and are NOT to be administered separately to the patient.

3. Since indium In-111 pentetreotide is eliminated primarily by renal excretion, use in patients with impaired renal function should be carefully considered.

4. To help reduce the radiation dose to the thyroid, kidneys, bladder, and other target organs, patients should be well hydrated before the administration of indium In-111 pentetreotide. They should increase fluid intake and void frequently for one day after administration of this drug. In addition, it is recommended that patients be given a mild laxative (e.g., bisacodyl or lactulose) before and after administration of indium In-111 pentetreotide (see Dosage and Administration section).

5. Indium In-111 pentetreotide should be tested for labeling yield of radioactivity prior to administration. The product must be used within six hours of preparation.

6. Components of the kit are sterile and nonpyrogenic. To maintain sterility, it is essential that directions are followed carefully. Aseptic technique must be used during the preparation and administration of indium In-111 pentetreotide.

7. Octreotide acetate and the natural somatostatin hormone may be associated with cholelithiasis, presumably by altering fat absorption and possibly by decreasing motility of the gallbladder. A single dose of indium In-111 pentetreotide is not expected to cause cholelithiasis.

8. As with any other radioactive material, appropriate shielding should be used to avoid unnecessary radiation exposure to the patient, occupational workers, and other persons.

9. Radiopharmaceuticals should be used only by physicians who are qualified by specific training in the safe use and handling of radionuclides.

Carcinogenesis, Mutagenesis, Impairment of Fertility

Studies have not been performed with indium In-111 pentetreotide to evaluate carcinogenic potential or effects on fertility. Pentetreotide was evaluated for mutagenic potential in an in vitro mouse lymphoma forward mutation assay and an in vivo mouse micronucleus assay; evidence of mutagenicity was not found.

Pregnancy Category C

Animal reproduction studies have not been conducted with indium In-111 pentetreotide. It is not known whether indium In-111 pentetreotide can cause fetal harm when administered to a pregnant woman or can affect reproduction capacity. Therefore, indium In-111 pentetreotide should not be administered to a pregnant woman unless the potential benefit justifies the potential risk to the fetus.

Nursing Mothers

It is not known whether this drug is excreted in human milk. Because many drugs are excreted in human milk, caution should be exercised when indium In-111 pentetreotide is administered to a nursing woman.

Pediatric Use

Safety and effectiveness in children have not been established.

ADVERSE REACTIONS

The following adverse effects were observed in clinical trials at a frequency of less than 1% of 538 patients: dizziness, fever, flush, headache, hypotension, changes in liver enzymes, joint pain, nausea, sweating, and weakness. These adverse effects were transient. Also in clinical trials, there was one reported case of bradycardia and one case of decreased hematocrit and hemoglobin.

Pentetreotide is derived from octreotide which is used as a therapeutic agent to control symptoms from certain tumors. The usual dose for indium In-111 pentetreotide is approximately 5 to 20 times less than for octreotide and is subtherapeutic. The following adverse reactions have been associated with octreotide in 3% to 10% of patients: nausea, injection site pain, diarrhea, abdominal pain/discomfort, loose stools, and vomiting. Hypertension and hyper- and hypoglycemia have also been reported with the use of octreotide.

DOSAGE AND ADMINISTRATION

Before administration, a patient should be well hydrated. After administration, the patient must be encouraged to drink fluids liberally. Elimination of extra fluid intake will help reduce the radiation dose by flushing out unbound, labelled pentetreotide by glomerular filtration. It is also recommended that a mild laxative (e.g., bisacodyl or

---

lactulose) be given to the patient starting the evening before the radioactive drug is administered, and continuing for 48 hours. Ample fluid uptake is necessary during this period as a support both to renal elimination and the bowel-cleansing process. In a patient with an insulinoma, bowel-cleansing should be undertaken only after consultation with an endocrinologist.

The recommended intravenous dose for planar imaging is 111 MBq (3.0 mCi) of indium In-111 pentetreotide prepared from an OctreoScan kit. The recommended intravenous dose for SPECT imaging is 222 MBq (6.0 mCi) of indium In-111 pentetreotide.

The dose should be confirmed by a suitably calibrated radioactivity ionization chamber immediately before administration.

As with all intravenously administered products, OctreoScan should be inspected visually for particulate matter and discoloration prior to administration, whenever solution and container permit. Preparations containing particulate matter or discoloration should not be administered. They should be disposed of in a safe manner, in compliance with applicable regulations.

Aseptic techniques and effective shielding should be employed in withdrawing doses for administration to patients. Waterproof gloves should be worn during the administration procedure.

Do not administer OctreoScan in TPN solutions or through the same intravenous line.

Radiation Dosimetry

The estimated radiation doses[1] to the average adult (70 kg) from intravenous administration of 111 MBq (3 mCi) and 222 MBq (6 mCi) are presented below. These estimates were calculated by Oak Ridge Associated Universities using the data published by Krenning, et al.[2]

Estimated Absorbed Radiation Doses after Intravenous Administration of Indium In-111 Pentetreotide[3] to a 70 kg patient

Organ	PLANAR		SPECT	
	mGy/111 MBq	rads/3 mCi	mGy/222 MBq	rads/6 mCi
Kidneys	54.16	5.42	108.32	10.83
Liver	12.15	1.22	24.31	2.43
Spleen	73.86	7.39	147.73	14.77
Uterus	6.34	0.63	12.67	1.27
Ovaries	4.89	0.49	9.79	0.98
Testes	2.90	0.29	5.80	0.58
Red Marrow	3.46	0.35	6.91	0.69
Urinary Bladder Wall	30.24	3.02	60.48	6.05
GI Tract				
Stomach Wall	5.67	0.57	11.34	1.13
Small Intestine	4.78	0.48	9.56	0.96
Upper Large Intestine	5.80	0.58	11.59	1.16
Lower Large Intestine	7.73	0.77	15.46	1.55
Adrenals	7.55	0.76	15.11	1.51
Thyroid	7.43	0.74	14.86	1.49
	mSv/111MBq	rem/3 mCi	mSv/222MBq	rem/6mCi
Effective Dose[4] Equivalent	13.03	1.30	26.06	2.61

1. Values listed include a correction for a maximum of 0.1% indium In-114m radiocontaminant at calibration.

2. E.P. Krenning, W.H. Bakker, P.P.M. Kooij, W.A.P. Breeman, H.Y.Oei, M. de Jong, J.C. Reubi, T.J. Visser, C. Bruns, D.J. Kwekkeboom, A.E.M. Reijs, P.M. van Hagen, J.W. Koper, and S.W.J. Lamberts, "Somatostatin Receptor Scintigraphy with Indium-111-DTPA-D-Phe-1-Octreotide in Man: Metabolism, Dosimetry and Comparison with Iodine-123-Tyr-3-Octreotide," The Journal of Nuclear Medicine, Vol. 33, No. 5, May 1992, pp. 652-658.

3. Assumes 4.8 hour voiding interval and International Commission on Radiological Protection (ICRP) 30 model for the gastrointestinal tract calculations.

4. Estimated according to ICRP Publication 53.

HOW SUPPLIED

The OctreoScan kit, NDC 0019-9050, is supplied with the following components:

1. A 10-mL OctreoScan Reaction Vial which contains a lyophilized mixture of:
   (i) 10 μg pentetreotide [N-(diethylenetriamine-N,N,N',N''-tetraacetic acid-N''-acetyl)-D-phenylalanyl-L-hemicystyl-L-phenylalanyl-D-tryptophyl-L-lysyl-L-threonyl-L-hemicystyl-L-threoninol cyclic (2→7) disulfide], (also known as octreotide DTPA),
   (ii) 2.0 mg gentisic acid [2,5-dihydroxybenzoic acid],
   (iii) 4.9 mg trisodium citrate, anhydrous,
   (iv) 0.37 mg citric acid, anhydrous, and
   (v) 10.0 mg inositol.

Before lyophilization, sodium hydroxide or hydrochloric acid may have been added for pH adjustment. The vial contents are sterile and nonpyrogenic. No bacteriostatic preservative is present.

2. A 10-mL vial of Indium In-111 Chloride Sterile Solution, which contains 1.1 mL of 111 MBq/mL (3.0 mCi/mL) indium In-111 chloride in 0.02 N HCl at time of calibration. The vial also contains ferric chloride at a concentration of 3.5 μg/mL (ferric ion, 1.2 μg/mL). The vial contents are sterile and nonpyrogenic. No bacteriostatic preservative is present.

In addition, the kit also contains the following items: (1) a 25 G x 5/8" needle (B-D, Monoject) used to transfer Indium In-111 Chloride Sterile Solution to the OctreoScan Reaction Vial, (2) a pressure sensitive label, and (3) a package insert.

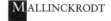

MALLINCKRODT

Mallinckrodt Medical, Inc.,
Mallinckrodt Nuclear Medicine Division
P.O. Box 5840
St. Louis, MO 63134

For orders, product information, and medical assistance, call us toll free at (800) 325-3688.

©1994 Mallinckrodt Medical, Inc.   MI22496   8/94